S0-AUS-168

DEDICATION

This book, *Diets For Healthy Healing,* is dedicated to all of us on the go: those who need an easier path to dealing with our health problems naturally. Those looking for a simpler way, that we can seamlessly weave into lives that leave us no time to be unwell.

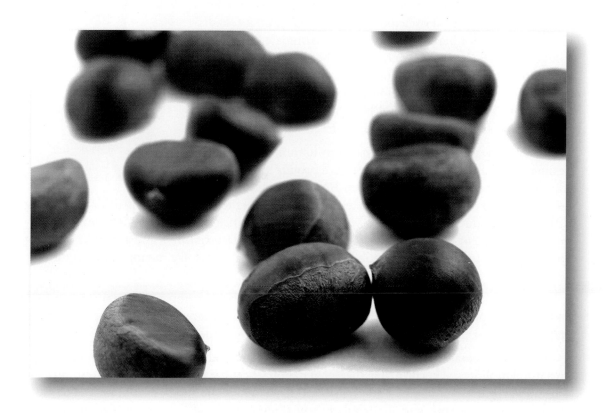

ACKNOWLEDGMENTS

Thanks to the dedicated publishing staff at Healthy Healing:

Michael Kohler, Sarah Abernathy, Leah Thomson, August Tarantino and Olga Mikheeva

for bringing out *Diets for Healthy Healing,* a new concept that they were somehow able

to weave with responsibility and professional detail into their already fully-packed jobs.

ABOUT THE AUTHOR

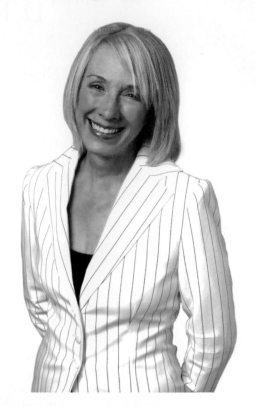

Long before natural foods and herbal formulas became a widely accepted method for healing, Linda Page was sharing her extensive knowledge with those who dared to listen.

Through what some would call an accident of fate but she calls a blessing, she was compelled to research alternative avenues of healing. Sequestered in a hospital with a life-threatening illness, watching her 5-foot frame wither to 69 pounds, her hair drop out, and her skin peel off, doctors told her they had no cure. With only a cursory knowledge of herbs, she began a frantic research process of testing herbal formulas and healing food combinations on herself. She read voraciously about herbal healing. Good friends shopped for herbs and she began to formulate the many compounds, which would eventually save her life, revitalize her health and restore beautiful new hair and skin. It was that incident that led her to seek her degrees in Naturopathy and Nutrition from Clayton College of Natural Health in Birmingham, Alabama, where she is now adjunct professor.

Linda's rewarding career as a leader in natural health and healing spans almost three decades. She is a prolific author and educator. Her best-selling book, *Healthy Healing™ – A Guide To Self-Healing For Everyone*, is used as a textbook at many higher educational institutions teaching natural health courses. She has also written other books including: *Cooking For Healthy Healing, How To Be Your Own Herbal Pharmacist, Party Lights, Detoxification* and a popular series of library books which address specific healing therapies for topics like menopause, weight loss, sexuality, colds and flu and cancer.

A master classical herbalist, she founded the herbal nutrition company, Crystal Star® in 1978 and she has formulated over 250 whole herb combinations. She received some of the first United States Patents for herbal formulations for her women's hormone balancing formulas.

Linda is in demand by the media and she has appeared weekly on CBS television with a report on natural healing; she is a principle speaker at national health symposiums and conventions; she is featured regularly in national magazines and newspapers; she appears on hundreds of radio and television programs and she regularly contributes to *WebMD* and other health websites. Currently, she is featured on the television program, "The World of Healthy Healing" airing on PBS television and she leads educational tours to destinations such as China, the southwestern US and Kauai, Hawaii.

Today, Linda delights in having come full circle. "I am so grateful that knowledge of healing through herbal formulas and good foods is becoming so widespread. I see it as an opportunity for people to seize the power to heal themselves. Knowledge is power. Whether one chooses conventional medicine, alternative healing avenues, or combines them both in a complementary process, the real prescription for healing is knowledge."

Linda has spoken before Congressional and Senate Committees on behalf of DSHEA and she continues to be a staunch advocate for the freedom of all to choose natural health protocols and products. She is a member of The American Naturopathic Medical Association, The California Naturopathic Association, The American Herbalist Guild, The American Botanical Council and The Herb Research Foundation.

OTHER BOOKS AND RESOURCES BY DR. LINDA PAGE

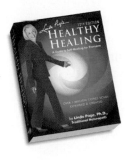

Healthy Healing, 12th Edition
The Ultimate Resource For Improving Your Health Naturally

- NEW! Product rating system revealing which products our test group found to be the most beneficial, fastest-acting, and most highly recommended.
- Over 80 NEW pages of the latest research including emerging ailments such as SARS, Syndrome X, and Stress-Related Weight Gain.
- NEW! Specific guidelines for using herbal therapy before and after surgery in order to ensure maximum healing.
- NEW! Information on Genetically Engineered Foods, and Drug-Herb-Nutrient Interactions.

In its first edition nearly 20 years ago, Dr. Linda Page's book, Healthy Healing, was the only one of its kind. Now updated and expanded, Healthy Healing is still the easiest to use bestselling natural health reference book on the market.

Customize your own personal healing program using natural therapies for more than 300 ailments through diet, whole herb supplements and exercise.

12th Edition, 664 Pages, Illustrated, 1884334-92-X SRP: $32.95   Spiral Bound Edition - 1884334-93-8 SRP: $35.95

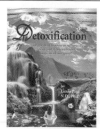

Detoxification
All You Need to Know to Recharge and Rejuvenate Your Body, Mind and Spirit!

- Step-by-Step Detox Charts
- Recommended Detox Products
- Extensive Review of Detox Spas in America
- Green Cuisine Recipes

More than 25 thousand new toxins enter our environment each year. Detoxification is a necessary commitment for staying healthy in a destructive world. In this complete guide of detailed instructions for detoxification and cleansing, Dr. Page shows you: what you can expect when you detox; what a good cleanse really does; how to direct a cleanse for best results; and much more!

264 Pages, Illustrated, 8 1/2 x 11, 1884334-54-7 SRP: $21.95

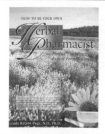

How To Be Your Own Herbal Pharmacist, Second Edition
108 Step-by-Step Healing Formulas!

- Making Herbal Cosmetics
- Using Herbal Remedies instead of Drugs
- Remedies for Children and Pets

Formulating herbal combinations is usually a deep dark secret between herbalists. Most books on herbs don't really show you how to combine herbs to address specific ailments. This fascinating book shows you how it's done, with detailed work pages, how to take the formula for best results, and much more!

2nd Edition, 256 Pages, Illustrated, 8 1/2 x 11, 1884334-78-4 SRP: $18.95

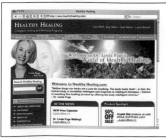

www.HealthyHealing.com
Your Complete Online Natural Healing & Wellness Resource.

The official website for Dr. Linda Page, Healthy Healing Publications and Crystal Star Herbal Nutrition.

- Extensive Crystal Star Product Information
- More than 16 books by Dr. Linda Page
- Dr. Linda Page Weblog
- Free Recipes, Self Tests, Therapy Plans and Articles
- Downloadable Catalogs, Audio Interviews and Educational Content

THIS BOOK CAN BE GREAT MEDICINE!

Food is a potent healer. Your diet can literally transform your body.

Wholesome food not only fuels your body, but it can also help solve your health problems. Your diet can keep your energy levels up and stress levels down; your skin, hair, and nails healthy; your complexion glowing; your eyes bright; and your bones and muscles strong. It can fine-tune mental awareness and prevent disease from taking hold. A poor diet and junk foods produce lethargy, illness, and indifference.

Good food is good medicine. It is the prime factor for changing your body chemically and psychologically. The food you eat changes your weight, your mood, the texture and look of your body, your outlook on life, indeed the entire universe for you… and therefore your future.

Eating right is the first step to the health and balance of your universe. This book is about getting back to the basics… because basics are basics (like classics are classics) for a reason.

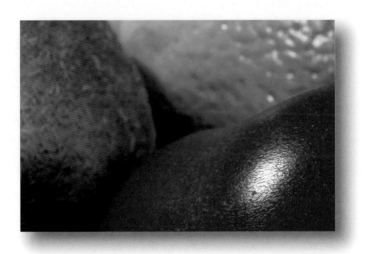

The book you hold in your hands is the culmination of twenty years of hard work. It's the result of an enormous amount of research in using foods as medicine. All the recipes and diet plans were tested again and again, first through the Rainbow Kitchen restaurant and juice bar I owned in the early eighties, to the diet programs I developed for Country Store Natural Foods and Crystal Star Herbal Nutrition, to the highly focused healing diets of today using foods as Nature's Perfect Pharmacy.

Through all this time, the results were clear and undeniable: foods and herbs (we have to remind ourselves that herbs *are* foods) can indeed heal—even serious diseases—sometimes dramatically. Foods and herbs can prevent some health problems from happening at all and many illnesses from developing further. The secret is using foods and herbs to change body chemistry. Only foods and herbs can do it, and *Diets for Healthy Healing* tells you how.

I believe the history of the world would have been entirely different if the human diet had been different. Our children are literally formed from, and become, the nutrients (or poisons) within us. Not only are we what we eat, our children are as well, before and after birth. The pattern for the immune system and inherited health of your children and grandchildren is laid down by you. It's all about choices and this book shows you the best choices for your healing path.

A personal letter to my readers…

Before our "modern age," food was pretty wholesome: people were close to their gardens and farms, to animals and natural resources. Today, it seems we live in more of a man-made jungle of food substances instead of foods—many of them highly processed, low in nutrients, full of fat, chemicals and sugars.

Our scientific culture relies totally on things like lab tests and substances that are man-made because they fit into our ability to understand. "Scientific" medicine attacks anything that can't be specifically isolated, broken down, peeled apart or synthesized. It discounts the value of something it can't understand, believing that a thing can't possibly work if we can't understand it.

It doesn't even matter if the natural, whole substance works. A "silver bullet" must be identified so that it can be synthesized and manufactured. Even advanced medical techniques, like genetic science, work this way.

We feel uncomfortable when something isn't logical… but nature isn't logical… people aren't logical…

The way natural healing and food medicines work sometimes isn't logical, either.

It just doesn't "fit" into the way western science sees and understands things. There's nothing wrong with the scientific method as long as we realize it isn't the only way… especially when we're dealing with an incredible, complex human being who is far more than a lab test or a blood panel.

I believe only the whole food can give the whole benefit.

Many plants only work in their whole form. While single plant elements can be tested and measured, a lab can only give a partial answer about a highly complex living thing. When we take one out of the literally hundreds of elements in a plant and say, "That's it, that's what this plant is good for," we lose. It's never the whole story. Healing foods and herbs are never just one plant for one problem.

Foods and herbs are so much more than a test or a scientific measurement. Plants are the only medicines I know of that treat the whole person, not just their symptoms.

I say, let foods and herbs do what they do so well: heal and balance from the inside out, naturally and safely. Use them in their whole form as medicinal foods.

Health for each of us is personal. To approach it impersonally, only through big business, science and government means that our health is bound to lose.

Linda Page

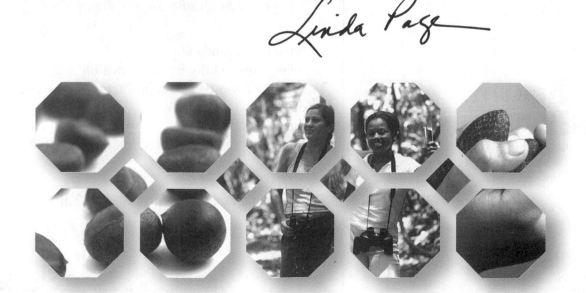

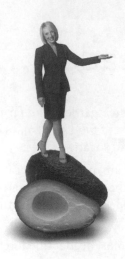

About the Cover

The cover of this book is meant to serve as a whimsical reminder of the enormous role that food plays in our lives. The image of Dr. Page balancing atop the avocado is symbolic of the concept that a healthy, well-balanced diet—while challenging to maintain—is the very foundation of a healthy, happy life.

Cover concept and design by Michael Kohler

This reference is to be used for educational information. It is not a claim for cure or mitigation of disease, but rather an adjunctive approach, supplying individual nutritional needs that otherwise might be lacking in today's lifestyle.

First Edition, October 2005.

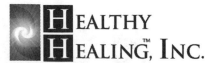

Copyright © October 2005 by Linda Page.
Published by Healthy Healing, Inc.
www.healthyhealing.com

Publisher's Cataloging-in-Publication
(Provided by Quality Books, Inc.)

Rector-Page, Linda G.
   Diets for healthy healing : healing diets for America's top 10 health problems / Linda Page. -- 1st ed.
   p. cm.
   Includes bibliographical references and index.
   ISBN 1-884334-83-0

1. Diet therapy. 2. Nutrition.   I. Title.

RM216.R3795 2005   615.8'54
                          QBI05-200120

How to Use this Book....

A healing diet is the first step to your best health. Good food can be great medicine!

All the advances made by modern medicine still don't address chronic diseases very well; they don't address disease prevention at all.

Sometimes food can be your best medicine… even for serious diseases. We tend to think that the healing powers of foods are subtle or mild, without the overwhelming potency of drugs. Yet healing doesn't always need to deal a hammer blow… even for serious problems.

As new research advances in the science of nutrition, there's an enormous thirst for information about how to use it. Most people are actively trying to eat better. Organic foods are mainstream today. But most people don't know HOW to use foods as medicine. *Diets for Healthy Healing* can help you navigate the healing path easily and effectively. After your initial diet is producing good results, use the sample recipes at the end of the chapter to help maintain good health, sound nutrition and system balance.

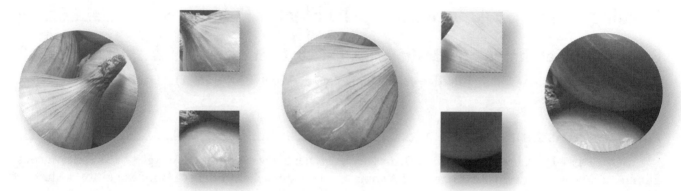

This book gives you everything you need to do it yourself, day by day, and succeed.

• Detailed STEP-BY-STEP DIETS for the top 10 health problems Americans face today.

• RECIPES for every health problem in the book that help you maintain good health.

• BONUS Diets for Beauty, Anti-Aging, and Children's Health

In the 1930s, at the height of the scientific love affair with orthodox medicine, the Nobel prize-winning doctor, Albert Schweitzer said, "the doctor of the future will be oneself." He saw the limitations of drugs and surgery-based healing. He knew that immune strength was the only real way to prevent disease.

Medicines from foods and herbs work just the opposite from drugs. They nourish the body and enhance the immune system. Drugs function outside the system, usually operating to overwhelm a harmful organism. Today's orthodox medicine is "heroic medicine," largely developed in wartime for emergency wartime requirements. It's a patching up system.

Yet, I feel we need both types of medicine. Drugs can arrest an emergency and stabilize your body to give your immune system a chance to take over.

Clearly, orthodox medicine has saved many lives. Just as clearly, natural medicine has prevented much illness. Whether you want to address a specific health condition or you have a family history of that has you focused on illness prevention, *Diets for Healthy Healing* is help when and where you need it. Use the healing diets in this book to put yourself on the path to the best health you've ever had!

Table of Contents

Healing Diets for America's Top 10 Health Problems............................9

Before You Get Started: A Basic Stress Detox Diet................................10

Body signs that show you may need to detoxify. Steps in a good detox program. 1) 3-Day Body Stress Cleanse. Recipes for your Stress Detox.

Allergies & Asthma: Healing and Control................................20

Diets: (1) 7-Day Chemical Pollutant Detox Diet   (2) Diet to Overcome Food Allergies   (3) Basic Mucous Elimination Diet for Seasonal Allergies and Asthma   (4) Asthma Control Diet Plan. Recipes for a Mucous Cleanse. Recipes For Allergy/Asthma Control.

Arthritis: Pain Relieving Diet 38

Diets: (1) A Three-Day Arthritis Cleansing Diet   (2) Arthritis Symptom Control. Key Recipes For an Arthritis Detox. Recipes for Arthritis Symptom Control.

Blood Sugar Imbalances: Diabetes and Hypoglycemia................................48

Diets: (1) Diabetes Control Diet   (2) Hypoglycemia Control Diet. Recipes for Sugar Control.

Cancer: Controlling and Rebuilding Health 64

Diets: (1) Cancer Diet Watchwords   (2) Macrobiotic Diet For Cancer Control   (3) Cancer Control & Prevention Diet   (4) Normalizing after Chemotherapy or Radiation. Recipes for Macrobiotic and Cancer Control.

Digestive Disorders: Ulcers, Heartburn, Irritable Bowel 84

Diets: (1) GERD (Gastroesophagael Reflux) Diet   (2) Enzyme-Rich Diet and Chart   (3) Diet to Rebuild Colon & Bowel Health.   (4) Diet to Heal Irritable Bowel. Recipes for Digestive Disorders and Colon/Bowel Healing.

Heart Disease, Stroke and High Blood Pressure................................108

Diets: (1) Heart Attack Recovery   (2) A Man's Heart Program   (3) A Woman's Heart Program   (4) Lowering Blood Pressure   (5) Lowering Cholesterol. Recipes for a Healthy Heart Diet.

Special Bonus Diets

Creating Your Own Food Pharmacy

What is a food pharmacy?

Your diet is one of the most powerful tools you can use for your health. The secret is using foods and herbs to balance body chemistry. Each one of us is entirely individual; our immune systems are individual to each of us. It would be impossible for a laboratory to *ever* develop a drug to activate immunity for everyone. Only something like foods or herbs, which are able to combine with each of us individually, operate at the deepest levels of our bodies, and work with our own enzyme activity, can do the job.

How can you get the most from your food pharmacy?

The foods you eat can accomplish almost every health and healing need. Studies show that people who eat plenty of vegetables have more than 50% less cancer risk than people who eat few vegetables. One National Cancer Institute spokesman said it is almost mind-boggling that common foods can be so effective against a potent carcinogen like tobacco! Even if your genetics and lifestyle are against you, your diet still makes a tremendous difference in your odds for better health and fast healing.

Medicines from foods and herbs work differently than drugs.

Ordinarily, you have to take more and more of a drug to get the same effect… in some cases creating dependency or tolerance. With herbal medicines, instead, you might start with a larger amount to stimulate your body's vital healing force, then reduce the amount you take as your healing program goes on and your body picks up its own work from the nutrients you have been giving it.

Today we're flooded with information (and misinformation) about nutrition. Yet, there's still a real need for people to learn what a healthy diet is and what it is not. Nutrition is both a science and an art of nourishing yourself. Sound nutritional knowledge can help you navigate through all the unhealthy foods and eating habits you may be faced with.

A recent Surgeon General's report notes that "diet-related diseases account for 68% of all deaths in America!" The study goes on to say that "a diet rich in plant foods protects against many common diseases in Western society," and that "a diet with low plant foods contributes to the development of common diseases, encouraging conditions under which disease factors can become active." The newest research shows that if we spent more time on cancer *prevention* rather than *treatment*, cancer deaths in the U.S. could drop by nearly a third. That translates into 100,000 fewer cancer cases and 60,000 prevented cancer deaths by 2015, largely from better food choices.

It seems that we've all been talking about diet and nutrition forever. Everyone's aware of the need to keep a clean, well-nourished body… right? This is simply not the case. The general diet today in our society still consists mainly of meat, dairy foods, highly processed foods, and only occasional fresh foods. Instead of a diet that easily supports us, our bodies are forced into stress procedures in order to process an overload of concentrated proteins, refined food substances and chemicals.

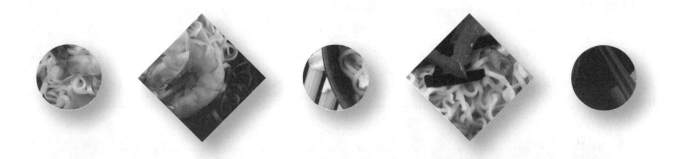

Diet overload means our bodies don't work well; organs and glands work overtime. Here are some of the diseases we get when we overload:

- **Diabetes and Hypoglycemia**
  (overload from refined carbohydrates)

- **Hardening of the Arteries and High Blood Pressure**
  (overload from fat and refined salt)

- **Degenerative Problems and Premature Aging**
  (overload from proteins, chemicalized and microwaved foods)

- **Chronic Poor Digestion**
  (overload of chemicalized foods, microwaved foods, alcohol, drugs and sugars)

- **Obesity** *(overload from all of the above)*

How can we remind ourselves in a positive way that we really are what we eat?

It's hard for anybody to make major diet changes with a "cold turkey" approach. Weight loss dieters know all too well that "all or nothing" plans don't work. Overnight changes are just too difficult to maintain. A gradual program works best. Keep yourself motivated with small improvements that show positive results and provide a framework for more changes. You'll be delighted when you start to see your energy level change, when you feel the first golden suffusion of well being as your body chemistry balances, when you get a taste of physical strength you haven't experienced in years.

Try this plan:

- Simplify your diet—reduce fried foods, meat and dairy, foods with chemicals.
- Buy the highest quality foods you can find—organically grown and GMO-free when you can.
- Read food product labels before you buy—your food decisions will be better. Note: most carb-free, fat-free, sugar-free choices are loaded with chemicals that can slow down your healing diet.
- Eat more foods that don't have ANY labels—like fresh fruit and vegetables, and whole grains. Promise yourself you'll limit microwaving foods because it destroys enzymes, the key to a strong digestive system.
- Eat a variety of foods. Some drastic detox or weight loss diets limit you to only one or two types of foods. I have tried diets like this. They provide limited nutrition. They wreak havoc on your body chemistry. They can be devastating to your health. The healthiest people eat a wide variety of low fat, fresh foods.
- A food reward program works. Eat a super healthy diet Monday through Friday, then relax your diet on weekends to eat a few of your favorites.
- Be gentle with yourself. Mark Twain said that a habit can't simply be tossed out the window. Escort it like an old friend, down the stairs one at a time, then out the door.

You can always use your food as medicine.

Healthy foods make all the difference, and they taste so good, fresh or prepared in easy recipes. Long gone are the days when health food has to taste like cardboard (a lot of it did in the early eighties). Use this book to find out about specific foods with constituents to help solve your health problems. Start integrating these healthy foods into your diet. Pretty soon, healthy foods will form the basis of your whole diet!

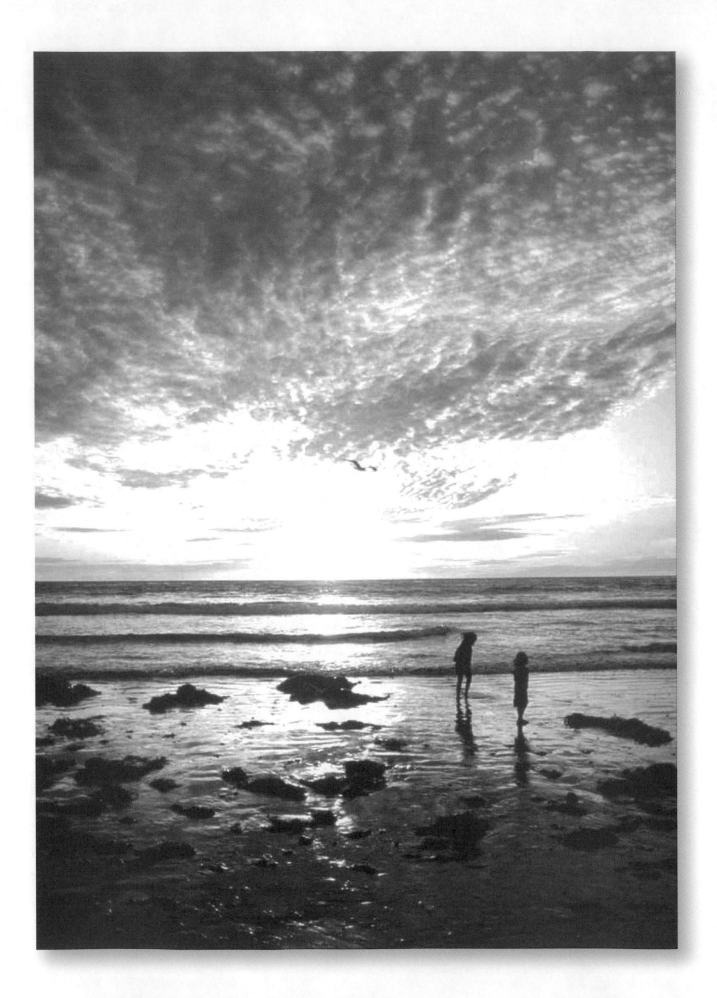

Diets for Healthy Healing

Healing Diets for America's Top 10 Health Problems

by Dr. Linda Page, Ph.D., Traditional Naturopath

Before You Get Started:
Try A Basic Stress Detox Diet

Do you need to detoxify?

A short cleansing diet at the start of a healing program can be critical to its success. Most of us suffer from some form of overload today. Cleansing your body of embedded pollutants and chemicals with a short purifying diet can dramatically boost your body's healing ability.

What is detoxification?

Detoxification is the normal body process of eliminating or neutralizing toxins through the colon, liver, kidneys, lungs, lymph and skin. Our bodies are naturally designed to detoxify us every day… automatically. It's a perfect natural set-up… just like our hearts beat and our lungs breathe, our metabolic processes constantly dispose of accumulated toxic matter. The catch is that today, body systems and organs that were once capable of cleaning out unwanted substances are now overloaded with toxic material from our environment.

We long for what we see as yesterday's pollution-free environment, whole foods and pure water. Yet, since humans are born with a "self-cleaning system," this ideal probably never existed. Our bodies try to protect us by surrounding dangerous material with mucous or fat so it won't trigger an immune reaction. For instance, foreign substances are stored in fatty deposits—a significant reason to keep your body fat low. Some people carry around up to 15 extra pounds of mucous that harbors this waste!

A detox program aims to remove the cause of disease before it makes us ill. It's a time-honored way to keep immune response high, elimination regular, circulation sound, and stress under control. In fact, a cleansing diet may be the missing link to disease prevention, especially for immune-compromised diseases like cancer, arthritis, diabetes and fatigue syndromes like candida.

Should you detoxify?

A regular detox program two or three times a year makes a big difference not only for health, but for the quality of our lives. Today Americans are exposed to chemicals of all kinds on an unprecedented scale. Industrial chemicals and their pollutant run-offs in our water, pesticides, additives in our foods, heavy metals, anesthetics, residues from drugs, and environmental hormones are trapped within the human body in greater concentrations than at any other point in history.

Chemicalized, genetically altered foods can radically alter our internal ecosystems—that's not even counting today's overloads of fat, sugar, caffeine and alcohol. Many chemicals are so widespread that we are unaware of them. But they have worked their way into our bodies faster than they can be eliminated, and are causing allergies and addictions in record numbers. More than 2 million synthetic substances are known, 25,000 are added each year, and over 30,000 are produced on a commercial scale. Only a tiny fraction are ever tested for toxicity. A lot of them come to us from developing countries that have few safeguards in place.

Look at some recent statistics…
• Air pollution alone now claims over 50,000 lives in the United States each year.
• 1.2 billion pounds of pesticides are dumped yearly; 78% are used in agriculture to produce our food.
• The World Health Organization implicates environmental chemicals in 60 to 80% of all cancers.

The chemical beat goes on...

The molecular structure of some chemicals interacts with human DNA, so long term exposure may result in genetic alteration that affects cell functions. Hormone-disrupting pesticides are linked to hormone problems, learning disorders, birth defects, still births and now breast cancer.

Chemical oxidation, the oxygen that "rusts" and ages us also triggers free radical activity, a destructive cascade of incomplete molecules that damages DNA and other cell components. If you didn't have a reason to reduce your animal fat intake before, here is a critical one: oxygen combines with animal fat in body storage cells and speeds up the free radical process.

As chemical toxins saturate our tissues, antioxidants and minerals in vital body fluids are reduced, so immune defenses are thrown out of balance, and allow immune compromised diseases like candidiasis, lupus, fibromyalgia, even arthritis (which now impairs over 50 million Americans).

What can we do?

A cleanse is one of the best ways to remain healthy in polluted surroundings. Not one of us is immune to environmental toxins, and we can't escape to a remote, unpolluted habitat. Keeping our body systems in good working order eliminates toxins quickly. Even if your diet is good, a body cleanse can restore your vitality against environmental toxins that pave the way for disease.

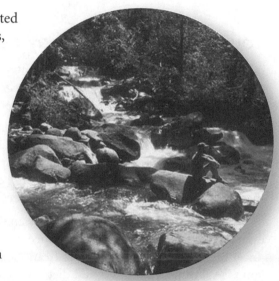

We can take a closer look at our own air, water and food, and keep a watchful eye on the politics that control our environment. Legislation on health and the environment follows two pathways in America... the influence of business and profits, and the demands of the people for a healthy habitat and responsible stewardship of the Earth. Technology is now seriously able to harm the health of our entire planet, even to the point of making it uninhabitable for life. Mankind and the Earth must work together—to save it for us all.

Is your body becoming toxic?

We all have different "toxic tolerance" levels. Listen to your body when it starts giving you those "cellular phone calls" of toxic body symptoms. If you can keep the amount of toxins in your system below your toxic level, your body can usually adapt and rid itself of them.

Body signs that tell you may need to detoxify.
- Frequent, unexplained headaches, back or joint pain (a sign of uric acid build-up) or arthritis?
- Chronic respiratory problems, sinus problems or asthma?
- Abnormal body odor, bad breath or coated tongue?
- Food allergies, poor digestion or chronic constipation with intestinal bloating or gas?
- Brittle nails and hair, psoriasis, adult acne, or unexplained weight gain over 10 pounds?
- Unusually poor memory, chronic insomnia, depression, irritability, chronic fatigue?
- Environmental sensitivities, especially to odors?
- Chronic stress, low energy, or unusual depression?

Lab tests like stool, urine, blood or liver tests, and hair analysis can also shed light on the need for a detox.

What benefits can you expect from a good detox?

A detox frees your body of clogging waste deposits, so you aren't running with a dirty engine or driving with the brakes on. Cleansing lets your body rebalance, so energy levels rise physically, psychologically and sexually, and creativity begins to expand. You start feeling like a different person—because you are. Your outlook and attitude change, because your actual cell make-up changes.

1. You'll clean your digestive tract of accumulated waste and fermenting bacteria.

2. You'll clear your body of excess mucous and congestion.

3. You'll purify your liver, kidney and blood, impossible under ordinary eating patterns.

4. You'll enhance mental clarity, impossible under chemical overload.

5. You'll be less dependent on sugar, caffeine, nicotine, alcohol or drugs.

6. You'll turn around bad eating habits... your stomach can reduce to normal size for weight control.

7. You'll release hormones that couple with essential fatty acids to stimulate your immune system.

You've decided your body needs a cleanse.

Ask yourself how long can you give out of your busy lifestyle to focus on a cleansing program so that all the processes can be completed. 24 hours, 2 or 3 days, or up to ten days? The time factor is important—you'll want to allocate your time ahead of time, to prepare both your mind and your body for the experience ahead.

Years of experience with detoxification have convinced me that if you have a serious health problem, a brief 3 to 7 day juice cleanse is the best way to release toxins from your body. Shorter cleanses can't get to the root of a chronic problem. Longer cleanses upset body equilibrium more than most people are ready to deal with except in a clinical environment. A 3 – 7 day cleanse can "clean your pipes" of systemic sludge—excess mucous, old fecal matter, trapped cellular and non-food wastes, or inorganic mineral deposits that are part of arthritis.

A few days without solid food can be an enlightening experience about your lifestyle. It's not absolutely necessary to take in only liquids, but a juice diet increases awareness and energy availability for elimination. Fresh juices literally pick up dead matter from the body and carry it away. Your body becomes easier to "hear," telling you via cravings what foods and diet it needs—for example, a desire for protein foods, or B vitamin foods like rice, or minerals from greens. This is natural biofeedback.

(Note: For hypoglycemics who experience severe sugar swings on juice cleanses, adding brown rice and organic fresh salads during the detox helps keep the body stable while still allowing you to get the cleansing benefits.)

A detox works by self-digestion. During a cleanse, the body decomposes and burns only the tissues that are damaged, diseased or unneeded, like abscesses, tumors, excess fat deposits, or congestive wastes. Even a relatively short fast accelerates elimination, often causing dramatic changes as masses of accumulated waste are expelled.

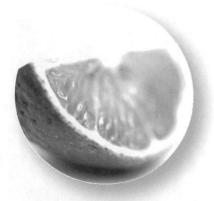 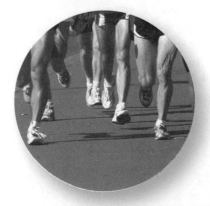 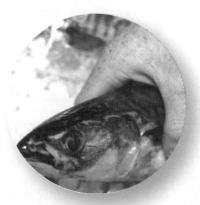

You will know your body is detoxifying if you experience a short period of headaches, fatigue, body odor, bad breath, diarrhea or mouth sores that commonly accompany accelerated elimination. However, digestion usually improves right away as do many gland and nerve functions. Cleansing also helps release hormone secretions that stimulate immune response and encourages a disease-preventing environment.

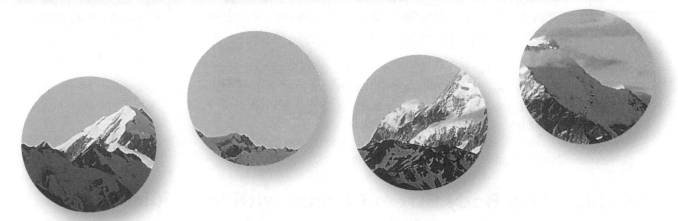

Is a water fast the fastest way to cleanse? I don't recommend it. Here's why:

Juice cleansing is a better evolution in detoxification methods. Popular since the 1960s, today experts agree that fresh vegetable and fruit juice cleansing is superior to water fasting. Fresh juices, broths and herb teas help deeply cleanse the body, rejuvenate the tissues and guide you to a faster recovery from health problems. A water fast is harsh and demanding on your body, even in times past before huge amounts of food and environmental toxins were part of the picture. Today, a water fast can be dangerous, because deeply buried pollutants and chemicals may be released into elimination channels too rapidly. Your body is essentially "re-poisoned" as the chemicals move through the bloodstream all at once. Sometimes, the physical and emotional stress of a water fast even overrides the healing benefits.

Vegetable and fruit juices are alkalizing, so they increase the healing effects, and neutralize uric acid and other inorganic acids better than water. Juices support better metabolic activity, too. (Metabolic activity actually slows down during a water fast because your the body tries to conserve dwindling energy resources.) Fresh juices don't disturb the detoxification process, because they're loaded with life giving enzymes that play a vital part in breaking down foreign matter like toxins as well as food. Best of all, they have a powerful effect on the body's recuperative powers because of their rich, easily absorbed nutrients.

A good detox program is in 3 steps: cleansing, rebuilding and maintaining

Step one: **Elimination.** Clean out mucous and toxins from the intestinal tract and major organs. Everything functions more effectively when toxins, obstructions and wastes are removed.

Step two: **Rebuild healthy tissue and restore energy.** With obstacles removed, activate your body's regulating powers to rebuild at optimum levels. Eat only fresh, simply prepared, vegetarian foods during the rebuilding step. Include supplements and herbal aids for your specific needs.

Step three: **Keep your body clean and toxin-free.** Modify your lifestyle habits for a strong resistant body. Rely on fresh fruits and vegetables for fiber (organic whenever possible), cooked vegetables, grains and seeds for strength, lightly cooked sea foods, GMO-free soy foods, eggs and low fat cheeses for protein, and a little dinner wine for circulatory health. Include supplements, herbs, exercise and relaxation techniques.

Cleanses come in all shapes and sizes. You can easily tailor a cleanse to your individual needs. Unless you require a specific detox for a serious illness, or recovery from a long course of drugs or chemotherapy, I recommend a short cleanse twice a year, especially in the spring, summer or early autumn when sunshine and natural vitamin D can help the process along. The easy detox program on the next two pages is a general cleanse that you can return to again and again, whenever your body needs a "wash and brush."

A body stress cleanse can start you off right

We're all overstressed today. A stress cleanse revitalizes your whole body. Just as you change the oil in your car to make it run smoother, and buy air and water filters to clean out environmental toxins, a stress cleanse clears the junk out of body pathways so that wholesome nutrients can get in to rebuild energy and strength. Highly processed "food" in today's supermarkets doesn't really have a lot that your body can translate into usable nutrients. Some "foods" like designer fake fats or hormone-treated animal foods may even contribute to illness.

Is your body showing signs that it needs a stress cleanse?

- Is your immune response low? Are you catching every bug that comes down the pike?
- Are you unusually tired? Do you feel mentally dull? Do you feel like you need a pick-me-up?
- Have you had bad body odor or bad breath lately?
- Are you under chronic stress or unusually depressed or irritable?
- Have you gained weight even though your diet hasn't changed?

Try this 3-Day Body Stress Cleanse with fresh juices

Start with a 3 day juice-liquid diet like this one and follow with 4 days of fresh foods. Eat plenty of fresh veggies and fruits, and fiber foods like whole grains and beans. Avoid trans fats, but get plenty of essential fatty acids from sea veggies, and herbs like ginger, borage or evening primrose oil. Drink plenty of water.

On rising: take a glass of 2 fresh squeezed lemons, and 1 tbsp. maple syrup in 8 oz. of water.

Breakfast: have a nutrient-dense Kick-Off Cleansing Cocktail: juice 1 handful fresh wheat grass or parsley (both rich in chlorophyll and antioxidants), 4 carrots, 1 apple, 2 celery stalks with leaves, ½ beet with top.

Mid-morning: have a glass of fresh carrot or fresh apple juice. Add 1 tbsp. of a green superfood like CRYSTAL STAR® ENERGY GREEN RENEWAL™ drink mix or PURE PLANET GREEN KAMUT.

Lunch: have a Salad-In-A-Glass: juice 4 parsley sprigs, 3 tomatoes, ½ bell pepper, ½ cucumber, 1 scallion, 1 lemon wedge.

Mid-afternoon: have a cup of CRYSTAL STAR® CLEANSING & PURIFYING™ tea, green tea or mint tea.

Dinner: have a warm Potassium broth for mineral electrolytes (page 16). Or Super Antioxidant Soup: 1 cup broccoli florets, 1 sliced leek, 2 cups peas, ½ cup sliced scallions, 4 cups chard leaves, ½ cup diced fennel bulb, ½ cup fresh parsley, 6 garlic minced cloves, 2 tsp. astragalus extract (or ¼ cup broken astragalus bark), 6 cups vegetable stock, pinch cayenne, 1 cup diced green cabbage, ¼ cup dry, chopped sea greens. Bring ingredients to a boil. Simmer 10 min. Let sit 20 minutes. Strain and use broth only.

Before bed: have a cup of warm miso soup with sea greens (any kind) snipped on top.

Choose 2 or 3 stress cleansing enhancer supplements to use during your cleanse:

- Cleansing boosters: CRYSTAL STAR® DETOX BLOOD PURIFIER™ caps with goldenseal stimulates the body to eliminate wastes rapidly, or CRYSTAL STAR® CLEANSING & PURIFYING™ tea.
- Cleansing nutritional support: NEW CHAPTER LIFE SHIELD or EARTH'S BOUNTY OXY-CLEANSE. When solid food is re-introduced, use NATURE'S SECRET ULTIMATE CLEANSE.
- Enzyme support: CRYSTAL STAR® DR. ENZYME 2: FAT & STARCH BUSTER™ or ENZYMEDICA PURIFY, or TRANSFORMATION EXCELLZYME.
- Antioxidants help remove toxins: SOURCE NATURALS ALPHA LIPOIC ACID, or BIOTEC CELL GUARD or RAINBOW LIGHT MULTI CAROTENE COMPLEX.
- Probiotics restore a friendly intestinal environment: JARROW FORMULAS JARRO-DOPHILUS+FOS or WAKUNAGA KYO-DOPHILUS or PREVAIL INNER ECOLOGY or GARDEN OF LIFE PRIMAL DEFENSE.
- Electrolytes dramatically boost energy: ALACER ELECTROMIX or NATURE'S PATH TRACE-LYTE LIQUID MINERALS.
- Green superfoods: CRYSTAL STAR® ENERGY GREEN RENEWAL™ drink; WAKUNAGA HARVEST BLEND.
- Detoxifying flower remedies: NATURAL LABS STRESS AND TENSION or NELSON BACH RESCUE REMEDY.

Bodywork techniques accelerate your cleanse:

- **Enemas:** Flushing your colon on the first and the last day of your stress detox quickly releases toxins.
- **Especially helpful:** Guided imagery, biofeedback and aromatherapy techniques.
- **Stretch:** Body stretch daily during your cleanse. Repeat 5 times.

   Stand tall; raise your hands above your head.
   Stretch your arms and fingers to reach for the sky.
   Move your hands and fingers as if you are climbing up into the sky.
   Rise on your toes as you reach; inhale deeply through your nostrils.
   Exhale slowly; gradually return to your starting position, arms loose at your sides.
   Follow your stretch with a brisk walk.
- **Breathing:** Deep, slow breathing removes stress, composes the mind, improves mood, increases energy.

   1. Take a full breath. Exhale, slowly. Slowly.
   2. Take another deep, full breath. Release slowly.
   3. And again.
   4. Maintain a quiet rhythm, exhaling more slowly than you inhale.
- **Massage:** A massage therapy treatment further removes toxins and stimulates cleansing circulation.
- **Yoga:** "Asanas" postures let energy to flow unimpeded in the body. Bikram classes are recommended.

Benefits you may notice as your body responds to a stress cleanse:

- Your digestion noticeably improves as your digestive tract is cleansed of accumulated waste.
- You'll feel lighter (most people lose about 5 pounds on this cleanse) and more energized.
- You'll feel less dependent on sugar, caffeine, nicotine, alcohol and drugs as your blood purifies.
- You'll feel healthier. Most people have noticeably better resistance to common colds and flu.
- You'll feel more mentally alert, less space-y, more emotionally balanced. Creativity begins to expand.
- You'll feel energized as your body rebalances. Energy levels rise physically, psychologically and sexually.

Remember these easy cleansing watchwords:

1. The day before you begin, eat green salads and fresh fruits, and drink plenty of healthy liquids, so that the upcoming body chemistry changes will not be uncomfortable. A gentle herbal laxative the night before helps.

2. Avoid all dairy products and cooked foods during this cleanse.

3. Drink 6 to 8 glasses of water daily to keep your body flushing out the toxins your tissues are releasing.

4. Focus your mind on internal cleansing—allow your energy to concentrate on inner vitality.

5. Bathe twice daily while cleansing, to remove toxins coming out on the skin. Dry brush your skin with a natural bristle brush for five minutes before a bath or shower, until skin is pink and glowing. Use a body scrub or natural "salt glow" for best results. Take an enema during the cleanse, to remove old, encrusted waste from the colon and to allow the juices to do their best work.

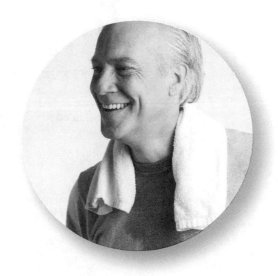

6. Take daily fresh air walks with deep breathing to enhance aerobic activity. Sunbathe early in the morning every day possible for increased purification and fortifying vitamin D.

Maintenance Recipes For Your Stress Detox Diet

Use these recipes on an ongoing basis once your initial healing diet is producing good results.

Potassium Juice

This recipe works for almost every health problem where cleansing is needed. It's the single most effective juice that I know for cleansing, neutralizing acids and rebuilding the body. It is a blood and body tonic that provides rapid energy and system balance.

Juice in the juicer:

3 carrots	3 stalks celery	½ bunch spinach
½ bunch parsley		

Add 1 – 2 tsp. Bragg's Liquid Aminos if desired. Makes 1 serving.

Nutrition per serving:	Vitamin E --------- 73 mg.	Cholesterol-------- 0	Potassium --------- 1602 mg.
Calories ----------- 136	Carbohydrates ---- 30 g.	Calcium ----------- 211 mg.	Sodium------------ 244 mg.
Protein ----------- 6 g.	Fiber ------------- 3 g.	Iron -------------- 2 mg.	Zinc -------------- 1 mg.
Vitamin C--------- 73 mg.	Trace Fats	Magnesium ------- 122 mg.	

Potassium Essence Broth

This recipe works for almost every health problem where cleansing is needed. Make this broth in a soup pot. It is an ideal source of minerals and electrolytes.

Cover with water in a soup pot:

4 carrots	3 ribs celery	2 potatoes (with skins)
½ bunch parsley	½ head cabbage	1 onion
½ bunch broccoli		

Simmer covered 30 minutes. Strain and discard solids. Add:

2 tsp. Bragg's Liquid Aminos or 1 tsp. miso	2" piece dry dulse

Store in the fridge. Makes a 2 day supply.

Nutrition per serving:	Vitamin E --------- 1 mg.	Cholesterol-------- 0	Potassium --------- 713 mg.
Calories ----------- 66	Carbohydrates ---- 15 g.	Calcium ----------- 84 mg.	Sodium------------ 32 mg.
Protein ----------- 4 g.	Fiber ------------- 6 g.	Iron -------------- 1 mg.	Zinc -------------- 1 mg.
Vitamin C--------- 39 mg.	Trace Fats	Magnesium ------- 53 mg.	

Purifying Vitamin C Flush

This recipe works for: Respiratory Infections, Immune Power, Childhood Diseases.

Juice:

1 cup strawberries, sliced	1 cup orange juice	1 kiwi, peeled
½ cup mango or pineapple chunks	¼" slice, peeled ginger root	¼ tsp. vitamin C crystals

Makes 2 servings.

Nutrition per serving:	Carbohydrates ---- 20 g.	Calcium ----------- 32 mg.	Zinc -------------- 1 mg.
Calories ----------- 91	Fiber ------------- 3 g.	Magnesium ------- 22 mg.	
Protein ----------- 2 g.	Fats---------------- 2 g.	Potassium --------- 404 mg.	
Vitamin E --------- 1.3 IU	Cholesterol-------- 0	Sodium------------ 32 mg.	

Diuretic Melon Mix

This recipe also helps Kidney Problems, Weight Control, High Blood Pressure. A morning drink for diuretic activity; take on an empty stomach 3 times daily.

Juice:

3 cups watermelon cubes	2 cups cantaloup cubes	2 cups honeydew cubes

Makes 1 quart.

Cleansing & Purifying Soup

This recipe also helps Asthma and Allergies, Compromised Immunity. May be used for the start of almost any healing diet.

Toast in a large pan until aromatic (about 5 minutes):

⅔ cup lentils	⅔ cup split peas	⅔ cup brown rice
2 cloves garlic, minced		

Add:

1 onion, chopped	1 carrot, chopped	1 rib celery, chopped
3 cups onion or veggie broth	3 cups water	1 tsp. turmeric powder
½ tsp. lemon-pepper seasoning	½ tsp. ginger powder	

Simmer gently for 1 hour, stirring occasionally. Makes 6 cups.

Nutrition per serving:	Vitamin E --------- 1 IU	Cholesterol-------- 0	Potassium --------- 446 mg.
Calories ----------- 341	Carbohydrates ---- 74 g.	Calcium ----------- 24 mg.	Sodium------------ 88 mg.
Protein ------------ 13 g.	Fiber ------------- 14 g.	Iron -------------- 1 mg.	
Vitamin C--------- 24 mg.	Fat---------------- 1 g.	Magnesium ------- 71 mg.	

Miso, Green Tea & Mushroom Healing Broth

This recipe works for: Illness Recovery, Compromised Immune Diseases.

In 1 cup water, steep:

2 tbsp. green tea leaves	2" piece of lemongrass	2 tbsp. sea greens, chopped

Add 3 cups dry shiitake mushrooms, soaked and slivered (save mushroom soaking water), and set aside.

In a medium pan, sauté the following:

1 tsp. olive oil	1 tsp. sesame oil
1 garlic clove, minced	½ small onion

Add 3 cups vegetable stock, bring to a boil and add:

¼ cup carrots, shredded	1 tbsp. miso paste	mushroom soaking water
¼ tsp. cayenne pepper		

Cook five minutes. Add green tea mixture and simmer gently 5 minutes. Makes 2 large servings.

Nutrition per serving:	Vitamin E --------- 1 IU	Cholesterol-------- 0	Potassium --------- 760 mg.
Calories ----------- 141	Carbohydrates ---- 31 g.	Calcium ----------- 98 mg.	Sodium------------ 154 mg.
Protein ------------ 9 g.	Fiber ------------- 6 g.	Iron -------------- 3 mg.	
Vitamin C--------- 25 mg.	Fat---------------- 1 g.	Magnesium ------- 79 mg.	

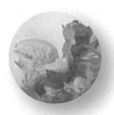

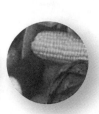
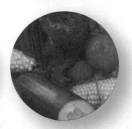

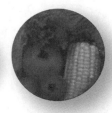

Stress Cleanse Veggie Juice

This recipe works for: Mental Energy, Liver/Organ Problems, Stress Exhaustion.

Juice:

1 small handful parsley	1 small handful watercress	2 stalks celery
1 carrot	½ bell pepper	1 tomato
1 broccoli floret		

Add ½ tsp. barley green powder. Makes 1 serving.

Nutrition per serving:	Vitamin E --------- 5 IU	Cholesterol-------- 0	Potassium --------- 1208 mg.
Calories ----------- 111	Carbohydrates ---- 24 g.	Calcium ----------- 141 mg.	Sodium------------ 145 mg.
Protein ------------ 6 g.	Fiber ------------- 8 g.	Iron -------------- 56 mg.	
Vitamin C--------- 195 mg.	Trace Fats	Magnesium ------- 67 mg.	

Apple Cleanse For Mucous Congestion

This recipe works for: Kidney Problems, Weight Control, High Blood Pressure.

Juice:

2 large apples, seeded	½ tsp. grated horseradish	2 tbsp. lemon juice

Makes 1 serving.

Immune Enhancer

This recipe also helps Immune Power, Immune Compromised Disease, Cancer.

Juice:

½ bunch parsley	1 garlic clove	6 carrots
3 stalks celery with leaves	2 tomatoes	1 bell pepper
a dash of hot sauce	4 romaine leaves	1 stalk broccoli
(or cayenne pepper)		

Add 1 tsp. miso paste mixed with a little water. Makes 2 drinks.

Nutrition per serving:	Carbohydrates ---- 27 g.	Calcium ----------- 70 mg.	Sodium------------ 128 mg.
Calories ----------- 126	Fiber ------------- 9 g.	Iron -------------- 2 mg.	Zinc -------------- 1 mg.
Protein ------------ 6 g.	Trace Fats	Magnesium ------- 42 mg.	
Vitamin C--------- 62 mg.	Cholesterol-------- 0	Potassium --------- 984 mg.	

Personal Best V-8

This recipe also helps Immune Power, Fatigue / Candida Syndromes, Anti-Aging. A high vitamin/mineral drink for normalizing body balance.

Juice:

6 – 8 tomatoes	3 – 4 green onions with tops	½ green pepper
(or 4 cups tomato juice)	2 carrots	2 ribs celery with leaves
½ bunch spinach, washed	½ bunch parsley	2 lemons, peeled,
		(or 4 tbsp. lemon juice).

Add: 2 tsp. BRAGG'S LIQUID AMINOS   ½ tsp. ground celery seed

Makes 6 glasses.

Sweep The Cobwebs Brain Booster

This recipe works for: Stress and Exhaustion, Brain Boosting, Anti-Aging.

Juice:

1 bunch parsley	4 carrots	1" piece of fresh or dried
2 stalks celery		burdock or ginseng root

Add 2 squirts of ginkgo biloba extract if desired. Makes 1 large drink.

Gland & Organ Cleanser

This recipe also works for Liver/Organ Problems, Skin Problems, Arthritis Diseases.

Juice:

4 apples	2 stalks celery	1 beet
1 bunch watercress	1 lemon	1 scallion
½ tsp. spirulina		

Makes 2 drinks.

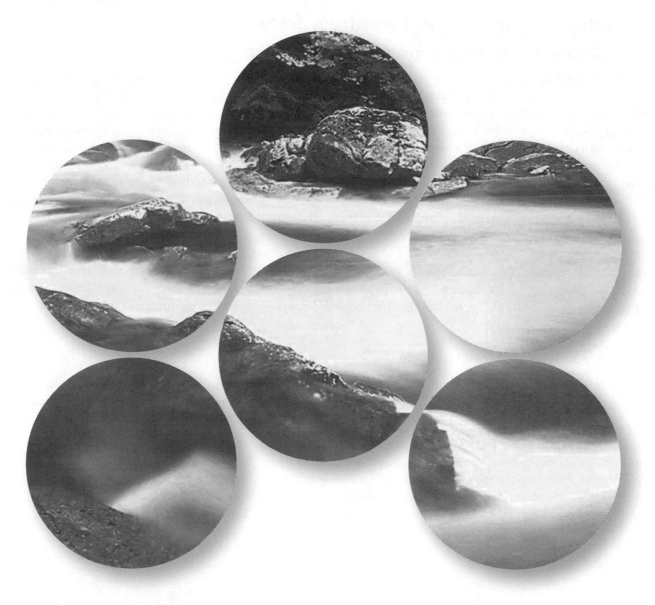

Allergies & Asthma:
Healing and Control

Allergies have become an epidemic of the 21st century. Once merely a nuisance, today more than 60 million Americans suffer from allergies—over 20% of our population! Environmental chemicals, acid rain, chemically treated and genetically altered foods, radiation levels, air and soil pollutants all add to the allergen load our bodies are faced with. Irresponsible use of antibiotics and steroid drugs taken over a long period of time for allergy symptoms can reduce immune response, and our ability to deal with allergens permanently. Allergy reactions are often an unrecognized cause of other illnesses, too—with problems like chronic sinusitis, cyclical headaches, epilepsy seizures, hypoglycemia, candida albicans infections and emotional over-reactions.

Substances that cause allergy reactions are called allergens. Most allergens produce congestion. Our bodies try to seal them off by forming a thick mucous shield and we get the allergy symptoms of sinus clog, stuffiness, headaches and red, puffy eyes. Our bodies may also try to throw them out through the skin causing rashes or boils, fever blisters, or a scratchy throat. Allergies can even alter personality, emotions, and one's sense of well-being.

Allergy origins fall into three main areas:

1. Allergies to seasonal environmental conditions.

Respiratory allergies affect up to 50 million people in the U.S. Allergies used to be defined as inappropriate immune responses to substances that *weren't* normally harmful—like cat hair, dust or wheat, or seasonal conditions like dust, pollen or spores. Today's dramatic rise in allergies is due to substances that *are* harmful, like environmental pollutants, secondhand smoke, and exhaust fumes. Stress and adrenal exhaustion, common problems in western societies set the stage for allergies by lowering immune response. Low enzymes and essential fatty acids are also usually involved. In response to all the sniffing and sneezing, the FDA recently approved over-the-counter sales of *(loratadine)* Claritin, an anti-allergy medication that is linked to animal liver tumors in high doses. Most drugstore medications for environmental allergies only mask symptoms, cause drowsiness and have a rebound effect. The more you use them, the more you need them. The newest ones are strong medicine… with strong side effects like rapid heartbeat. Even older antihistamines can be dangerous. *Diphenhydramine* (Benadryl) impairs driving performance more than alcohol. Steroid drugs for hayfever allergies, if taken for long periods, do not cure and often make the situation worse by depressing immune defenses, and impeding allergen elimination. More worrisome, environmental allergens frequently interact in the bodies of allergy sufferers, activating and aggravating other irritants. Then, even the most powerful drugs do not relieve symptoms.

Do you have seasonal allergies?

Respiratory allergies to environmental allergens like air pollutants, and seasonal allergens to dust, pollen, spores and mold, are called Type 1 allergies. This type of allergy develops more easily if your body has excess mucous accumulation to harbor the allergen irritants.

Spore and pollen allergens produce congestion, making you feel symptoms of sinus clog, stuffiness, headaches and puffy eyes. Sometimes your body throws this excess off through the skin, and you get skin irritations or a sore throat. An allergic response to spores and pollen may cause a histamine release that swells nasal passages and membranes, producing symptoms like runny, itchy nose and eyes, sneezing, coughing attacks, bronchial and sinus infections, skin rashes, asthma, insomnia, menstrual disorders and hypoglycemia.

Signs that you have a Type 1 allergy to environmental or seasonal allergens:

- Do you have chronic lung, bronchial and sinus infections with itchy, watery nose and eyes?
- Do you get frontal headaches with sneezing, coughing attacks and sore, scratchy throat?
- Does your face swell up, with an itchy rash on the skin? Do you have an itchy skin rash on your arms or torso?
- Do you have trouble sleeping? Do you have dark circles under your eyes that don't go away with sleep?
- Do you have PMS, unusual menstrual pain and congestion?
- Do you have hypoglycemia? Candida albicans yeast overgrowth? Learning disabilities?

2. Allergies to chemicals and contaminants.

We're exposed every day to more chemicals than any generation in history. One-third of Americans have sensitivities to chemicals! Allergic reactions to them are multiplying. Multiple Chemical Sensitivity (MCS), an illness now called a "silent epidemic," affects up to 15 million Americans. Irritants range from petrochemicals and estrogenic chemicals, to paints and household cleaners. Benzene, fluoride, formaldehyde, and carcinogens from carpeting and dry cleaning affect our brains. Other culprits include: gas stoves, chlorine bleach, laundry detergent (for less chemicals, try T-Wave Cleaning Capsules), fabric softener, nail polish remover, synthetic perfumes, moth balls and insect repellents. Sick buildings, Gulf War syndrome, nerve damage and attention deficit disorders are other types of chemical allergies in a growing list. Our bodies use up enormous amounts of nutrients trying to detoxify from these chemicals—nutrients that could be used to keep us happy and healthy.

Repeated chemical exposures set off rampant free radical reactions, as well as allergic responses. (Histamine reactions like itching, sneezing and runny nose are related to free radical damage to liver function from chemicals and pollutants.) Research shows 60% of people with chemical sensitivity have a vitamin B6 deficiency; 30% have a vitamin C deficiency; and 30% are deficient in vitamins B1, B2, B3, and B5. While many physicians do not recognize MCS as an official disorder, natural health practitioners regularly treat it with encouraging results.

Allergies to chemicals and contaminant allergens are called Type 2 allergies. Reactions to chemicals are frequently a defense mechanism, the body's attempt to isolate an offending substance by storing it in fatty tissue. An allergic reaction of this type only occurs after *the second exposure* to the irritant when your body's histamine response is alerted. Repeated exposures set off massive free radical reactions as the body's contaminant toleration levels are reached; toxic overload results and a severe allergic reaction sets in. Not only does chemical overload from the environment cause allergic reactions, it also impairs the body's immune response to them. Worse, chemical sensitivities initiate other allergy reactions, so that the sufferer becomes allergic to nearly everything else. Drug reactions mimic allergy reactions but usually don't involve the immune system (IgE antibodies).

Need an MD who practices environmental medicine? Check out www.aaem.com or call 316-684-5500.

Signs that you may have a Type 2 allergy to chemicals and contaminants:

- Unexplained migraine headaches? Usually with nausea or diarrhea?
- Frequent skin rashes for no explained reason?
- Feel "under the weather" no matter how much sleep you get? Are your ears ringing, especially at night?
- Frequent colds and flu, or chronic respiratory inflammations and low immune response to them?
- Frequently moody and depressed for no reason?
- Gained or lost weight recently for no reason? (Chemical allergies may cause abnormal metabolism.)
- Do you have chronic musculoskeletal pain or fibromyalgia?
- Do you have an autoimmune condition like M.S., rheumatoid arthritis, Hashimoto's thyroiditis, lupus?
- Do you use pesticides in your house or yard?
- Are you regularly exposed to toxic metals, chemicals or minerals at work?
- Have you ever had breast implants?
- Do friends and family tell you that your personality changes?
- Are you often spacey? Is your brain foggy, your mind sluggish? Is your memory unusually bad?
- Do you have a child that's chronically hyperactive or who has difficulty learning?

7-Day Chemical Pollutant Detox Diet

A good way to begin fortifying the immune system, especially if you're feeling noticeably tired, have had several exposures to chemical pollutants, or frequent infections, is to go on a simple, detox diet for 7 days. A pollution cleansing detox re-establishes normal body chemistry, gives your body a break from processing cooked or heavy foods, and releases hormone secretions that stimulate the immune complex and help restore its action.

For best results from your pollutant-heavy metal cleanse:

A heavy metal, pollutant detox is one of the most likely cleanses for a "healing crisis" to occur. You may feel head-achy, with a slight upset stomach as toxins release. The feelings should pass quickly, usually within 24 hours. I don't recommend an all-liquid diet if you're trying to cleanse heavy metals or chemicals. They may enter the bloodstream too fast and heavily for your body to handle safely. Eat solid *cleansing foods* instead to release the toxins more slowly and safely like cruciferous vegetables—broccoli, cabbage and cauliflower—to help flush out environmental estrogens in meats and pesticides.

- Drink 8 – 10 glasses of bottled water each day to clear toxins more rapidly.
- Chlorophyll is the most powerful detoxifier in nature. Use green veggie drinks and green superfoods.
- Sea greens are powerful releasers of chemicals, heavy metals and radiation from the body. Sprinkle 2 tbsp. daily on any food during your cleanse. Keep sea greens high on your immune list with 6 pieces of sushi a week.
- Fresh fruit and vegetable juices maximize your body's immune power.

Key juices for immunity:
  - Garlic, tomatoes, celery and carrots: (antibacterial and antifungal properties).
  - Alfalfa sprouts, apples and celery: (an ideal source of cleansing protein). Sprouts are rich in vitamin A, B-complex, C, D and E, enzymes, essential fatty acids and antioxidant minerals, natural immune strengtheners, apples and celery improve lymphatic health by drawing toxins out of your tissues to be flushed away.
  - Potassium juice with beets, spinach, carrots and parsley (for liver function).
  - Banana, strawberry or blueberry (vitamin C and potassium).
  - Add ¼ tsp. of a potent acidophilus complex to each juice during your chemical detox diet cleanse to stimulate friendly G.I. flora, and build enzyme strength, a key factor of strong immunity.

The night before (and several times during your detox) have an immune boosting broth. Mix miso, onions, garlic, shiitake mushrooms, and astragalus root, (an immune-boosting Chinese herb from the health food store). The miso represses carcinogens and neutralizes toxins. The onions and garlic fight off pathogens. The shiitake mushrooms (easy to find today in gourmet stores) help stimulates interferon in the body.

On rising: take 2 tbsp. cranberry concentrate in water with ½ tsp. Vitamin C crystals; or CRYSTAL STAR® GREEN TEA CLEANSER™; or blend 2 tsp. lemon, 1 tsp. honey, 1 cup water and 1 tsp. acidophilus in 8 oz. of aloe vera juice.

Breakfast: a fresh carrot juice or veggie juice (see above) with 1 tbsp. green superfood like CRYSTAL STAR® ENERGY GREEN RENEWAL™ mix or SUN WELLNESS CHLORELLA, and whole grain muffins or rice cakes with kefir cheese; or a cup of plain yogurt blended with a cup of fresh fruit, walnuts, and ½ tsp. acidophilus.

Mid-morning: take a cup of green tea, with ½ tsp. ascorbate vitamin C crystals; or a fresh vegetable juice with 1 tbsp. green superfood like NUTRICOLOGY PRO-GREENS WITH EFAS, or ETHICAL NUTRIENTS HARVEST BLEND.

Lunch: a salad with lemon-flax oil dressing; or miso soup with sea greens and brown rice; or steamed veggies with brown rice and sea greens; and green tea with ½ tsp. vitamin C and ½ tsp. acidophilus powder.

Mid-afternoon: have carrot juice with 1 tbsp. green superfood like Crystal Star® Energy Green Renewal™ drink or a tonic broth (see above).

Dinner: have a baked potato with Bragg's Liquid Aminos and a fresh salad with lemon-flax dressing; or a black bean or lentil soup; or a Chinese steam/stir fry with vegetables, shiitake mushrooms and brown rice.

Before Bed: an 8 oz. glass of aloe vera juice with ½ tsp. vitamin C or a cup of green tea.

Choose 2 or 3 supplements that can enhance and accelerate your program:

- **Pollutant-heavy metal cleansers:** Crystal Star® Toxin Detox™ caps or Detox Blood Purifier™ caps for 3 months. Oral chelation Metabolic Response Modifiers Cardio-Chelate; Golden Pride Formula One w/ EDTA. For radiation poisoning: vitamin C powder with bioflavonoids ½ tsp. every hour to bowel tolerance.
- **Enzymes:** Protease binds to heavy metals, sparing metabolic enzyme destruction. Transformation Purezyme (high doses effective in lowering mercury toxins); or Crystal Star® Dr. Enzyme™.
- **Liver enhancers:** Alpha Lipoic Acid 600 mg. daily for 2 months; Jarrow Formulas Alpha Lipoic Acid or Glucotize by MRI; Crystal Star® Liver Renew™ caps or Liver Cleanse Flushing™ tea; or Planetary Bupleurum Liver Cleanse tabs or Dandelion extract; Evening Primrose oil caps 4 daily; Biostrath Liquid Yeast.
- **Antioxidants defeat pollutants:** Carnitine 1000 mg. 3x daily for 1 month; NAC (N-acetyl-cysteine) 500 mg. 3x daily; CoQ-10, 60 mg. 4x daily; Nutricology germanium 150 mg. daily. Beta carotene 150,000IU with extra lycopene 5-10 mg.; PCOs from grapeseed or white pine 100 mg. 3 daily; Vitamin E 400IU with selenium 200 mcg.; Glutathione 100 mg. daily; Microhydrin available at royalbodycare.com; Ethical Nutrients Zinc Status; Source Naturals Chem-Defense caps; Biotec Cell Guard 8 daily.
- **Build strong immune defenses with herbal immune enhancers:** Astragalus extract; Propolis extract or lozenges; Garlic 6 – 8 caps daily; Echinacea extract; Cat's Claw caps; Siberian eleuthero extract caps; Spirulina 2 tsp. daily, or Pure Planet 100% Spirulina tabs; C'est si Bon Chlorenergy daily for chemical toxins.

Bodywork techniques jump start healing and keep it going:

- Protect against radiation syndromes: avoid foods labeled irradiated or electronically pasteurized.
- Avoid as much as possible: smoking and secondary smoke, pesticides and herbicides, phosphorus fertilizers, fluorescent lights, aluminum cookware, deodorants and antacids. Use vinegar, baking soda and salt as cleansers instead of commercial products if you are very sensitive.
- Protect yourself from EMF fields: avoid non-filtered computer screens, cell phones, electric blankets, microwave ovens. (Don't use plastic wrap in the microwave, its heat can drive the molecules into the food.)
- Do deep breathing exercises on rising, and in the evening on retiring to clear the respiratory system.
- Use Earth's Bounty O$_2$ Spray on soles of feet every 2 days to keep tissue oxygen high.
- Seek out trees to live around. Trees produce oxygen and remove many air pollutants. Invest in an air filter. Pay attention to unhealthy air alerts; stay indoors if you have chemical sensitivities.
- Take a hot seaweed bath, like Crystal Star® Hot Seaweed Bath™ or a sauna once a week to accelerate toxin release. Use a dry skin brush before and after the bath or sauna to remove toxins coming out on the skin.
- Stimulate immunity with 20 minutes of early morning sunlight every day. Avoid excessive sun. A sunburn depresses immunity.
- Get quality rest: immune power builds most during sleep.

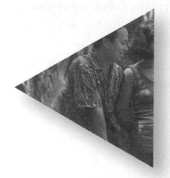
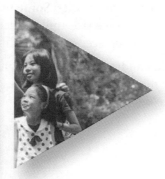
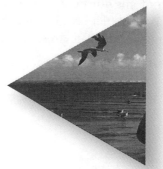
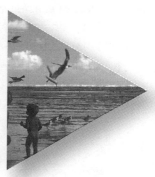

3. Allergies to foods and food additives.

Food intolerances are often confused with food allergies. A food allergy is an antibody reaction—an *immune system* response to a food your body sees as a pathogen or parasite. A food intolerance is a *non-immune* reaction, usually an enzyme deficiency to digest a certain food. For example, people with a lactose intolerance experience the bloating, cramping and diarrhea of an allergy reaction, but the symptoms are really due to a deficiency of the enzyme lactase, which helps digest milk sugar. Lactose intolerance affects between 30 and 50 million Americans, a full 75% of African Americans and over 90% of Asian Americans. Celiac disease, a sensitivity to gluten, a wheat protein, affects about 20% of Americans.

Food sensitivities of all kinds are growing as people are more exposed to chemically altered, genetically-modified, enzyme-depleted foods. Low enzyme activity means food assimilation is only partial, leaving large amounts of undigested fats and proteins that the immune system treats as potentially toxic. Prostaglandins, leukotrienes, and histamines enter the bloodstream in an immune response and allergy reactions occur.

You're highly likely to experience allergic reactions if you eat a lot of fast foods. Fast foods are often loaded with food additives—nitrites, aspartame, MSG and sulfites. Chemically altered, sprayed, or injected foods also put your body under a lot of stress—it shows up in low gastric pH, leaky gut syndrome or candida albicans yeast overgrowth. Watch your diet closely if you're a frequent traveler. Jet lag stress, insufficient sleep, unusual or unfamiliar foods, chemically sprayed or adulterated foods all lay the groundwork for allergic reactions.

Find out which foods you're allergic to with Coca's Pulse test

Coca's Pulse Test can help you find and eliminate foods that harm. Dr. Arthur Coca, an immunologist, discovered that when people eat foods to which they are allergic, there is a dramatic increase in heartbeat—20 or more beats a minute above normal. Since pulse rate is normally remarkably stable, unaffected by digestion, ordinary physical activities or normal emotions, Cocoa theorized that unless a person is ill or under great stress, pulse rate deviation is probably due to an allergy.

Coca's Pulse Test:

1. Take your pulse when you wake in the morning. Using a watch with a second hand, count the number of beats in a 60-second period. A normal pulse is 60-100 beats per minute.

2. Take your pulse again after eating a suspected allergy food. Wait 15 to 20 minutes and take your pulse again. If your pulse rate has increased more than 10 beats per minute, omit that food from your diet.

A Three-Day Food Allergy Cleansing Diet

Diet change and herbal supplements are the best and quickest means of overcoming food intolerances, and restoring digestive tract and immune system integrity. A food elimination-rotation diet has become well known for identifying suspected allergen foods, especially for those patients who are overweight, have candida, sluggish thyroid or hypoglycemia. In medical allergy treatment, much time is spent trying to find the offending foods. You can speed up the process by eliminating common food allergens first—like wheat, dairy foods, chocolate, eggs, sugar, corn, yeast and sprayed foods. Tune in to your personal diet history and try to eat ONLY the foods you *least* suspect of causing symptoms during the elimination phase of the diet. **Some normally safe food choices:** rice milk, almond milk, non-gluten flat breads or quick breads, brown rice, millet, buckwheat, amaranth, quinoa, date sugar, maple syrup, almond butter, sesame butter, and egg replacer made from flax or arrowroot.

Note about kids' allergies: Food allergies are common in children; many result from feeding babies meats and commercial dairy foods before 10 – 12 months. Babies do not have the right enzymes to digest these foods. Feed mother's milk, rice milk or goat's milk for 10 months to avoid food allergies.

The simple, short 3-day cleanse below is designed to rid your body of food allergens. You can also use it as the basis of a food rotation diet to determine your personal sensitivities. Introduce suspected foods in small amounts, one at a time. Most people notice a difference right away.

On rising: squeeze 2 fresh lemons in a glass of water with 1 packet of Sun Wellness Chlorella granules.

Breakfast: take a glass of cranberry-apple or papaya juice; or non-sweet fruits like pineapple or kiwi.

Mid-morning: a Personal Best V-8 (page 18), or Pure Planet Just Barley, or Crystal Star® Energy Green Renewal™ drink; and some fresh vegetable snacks with a little sesame salt.

Lunch: a glass of pineapple/coconut juice for protein; or a fresh carrot juice, with a green salad and lemon-olive oil dressing.

Mid-afternoon: take a cup of alkalizing herb tea, like green tea, catnip, alfalfa-mint, or peppermint tea.

Dinner: have a small green salad with lemon-olive oil dressing; or a glass of apple-alfalfa sprout juice.

Before bed: a relaxing tea, like chamomile or scullcap tea; or a glass of pineapple/papaya, or apple juice.

Notes:
- Drink 6 glasses of water daily to flush allergens through your system.
- Take 2 tbsp. apple cider vinegar with honey at each meal if desired to acidify saliva.
- Be sure, for these three days, that you eat only organically grown, fresh foods—no processed foods that might have fillers, additives or hidden sugars or chemicals.

Diet to Overcome Food Allergies and Sensitivities

Use this diet for 30 days or more to rebalance, alkalize and energize. It is dairy and gluten free, and does not include other common allergens, like corn, yeast, soy, mushrooms, eggs, refined sweeteners, or shellfish, currently at risk of contamination. It is rich in minerals and enzyme-producing foods, and uses good food combining techniques for optimal absorption. Be sure you're omitting any foods containing sulfites, nitrates, nightshade plant derivatives (like tobacco), colorants, preservatives and additives.

See the COOKING TIPS SECTION, page 237 for foods you can use in place of those that cause problems.

On rising: take a glass of lemon juice with 1 tsp. maple syrup; or cranberry juice with a little honey and ginger; or add New Chapter Ginger Wonder syrup to any drink to help block inflammation.

Breakfast: take a supplement drink like All One Multiple Vitamin And Mineral drink, or a superfood high vitamin C drink, like Jarrow Gentle Fibers drink to guard against leaky-gut; or some oatmeal or wheat-free grain cereal with apple juice or yogurt, and 1 tbsp. maple syrup.

Mid-morning: have a green drink (page 18), or Crystal Star Energy Green Renewal™ drink, or Green Foods Green Magma Drink; or a glass of fresh carrot juice; and a cup of light noodle soup with sea greens snipped on top and perhaps some cubes of almond cheese.

Lunch: have a green salad with a light dressing, and a cup of vegetable or onion soup; or some steamed vegetables and a baked potato with yogurt or kefir cheese topping; or a fruit salad with cottage cheese.

Mid-afternoon: a glass of apple juice, or an alkalizing herb tea, like a hibiscus cooler, or alfalfa/mint tea.

Dinner: have a stir-fry with greens, rice noodles, and a sweet and sour sauce; or a baked or grilled salmon or sea bass with brown rice and peas; or a large salad with nut and seed toppings and a yogurt dressing; or a baked vegetable casserole with a cup of black bean or lentil soup; or roast turkey slices from free-run organic turkeys, with a salad and baked potato with rice cheese on top. A little white wine (a cultured food) is fine before meals.

Before bed: have a glass of apple, pineapple or papaya juice; or a cup of miso soup with sea greens.

Notes:
- Weight gain is an insidious effect of food allergy. Eliminate wheat to stop allergy-related weight gain.
- Eat plenty of fresh vegetables, fruits, fruit and veggie juices, sea greens, whole grains, seeds and beans.
- Add ½ tsp. spirulina or chlorella granules to any juice or drink during the day to neutralize allergens.
- Cultured foods like yogurt help digestive flora; use unsaturated vegetable oils. Drink bottled water.
- Eat relaxed. Tension and stress reduce your body's ability to deal with allergens. Eat smaller meals.

Choose 2 or 3 supplements to enhance and accelerate your program:
- **Cleanse the G.I. tract:** CRYSTAL STAR® BITTERS & LEMON CLEANSE™, green tea, aloe vera juice each morning.
- **Produce antihistamines:** CRYSTAL STAR® ANTI-HST™ or BAYWOOD DR. HARRIS ORIGINAL ALLERGY FORMULA caps; CoQ-10 60 mg. 3x daily.
- **Reduce allergic reactions:** EUROPHARMA SNEEZE-EZE (especially for eczema caused by food allergies); CC POLLEN ALLER-BEE-GONE, MSM 1000 mg. 2x daily; CRYSTAL STAR® DR. VITALITY™ caps with green and white tea; Omega-3 flax oil with meals for essential fatty acids (EFAs).
  - For gluten intolerance: CRYSTAL STAR® CANDIDA YEAST DETOX™ caps especially if there is unexplained weight gain and bloating; BIO-ALLERS FOOD ALLERGY-GRAIN.
  - For lactose intolerance: Lactaid drops or tablets; COUNTRY LIFE DAIRY-ZYME; PREVAIL DAIRY ENZYMES.
- **Add a digestive & proteolytic enzyme formula:** Use a full spectrum digestive enzyme like CRYSTAL STAR® DR. ENZYME 2: FAT & STARCH BUSTER™ caps, and a protease formula like TRANSFORMATION PUREZYME. Quercetin 500 mg. daily between meals with bromelain 500 mg. 3x daily for antioxidant activity plus enzymes.
- **Add probiotics:** Acidophilus before meals; aloe vera juice with 2 tsp. bee pollen granules after meals for best enzyme activity. For a sour stomach: add lime juice and a pinch ginger.
- **Herbal enzymes boost immunity/normalize digestion:** Milk thistle seed extract; Dandelion root-nettles tea; Echinacea-goldenseal root caps; GAIA SWEETISH BITTERS; or add a tsp. of NEW CHAPTER GINGER WONDER SYRUP to water and take before and after meals.

Bodywork techniques jump start healing and keep it going:
- **Diagnose:** Use Coca's Pulse Test to identify allergens. (See page 24.) Both skin-prick and RAST tests used by many allergists often misdiagnose food allergies unless a rotation/re-introduction diet is also used.
- NAET (Nambudripad Allergy Elimination) combines muscle testing, acupuncture and chiropractic techniques to help eliminate allergies and sensitivities. Many allergy sufferers report good results.
- **Enema:** Consider a garlic-catnip enema to cleanse the digestive tract and balance colon pH.
- **Avoid caffeine, aspirin, and cortisone drugs.** Each of these can damage the stomach and intestinal walls, and cause gastritis and ulcers.
- **No smoking before meals.** Nicotine magnifies allergies almost more than any other substance.
- **No fluids with meals:** especially don't drink sodas or carbonated drinks. Phosphoric acid binds up many digestive enzymes.

Asthma Control Diet

Asthma, inflammation of the bronchial tubes, is a severe respiratory allergy reaction. Since 1980, asthma has increased by 75% in America, with a 50% rise in the last decade, mainly due to more environmental pollutants. It now affects 4% of the U.S. population, about 18 million people, 2.5 million of whom have needed emergency treatment. More alarming, a new study by The Pew Environmental Health Commission concludes that 29 million people will have asthma by 2020! Asthma is the leading serious, chronic illness in children under ten, (2:1 ratio of boys to girls), with a death rate of about 5,000 kids a year. Children have smaller lungs and bronchial tubes, and less breathing reserves during an asthma attack than adults. They also have more cold and flu infections that trigger asthma attacks. Heredity, diet and lifestyle are all involved with asthma's development and severity. A child whose mother has asthma is more likely to develop it than other children. Some studies show a greater risk of asthma with childhood vaccinations.

Some scientists believe that America's high rates of asthma are a result of a marked decrease in vitamin C antioxidants. Unlike other mammals, humans can't manufacture vitamin C on their own; we must obtain it from eating vitamin C rich foods or taking vitamin C supplements. An asthmatic's difficult breathing, choking, wheezing, coughing is actually a failure to *exhale*, not inhale. In asthma, the lung airways become red, swollen and full of thick mucous. A person with healthy lungs can empty air in about 2 – 3 seconds. An asthmatic's lungs take 6 – 7 seconds! Bronchial spasms constrict airways. The inflamed, constricted airways react, often progressively, to asthma triggers (see below). Drug-free natural therapies can help reduce the need for medication. Still, emergency medical measures may be necessary to arrest severe asthma attacks which can be life threatening.

Why has asthma risen almost 50% in the last decade?

Environmental toxins are becoming a clear cause for the rise in asthma attacks. Toxin build up in the body is a common trigger for allergy or asthma symptoms. We take in chemical contaminants as we breathe. We take in more chemicals from pesticides and additives in our foods, and chemical toxins in our water. Releasing toxic accumulations makes a big difference. **The average American eats his or her own weight in chemicals each year!**

Asthma is an immune deficient illness. Some naturopaths see the huge increase in prescription drug use over the last decade as a clear factor in asthma because it means more immune suppression. Even simple medications like aspirin may provoke asthma; and NSAIDS may aggravate asthma because they can elevate leukotrienes involved in allergic reactions. The over use of asthma drugs may be playing a role in the upswing of attacks, too. Prescription bronchodilators and inhalers for asthma work short-term, relaxing constricted airways during an attack. When overused, these drugs can lose their effectiveness and cause side effects like tremors, dizziness, nausea, even strokes. Bronchodilators relieve symptoms temporarily, but they don't address asthmatic inflammation. Inhaled corticosteroid drugs can help prevent asthma attacks and minimize severity. However, using steroid inhalers long term may increase risk for glaucoma, cataracts and interfere with normal growth in children. Most inhalers also contain chlorofluorocarbons (CFCs) linked to the depletion of the Earth's protective ozone layer.

- Be very cautious when switching from oral steroid drugs to the new inhaled steroid drugs (like FLOVENT) to treat asthma symptoms. The new inhaled steroids are less active than oral steroid drugs. A warning now appears in the PDR advising caution because deaths due to adrenal insufficiency have occurred in some patients who switched their medication abruptly.

- Food sensitivities play a major role in asthma attacks. The food allergy-asthma link has long been established, especially from triggers like foods with (MSG) and sulfiting agents used widely in wine, beer and snacks. New food colorants and additives are on the rise. Avoid high gluten breads, oily and fried foods, soft drinks and sugary foods that contain a lot of these additives. Reduce salt. Asthma is common when salt intake is high. Avoid dairy products; they generate the most mucous. Limit animal foods in general. Leukotrienes that contribute to asthma reactions are derived from arachidonic acid found only in animal products.

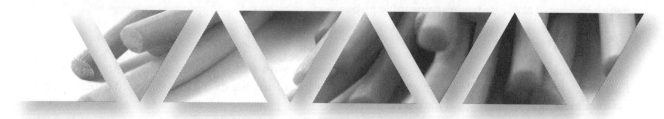

Is your body overloaded with mucous congestion?

Your body needs some mucous. We're taught that mucous is a bad thing because it obstructs our breathing during a sinus infection, asthma or a cold. But mucous is also a body lubricant and an important body safeguard. We take about 22,000 breaths a day. Mucous gathers up irritants like dirt, pollen, smoke and pollutants we take in to protect mucous membranes in the respiratory system. Foods that putrefy quickly in your body like meat, eggs and dairy products are those most likely to produce excess mucous. These foods also slow down transit time through your gastrointestinal tract. Some of us carry around as much as 10 – 15 pounds of excess mucous!

Is your body showing signs that it needs a mucous cleanse?

• Your breathing is labored. You have a chronic wheeze or cough. You have difficulty exhaling.
• You have chronic bronchitis or sinus congestion, with a runny nose and sneezing.
• You use over-the-counter drugs for allergy or asthma (which often drives congestion deeper into lungs).
• Allergies and asthma usually mean excess mucous in the colon, too, so you may experience constipation.
• You catch every infection going around, (excess mucous is a breeding ground for infectious microbes).

Basic Mucous Elimination Diet for Seasonal Allergies and Asthma: A 3 – 4 day nutrition plan

Diet changes and taking therapeutic herbs are the most beneficial and quickest means of controlling allergies and asthma. A short 3 or 4 day mucous elimination diet is a good way to start relieving allergy and asthma reactions because it rids the body of excess mucous build-up, paving the way for nutritional changes to take effect.

The night before your mucous elimination diet...

Mash 4 garlic cloves and a large slice of onion in a bowl. Stir in 3 tbsp. honey. Cover, let soak for 24 hours; remove garlic and onion and take only the honey/syrup infusion—1 tsp. 3x daily.

The next day...

On rising: take 2 squeezed lemons in water with 1 tbsp. maple syrup.

Breakfast: have a water-diluted grapefruit juice or pineapple juice as natural expectorants with 1 tbsp. green superfood, like CRYSTAL STAR® RESTORE YOUR STRENGTH, BARLEANS GREENS or NATURE'S SECRET ULTIMATE GREEN; take 2 or 3 garlic capsules and ¼ tsp. ascorbate vitamin C or Ester C powder in water.

Mid-morning: have a glass of fresh carrot juice with 1 tsp. BRAGG'S LIQUID AMINOS added; or spring water with 3 sprays of CRYSTAL STAR® D-CONGEST™ extract, an expectorant to aid mucous release, or YOGI BREATHE DEEP tea, to help in oxygen uptake.

Lunch: have a vegetable juice like V-8, or a Potassium Drink (page 16); or make a Mucous Cleansing Tonic by juicing: 4 carrots, 2 celery stalks, 2 – 3 sprigs parsley, 1 radish and 1 garlic clove.

Mid-afternoon: have a green veggie drink (page 18), or a tsp. of SUN WELLNESS CHLORELLA granules in water; or a sea greens drink like CRYSTAL STAR® ENERGY GREEN RENEWAL™.

Dinner: take a hot miso, green tea broth (page 17), add 1 tbsp. nutritional yeast. Add a small fresh salad the last night of the cleanse.

Before Bed: have apple or papaya/pineapple juice.

The day after that...

Have toasted muesli or whole grain granola for breakfast, with a little yogurt or apple juice; a small fresh salad for lunch with lemon/oil dressing; a fresh fruit smoothie during the day; a baked potato drizzled with flax or olive oil and a light soup or salad for dinner.

Benefits of a mucous elimination cleanse:

• Chest congestion clears as the non-mucous forming diet begins to work.
• Bronchial inflammation and a chronic cough are relieved as the cleanse progresses.
• Chronic lung and throat mucous are broken up and released.
• Mucous from the colon is often expelled in a series of ropy, slimy stools.
• Discomfort from colds or flu, allergies or asthma clears faster.

Pointers for best results from your mucous cleanse:

- Herbal teas are a good choice. They act as premier bronchodilators and antispasmodics to open congested airspaces and break up mucous. They soothe bronchial inflammation and coughs. They are expectorants to remove mucous from the lungs and throat.
- Drink 8 glasses of water each day of your cleanse to thin mucous and aid elimination.
- Eliminate junk foods, fried foods, pasteurized dairy foods, and refined foods; they are a breeding ground for continued congestion.
- Eat plenty of fresh enzyme-rich foods. They form little mucous and they are the easiest to digest.

Choose 2 or 3 supplements to enhance and accelerate your cleansing program:

Deep body cleanser for intestinal tract and lungs: NATURE'S WAY 5 SYSTEM CLEANSE caps after juice cleansing help pull and clear intestinal mucous and mucous congestion from the respiratory system. NATURE'S SECRET ULTI-MATE RESPIRATORY CLEANSE works especially well for long-standing respiratory-mucous congestion problems.

Mucous cleansers: CRYSTAL STAR® D-CONGEST™ SPRAY was specially formulated for mucous release; HERBS ETC. LUNG TONIC helps loosen and remove mucous; BAYWOOD DR. HARRIS' ORIGINAL ALLERGY FORMULA has herbal anti-histamines and enzymes which digest excess mucous secretions, allowing the body to safely eliminate them.

Herbs to relieve stuffiness: mullein loosens and expels mucous; slippery elm removes excess mucous, soothes mucous membranes; sage helps mucous discharge; white pine, an antioxidant expectorant, reduces mucous. CRYSTAL STAR® ANTI-HST™ for histamine reactions.

Herbal aromatherapy oils help clear mucous: Eucalyptus (inhale) - antiviral action works on respiratory tract to loosen mucous - treats asthma, bronchitis and sinusitis. Tea tree oil (inhale) - antiviral, antibacterial decongestant. Oregano oil (inhale) - antiviral and antibacterial properties help eradicate lung infection.

Better oxygen uptake: YOGI BREATHE DEEP tea; or 10,000 mg. ascorbate vitamin C crystals with bioflavonoids daily the first three days (just dissolve ¼ tsp. in water or juice throughout the day, until the stool turns soupy, and tissues are flushed). Take 5,000 mg. daily for the next four days..

Enzyme and Probiotics maintain proper mucous levels: PURE ESSENCE LABS ALLER FREE; TRANSFORMATION ENZYME GASTROZYME relieves bouts of mucous congestion. UAS DDS-PLUS WITH FOS; JARROW JARRO-DOPHILUS.

Bodywork techniques are pivotal to increase oxygen use in the lungs and tissues.

- **Release mucous fast:** Take 1 tsp. fresh grated horseradish in a spoon with lemon juice.
- **Enema:** Take an enema the first and last day of your fasting diet to thoroughly clean out excess mucous.
- **Irrigate:** A colonic offers a more thorough colon cleanse.
- **Exercise:** Take a brisk walk each day of your cleanse, breathing deeply to help the lungs eliminate mucous.
- **Massage therapy with percussion:** a percussion massage loosens mucous. Most people have several congestion-releasing bowel movements and expectoration incidences within 24 hours after massage therapy.
- **Compress:** Apply wet ginger-cayenne compresses to the chest to increase circulation and loosen mucous.
- **Bathe and Sauna:** Take a hot sauna or a long warm bath with a rubdown to stimulate circulation and help loosen mucous congestion. Add to your bath 5 drops of eucalyptus, tea tree oil or oregano oil.
- **Deep Breathing Exercise:** Do this deep breathing exercise often during your cleanse to remove stress, compose your mind, improve your mood and increase your energy: Take a deep, full breath: engage the diaphragm so that the lungs are filled to capacity. Exhale it slowly… slowly. Take another deep, full breath. Release slowly. And again. Maintain a quiet rhythm, exhaling more slowly than you inhale.

Maintenance Recipes For Your Mucous Elimination Cleanse

Use these recipes on an ongoing basis once your initial healing diet is producing good results.

Ginger - Lemon Cleanse For Allergies

Juice:

1" slice fresh ginger root	6 carrots with tops	1 lemon
1 apple, cored		

Makes 2 drinks (a day's supply).

Ever Green Drink

A personal favorite for taste, mucous release and enzymatic action.

Juice:

1 apple (with skin)	1 tub (4 oz.) alfalfa sprouts	½ fresh pineapple (skinned/cored)
1 tsp. spirulina or chlorella	4 sprigs fresh mint	

Makes 1 drink.

Onion - Miso Antibiotic Broth

1 onion, chopped	1 stalk celery (with leaves)	4 tbsp. miso
½ tsp. sesame oil	1 qt. vegetable broth	2 green onions, chopped

Sauté onion in sesame oil for 5 minutes. Add celery and sauté for 2 minutes. Add vegetable broth and simmer, covered, for 10 minutes. Add miso and green onions and remove from heat. Whirl in blender.

Makes 6 small bowls of broth.

Body Balancing Apple Broth

This broth also alkalizes body pH and helps lower serum cholesterol.

½ red onion chopped	1 small red bell pepper	2 tbsp. parsley, chopped
2 cloves garlic, minced	2 tart apples, cored	2 cups KNUDSEN'S LOW SODIUM
1 tsp. grapeseed oil	1 lemon, partially peeled	VERY VEGGIE-SPICY JUICE

Sauté onion and garlic in the grapeseed oil for 5 minutes. While sautéing, in a blender combine the bell pepper, apples, lemon, parsley and VERY VEGGIE-SPICY JUICE. Add onion mix to blender and purée. Return to the stove and heat gently. Take hot. Makes 4 servings.

Mucous Cleansing Chicken Soup

Your grandmother was right. Hot chicken broth has immune stimulants and really does clear chest congestion fast.

3 cups homemade chicken broth	2 thin slices ginger	½ cup fresh pea pods
½ cup bean sprouts	2 tbsp. soy sauce	½ cup Chinese cabbage, shredded
1 cup chicken, cooked & shredded	½ cup carrots, sliced	

In a soup pot, combine chicken broth and bean sprouts and bring to a simmer. Add chicken, ginger, soy sauce and carrots. Simmer 10 minutes. Add pea pods and cabbage and heat for another 3 minutes. Serve with a dash of light soy sauce or BRAGG'S LIQUID AMINOS. Makes 2 large bowls of soup.

Asthma Control Diet Plan

You can start with this 3-day nutrition plan, or use it after your Mucous Elimination Cleanse (page 28). Note: During an asthma attack, eat only fresh foods. Include fresh apple or carrot juice daily.

The night before your asthma diet...

Make a syrup of pressed garlic juice, cayenne, olive oil and honey. Take 1 tsp. each day of your diet as a liver cleansing, bile stimulant for fatty-acid metabolism.

On rising: take a glass of fresh apple, grapefruit juice or cranberry juice; or lemon juice in hot water with 1 tsp. honey; or a glass of apple cider vinegar, hot water and honey.

Breakfast: take a hot Potassium Broth (page 16); or CRYSTAL STAR® RESTORE YOUR STRENGTH™ drink; or apple juice with 1 tsp. SUN WELLNESS CHLORELLA. Add 3 garlic caps and ¼ tsp. Ester C powder with bioflavs in water.

Mid-morning: have a glass of fresh carrot juice; and/or a cup of comfrey/fenugreek tea.

Lunch: have a hot vegetable, miso or onion broth, or CRYSTAL STAR® RESTORE YOUR STRENGTH™ drink. Add 3 garlic caps and ¼ tsp. ascorbate vitamin C or Ester C powder with bioflavonoids in water.

Mid-afternoon: have an alfalfa/mint or CRYSTAL STAR® GREEN TEA CLEANSER™; or a fruit or vegetable juice.

Dinner: have a hot veggie broth, or miso soup with sea greens snipped on top; or a glass of carrot juice with 1 tbsp. BARLEAN'S GREENS. Add 3 garlic caps and ¼ tsp. Ester C powder with bioflavonoids.

Before Bed: take another hot water, lemon and honey drink; apple or cranberry juice.

Pointers for best results:

• Eat fish, like salmon, swordfish, halibut, etc; they contain Omega-3 fatty acids that help control asthma.
• You must avoid all food additives to control asthma. Check package labels on every food you buy.
• Water makes a big difference. There is a link between dehydration and excess histamine production. Eight to ten glasses a day noticeably thins mucous secretions.
• Add green leafy veggies: their magnesium relaxes bronchial muscle spasms.
• Take daily vitamin C; low vitamin C is linked to asthma.
• Focus on recipes that are low in fats, dairy free and full of enzyme-rich vegetables.

Choose 2 or 3 supplements to enhance and accelerate your program:

Note: Herbal combinations are some of the best choices. They help neutralize allergens, increase oxygen uptake, encourage critical adrenal activity and allow better sleep while addressing the underlying allergy cause.

• **Deep lung cleansers:** NATURE'S SECRET ULTIMATE RESPIRATORY CLEANSE; Use NATURE'S WAY 5 SYSTEM CLEANSE caps after juice cleansing to help pull and clear intestinal and lung mucous congestion.
• **Clear mucous, control spasms:** CRYSTAL STAR® STRESS OUT™ MUSCLE RELAXER drops (work fast, sometimes within 25 minutes to ease spasms) or CRYSTAL STAR® MUSCLE RELAXER™ caps; CoQ10 200 mg.
• **Minimize allergic reactions:** Futurebiotics MSM 400 mg. twice daily. Ease stress—the most common asthma trigger for children—with Reishi mushroom drops in water. Multiple reactions: una de gato drops.
• **Antihistamines for asthmatics:** CRYSTAL STAR® ANTI-HST™ caps; Quercetin 2000 mg. daily, with Bromelain 1000 mg.; Vitamin C up to 8000 mg. daily with bioflavs.; Vitamin E 400IU with selenium 200 mcg. or EIDON SELENIUM liquid; NAC (n-acetyl cysteine), 600 mg. twice a day.
• **For acute attacks:** Lobelia extract under the tongue relaxes chest constriction (highly recommended, dilute for kids); or sniff an anti-spasmodic oil like lavender, rosemary, or anise.
    - **Bronchodilators:** Ginkgo Biloba extract 50 mg. 3x daily; magnesium 800 mg. daily. Ayurvedic: Coleus Forskholii or Cordyceps sinensis; *Note:* Bronchodilating drugs deplete B6; a high quality B-complex daily like NATURE'S SECRET ULTIMATE B works well. Evening Primrose oil reduces inflammation 2000 mg. (adults).
    - **Bronchodilators for kids:** Calcium 500 mg., Magnesium 250 mg., or FLORADIX MAGNESIUM liquid for bronchodilating help. B12 2000 mcg. every other day, Vitamin C 1000 mg., B-complex 50 mg.

- **Normalize adrenal and immune response:** CRYSTAL STAR® ADRENAL ENERGY BOOST™ capsules; Astragalus-echinacea extract; TRANSFORMATION PUREZYME protease.
- **Ease cough, release mucous:** HERBS ETC. LUNG TONIC; CRYSTAL STAR® D-CONGEST™ drops; YOGI BREATHE DEEP TEA; ZAND DECONGEST HERBAL; Wild cherry syrup; Echinacea-goldenseal extract. Apply a hot ginger compress to the chest, then use light percussion on the back to release mucous faster.
- **Asthma stress remedies:** NATURAL LABS DEVA FLOWERS ALLERGIES/ASTHMA; NELSON BACH RESCUE REMEDY.

Bodywork techniques increase oxygen use in the lungs and tissues.

- **Enema:** Take an enema the first and last day of your mucous elimination diet to thoroughly clean out excess mucous. Or, have a colonic for a more thorough colon cleanse.
- **Vaporizer:** Use one of these aromatherapy oils to help clear mucous congestion in the lungs (inhale from vaporizer or from steam when mixed into hot water). Add to your bath 5 drops of eucalyptus or tea tree oil. Eucalyptus: antiviral action works to loosen mucous—treats asthma, bronchitis and sinusitis. Tea tree oil: antiviral and antibacterial decongestant.
- **Chest compress:** Apply wet ginger/cayenne chest compresses to increase circulation and loosen mucous.
- **Massage therapy with percussion:** a rubdown stimulates circulation and loosens mucous. Most people have several congestion-releasing bowel movements within 24 hours after massage therapy.

For more information on this topic, visit www.healthyhealing.com

Maintenance Recipes For Your Allergy-Asthma Control Diet

Use these recipes on an ongoing basis once your initial healing diet is producing good results.

Breakfast

Immune Support Breakfast

In a large bowl, mix together:

2 cups rolled oats	2 cups rolled barley	1 cup toasted sunflower seeds
½ cup dried cherries	½ cup dried blueberries	2 cups oat bran
1 cup chopped almonds	½ cup lecithin granules	½ cup ground flax seeds
½ cup raisins		

Make up and store airtight. Use about ½ cup dry mix per serving. Soak amount you need in vanilla rice milk or apple juice to moisten.

Breakfast Blueberry Crisp

2 cups brown rice, cooked	2 tbsp. honey	2 bananas, sliced
¾ cup rice milk	1 tbsp. grapeseed oil	2 cups blueberries, fresh or frozen
2 tbsp. brown sugar	1 tsp. cinnamon	

Preheat oven to 350°F. Combine rice, rice milk, brown sugar, honey, grapeseed oil and cinnamon. Fold in bananas and blueberries. Put into an 8" square baking pan and cover with foil. Bake 30 minutes. Cool slightly before serving. Makes 4 – 6 servings.

Non-Dairy Apple Raisin Oatmeal

2 cups water	banana slices	1 tbsp. honey
1 cup oatmeal	raisins	½ cup apple juice

Bring water to a boil. Add oatmeal and stir for 4 – 5 minutes. Remove from heat. Divide in two bowls. Top with banana slices and raisins. Drizzle with honey and apple juice. Serves 2.

Healing drinks

Non-Dairy Morning Drink

In a blender, blend:

1 cup strawberries or kiwi chunks	1 banana, sliced	1 cup apple juice
1 cup fresh papaya or pineapple chunks	1 cup apple juice	1 tbsp. bee pollen granules
	8 oz. RICE DREAM, vanilla rice milk, or vanilla yogurt	2 pinches ginger powder

Makes 2 servings.

Nutrition per serving:			
Calories ----------- 153	Vitamin E --------- 1 IU	Cholesterol-------- 0	Potassium --------- 515 mg.
Protein ------------ 4 g.	Carbohydrates ---- 32 g.	Calcium ----------- 27 mg.	Sodium------------ 20 mg.
Vitamin C--------- 44 mg.	Fiber ------------- 3 g.	Iron -------------- 2 mg.	
	Fat---------------- 2 g.	Magnesium ------- 46 mg.	

Cran-Apple Frost

Blend until smooth:

2 cups cranberry juice	2 cups apple juice	2 small frozen bananas, in chunks
2 tbsp. honey	¼ cup RICE DREAM or vanilla rice milk	1 tbsp. lemon juice
4 ice cubes		

Top with nutmeg and cardamom sprinkles. Makes 3 tall drinks.

Restoration Tonic

You can feel it release the congestion right away. Revitalizes your brain and body if you have a hangover. Works every time.

Mix in the blender:

48 oz. can tomato juice	1 cup green, yellow, and red onions, mixed and chopped	2 ribs celery, chopped
1 bunch parsley, chopped		2 tsp. hot pepper sauce
2 tbsp. fresh basil, chopped (or 2 tsp. dried)	½ tsp. fennel seeds	1 tsp. rosemary leaves
1 tsp. light soy sauce		1½ cups water

Pour into a large pot. Bring to a boil and simmer for 30 minutes. Store in the refrigerator. Makes 8 rejuvenating drinks. Serve chilled or steaming hot.

Nutrition per serving:			
Calories ----------- 46	Vitamin E --------- 1 IU	Cholesterol-------- 0	Potassium --------- 422 mg.
Protein ------------ 2 g.	Carbohydrates ---- 11 g.	Calcium ----------- 39 mg.	Sodium------------ 88 mg.
Vitamin C--------- 54 mg.	Fiber ------------- 2 g.	Iron -------------- 1 mg.	
	Trace Fats	Magnesium ------- 25 mg.	

Tomato Hammer

Stir in a pitcher:

3 cups tomato juice	2 tbsp. lime juice	2 tsp. worcestershire sauce
1 tsp. bottled horseradish	½ tsp. celery salt	¼ tsp. hot pepper sauce

Cover and chill thoroughly. Serve with a short celery spear with leafy top. Makes 4 servings.

Nutrition per serving:	Vitamin E --------- 1 IU	Cholesterol -------- 0	Potassium --------- 499 mg.
Calories ----------- 39	Carbohydrates ---- 10 g.	Calcium ----------- 38 mg.	Sodium------------ 198 mg.
Protein ----------- 2 g.	Fiber -------------- 2 g.	Iron -------------- 1 mg.	Vitamin A --------- 540 IU
Vitamin C--------- 38 mg.	Trace Fats	Magnesium ------- 24 mg.	

Soups, salads, appetizers

Creamy Spinach Soup

1 large onion, chopped	3 zucchini, thickly sliced	cracked black pepper
1 cup white wine	1 tbsp. BRAGG'S LIQUID AMINOS	toasted, salted pine nuts
3 potatoes, peeled and chopped	1 small bag baby spinach	or pumpkin seeds

Place onion in a soup pot with 1 cup water. Simmer for 3 minutes. Add 4 more cups water, white wine, potatoes, zucchini and BRAGG'S LIQUID AMINOS. Bring to a boil, reduce heat, cover and simmer for 30 minutes. Add baby spinach and cracked black pepper to taste. Immediately remove from heat. Purée soup in batches in blender. Return to pan; heat gently for 2 minutes. Serve hot, topping with plenty of toasted, salted pine nuts or pumpkin seeds. Makes 6 servings.

Nutrition per serving:	Vitamin E --------- 1 IU	Cholesterol -------- 0	Potassium --------- 682 mg.
Calories ----------- 161	Carbohydrates ---- 21 g.	Calcium ----------- 59 mg.	Sodium------------ 167 mg.
Protein ----------- 6 g.	Fiber -------------- 5 g.	Iron -------------- 3 mg.	Vitamin A --------- 213 IU
Vitamin C--------- 21 mg.	Fat ---------------- 4 g.	Magnesium ------- 103 mg.	

Sesame Chicken Salad with Pea Pods

8 oz. snow peas, trimmed	2 cloves garlic, minced	1½ tbsp. brown rice vinegar
¼ cup green onions, sliced	3 tbsp. lemon juice	3 cups chicken, cooked & shredded
2 tbsp. sesame seeds	1½ tbsp. tamari	1 cup diced celery
4 tbsp. olive oil	1 tbsp. fresh ginger, minced	⅓ cup fresh cilantro, chopped

Blanch snow peas and green onions in boiling water for 1 minute only. Rinse under cold water to set color. Set aside. Dry-roast sesame seeds in a skillet until golden. Toss 2 tsp. of the seeds with the snow peas. Add olive oil to remaining sesame seeds and sauté until fragrant with garlic, lemon juice, tamari, ginger and brown rice vinegar. To the sauce, add snow pea mixture, chicken, celery and cilantro, then toss. Chill and serve over greens. Makes 6 small salads.

Nutrition per serving:	Vitamin E --------- 1 IU	Cholesterol -------- 80 mg.	Potassium --------- 497 mg.
Calories ----------- 294	Carbohydrates ---- 13 g.	Calcium ----------- 47 mg.	Sodium------------ 168 mg.
Protein ----------- 35 g.	Fiber -------------- 3 g.	Iron -------------- 2 mg.	Vitamin A --------- 19 IU
Vitamin C--------- 11 mg.	Fat ---------------- 12 g.	Magnesium ------- 65 mg.	

Kiwi Carpaccio With Lemon-Lime Dressing

3 tbsp. honey	2 tbsp. lime juice	½ pint raspberries
3 tbsp. lemon juice	6 kiwi, peeled and thinly sliced	

Warm honey, lemon juice and lime juice in a saucepan; stir until combined. Set aside to cool. Arrange kiwi slices in a spiral to cover four chilled salad plates. Scatter raspberries over each plate and pour dressing over fruit. Make 4 appetizer salads.

Hawaiian Guacamole

Mash and mix:

1 large avocado	½ cup plain low-fat yogurt	1 – 2 tbsp. chunky salsa
1 – 2 tsp. lemon juice	2 – 3 tsp. BRAGG'S LIQUID	or picante sauce
2 dashes SPIKE or other	AMINOS or light soy sauce	
herbal seasoning salt		

Amounts vary depending on size of the avocado. Taste as you add seasonings. Makes about 1½ – 2 cups.

Yogurt Sauce And Dip

Combine in a blender, then chill:

½ cup plain yogurt	2 tbsp. low fat soy mayonnaise	2 tbsp. fresh cilantro or parsley
1 tsp. grated lemon zest	½ tsp. garlic-lemon seasoning	

Goes well with veggies, baked potatoes, broiled fish, rice crackers, and chips.

Nutrition per serving:	Vitamin E --------- 1 IU	Cholesterol-------- 3 mg.	Potassium --------- 173 mg.
Calories ----------- 85	Carbohydrates ---- 16 g.	Calcium ----------- 119 mg.	Sodium------------ 73 mg.
Protein ------------ 3 g.	Trace Fiber	Trace Iron	Vitamin A --------- 29 IU
Vitamin C--------- 7 mg.	Fat ---------------- 2 g.	Magnesium ------- 13 mg.	

Piquant Sauce for Steamed Veggies

2 tbsp. grapeseed oil	2 tbsp. miso paste	3 tbsp. balsamic vinegar
1 shallot, minced	2 cups water	2 tsp. fresh parsley, chopped
2 tbsp. whole wheat flour	½ tsp. lemon-pepper	2 tbsp. sweet pickle relish

Make a brown miso sauce in a hot skillet: Stir grapeseed oil, shallot and whole wheat flour until combined. Add miso paste, water and lemon-pepper. Stir until slightly thickened. Remove from heat. Add balsamic vinegar, parsley, and sweet pickle relish. Makes 4 servings.

Balsamic Onions

2 red onions, sliced	2 – 3 tbsp. balsamic vinegar	½ tsp. pepper
2 yellow onions, sliced	1 tsp. dry thyme	
4 tbsp. olive oil or organic chicken broth		

Sauté red onions and yellow onions in olive oil or chicken broth until aromatic, about 5 minutes. Add balsamic vinegar, thyme, and pepper. Chill for at least an hour. Serve over very tart greens like escarole, frisee or arugula. Makes 4 – 6 servings.

Quick Dairy-Free Savories

1 package thin, savory rice crackers	rice cheddar cheese red bell pepper, minced	green onion, minced hot pepper sauce

Spread crackers on a baking sheet. Cut slices of cheese into small squares. Lay slices on top of crackers and top with bell pepper and green onion. Sprinkle with hot pepper sauce and broil until bubbly.

Entrées

Baked Tofu Kabobs

1 lb. extra firm tofu	8 whole button mushrooms	3 tbsp. sherry
1 peeled cubed eggplant	1 red onion, cut in chunks	2 tbsp. tamari
1 red bell pepper	4 tbsp. Italian vinaigrette	1 tbsp. dijon mustard

Run skewers under a broiler for 30 seconds to "charcoal" kabobs. Blanch tofu in boiling water for 5 minutes. Cut in large cubes. Marinate tofu cubes for 1 hour in your favorite marinade. (See previous pages for suggestions.) Marinate eggplant, bell pepper, mushrooms, and red onion for 1 hour in Italian vinaigrette, sherry, tamari and dijon mustard. Alternate tofu cubes with the veggie cubes on the skewers. Bake on oiled sheets, or on a barbecue grill until tender. Makes 6 skewers.

Fresh Corn Chowder With Chicken and Popcorn

This soup is a complete meal.

8 large ears of fresh corn	½ red bell pepper, diced	2 cups organic chicken, cooked & diced
1 yellow onion, chopped	15 oz. can whole corn kernels	1 tbsp. tarragon, chopped
2 tbsp. soy bacon bits	1 cup plain yogurt	1 tbsp. thyme, chopped
2 tbsp. grapeseed oil	4 cups organic chicken broth	popped popcorn
1 large russet potato, peeled & cubed		

Use a serrated knife to strip fresh corn kernels from their cobs. Set aside. In a soup pot, sauté the yellow onion and soy bacon bits in the grapeseed oil for 5 minutes. Add the potato and bell pepper; sauté 5 minutes more. Add the fresh corn and sauté 5 minutes more. Place the canned corn and yogurt into a blender, purée, and add to the soup pot. Cover pan; simmer 5 minutes. Add chicken broth, diced chicken, tarragon and thyme. Partially cover pan; simmer until potatoes are tender, about 15 minutes. Season with sea salt and pepper. Ladle into bowls and sprinkle with plenty of popcorn. Makes 6 servings.

Leek and Mustard Tart

rye crackers	½ tsp. sesame salt	3 oz. feta cheese, crumbled
cheddar-type rice cheese	¼ tsp. ground black pepper	2 tbsp. chives, chopped
1 lb. leeks, white parts, sliced	½ cup plain low fat yogurt	2 tbsp. soy bacon bits
2 tbsp. olive oil	½ cup low fat cream cheese	
½ cup white wine	2½ tbsp. Dijon mustard	

Preheat oven to 375°F. Cover a 9" tart or quiche pan with crushed rye crackers. Sprinkle crackers with cheddar-type rice cheese. Sauté leeks in olive oil for 5 minutes. Add white wine; simmer 10 minutes. Season with sesame salt and pepper. Scrape into tart pan. Combine yogurt, cream cheese, mustard and feta cheese and beat until smooth. Pour over quiche. Sprinkle chives and soy bacon bits over the top. Bake until top is firm-golden, about 30 minutes. Let sit 5 minutes and slice. Makes 8 servings.

Tempeh Burrito Wraps

4 soft whole wheat tortillas   2 red onions, sliced   1 cup baby spinach
8 oz. tempeh, cut into strips   barbecue sauce

Preheat the broiler. Place tempeh and onions in a baking dish. Slather with a natural barbecue sauce, let sit for 10 minutes, then place under the broiler until brown. Assemble wraps: spread baby spinach down center of each tortilla. Divide tempeh mix on top of spinach; roll up tucking in sides as you roll to form a bundle. Slice in half. Makes 4 servings.

Healthy dessert options

Light Orange Soufflé with Raspberry Sauce

4 egg yolks   ½ cup water   cream of tartar
½ cup fructose   grated zest of 1 orange   2 cups raspberries
¼ cup unbleached flour   ½ cup orange juice   3 tbsp. sugar-free raspberry jelly
1 cup plain low fat yogurt   6 egg whites   2 tbsp. orange juice

Preheat oven to 375°F. Make soufflé in the top of a double boiler over hot water. Blend egg yolks and fructose until thick and creamy. Stir in flour, yogurt, water and orange zest. Cook over low heat stirring, until mixture boils. Let cool, stirring gently every few minutes. Add ½ cup orange juice. Whip egg whites to stiff peaks and fold into orange sauce with a pinch of cream of tartar. Turn into a lecithin-sprayed 2 qt. straight-sided soufflé dish. Bake for 30 minutes until light and puffy. While soufflé bakes, make the raspberry sauce in a sauce pan: stir and heat raspberries, raspberry jelly, 2 tbsp. orange juice until blended. Chill and pour over cold soufflé. Makes 6 servings.

Orange Gingerbread

¾ cup water   ½ cup unsulphured molasses   2½ cups whole wheat flour
1 egg   ½ cup maple syrup   1 tsp. baking soda
⅓ cup orange juice   5 tbsp. grapeseed oil   2 tsp. crystallized ginger, minced
1 tbsp. orange peel   5 tbsp. melted butter   1 tsp. cinnamon

Preheat oven to 350°F. Use a 9" x 9" lecithin-sprayed baking pan.

Mix wet ingredients: water, egg, orange juice, orange peel, molasses, maple syrup, grapeseed oil, butter. Mix dry ingredients: flour, baking soda, ginger, cinnamon.

Combine the two mixtures together just to moisten. Turn into baking pan; bake for 35 – 40 minutes until an inserted toothpick comes out clean. Center should still be moist. Serve warm or cool. Makes 12 pieces.

Nutrition per serving:

Calories ----------- 216	Vitamin E --------- 3 IU	Cholesterol -------- 20 mg.	Potassium --------- 490 mg.
Protein ----------- 4 g.	Carbohydrates ---- 3 g.	Calcium ----------- 164 mg.	Sodium ------------ 111 mg.
Vitamin C --------- 3 mg.	Fiber -------------- 3 g.	Iron -------------- 4 mg.	Vitamin A --------- 63 IU
	Fat ---------------- 9 g.	Magnesium ------- 68 mg.	

Strawberries Balsamico

Mmmmmmm.

2 baskets of strawberries   3 tbsp. balsamic vinegar   1 tsp. stevia flakes, or 10 drops
     stevia liquid extract

Cut strawberries in half. Toss with balsamic vinegar and stevia flakes (or stevia liquid extract). Makes 8 servings.

Arthritis:
Pain Relieving Diet

The term arthritis (joint inflammation), refers to over 100 diseases that attack joints and connective tissue. Degenerative joint and rheumatic diseases include gout, lupus, ankylosing spondylitis (arthritic spine), psoriatic arthritis (skin and nail arthritis), infective arthritis (bacterial joint infection), fibromyalgia and rheumatism. Today more than 40 million Americans are afflicted by one or more of these crippling conditions, now the leading cause of disability in the U.S. Arthritis affects up to 80% of people over 50. Experts say arthritis cases are rising too… over 60 million people in the U.S. will be afflicted in the next two decades. Add to that, people suffering from arthritis-like diseases—gout, bursitis, tendonitis and lupus, and the figure becomes staggering.

Arthritis isn't a simple disease. It affects not only bones and joints, but also blood vessels, kidneys, skin, eyes, brain and immune response. Unfortunately, NSAIDs (non-steroidal anti-inflammatory drugs), commonly used to relieve arthritis pain, send 76,000 people to the hospital and kill 7,600 people each year! Merck has now even pulled its new COX 2 inhibiting drug, Vioxx, from the market because of link to blood clots, heart attacks and stroke. Celebrex and Naproxen (Aleve) have documented links to cardiovascular risks, too.

Natural therapies address the causes of arthritis while reducing pain. Some, like glucosamine, actually help rebuild joints and prevent further destruction. Natural treatment relies on improved nutrition to create an environment for the body to support its own healing functions. Even in advanced inflammation and joint degeneration, diet change can affect improvement. I have personally seen notable reduction of swelling and deformity in long-standing cases. Further, COX-2-inhibiting herbs like ginger, turmeric and rosemary can effectively reduce arthritis inflammation without causing intestinal damage or cardiovascular risks.

Even though the medical focus of diagnosis has been on organic mineral (especially calcium) depletion as a cause of arthritis, I find that hormone imbalance and adrenal exhaustion are the keys to repair. **Vigorous diet therapy is the most beneficial thing you can do to control the causes and improve the symptoms of arthritis.** Arthritic conditions are degenerative processes that take years to develop. Small or subtle changes are not successful in reversing them. Additional actions you can take for noticeable benefits are seaweed baths, an arthritis sweat bath (pg. 41), and morning sunbaths for Vitamin D and better calcium use.

Important note: Arthritis is unique in its close ties to emotional health.

Negative emotional resentments and obsessive-compulsive actions aggravate arthritis. Emotional stress frequently brings onset of the disease. Most arthritis sufferers have a marked inability to relax (relaxation techniques are essential to arthritis healing). Many have a negative attitude toward life that locks up their body's healing ability. Relaxation therapies like yoga, meditation, and massage therapy are beneficial for recovery. Writing about stressful or traumatic life experiences has been shown to help rheumatoid arthritis sufferers.

Do you have signs of arthritis?
• Are you stiff when you get up in the morning?
• Do you have marked redness and swelling in your fingers, shoulders or neck when it's cold and damp?
• Are your joints starting to crack and pop?
• Do you have back or joint pain when you move? Does it get worse with prolonged activity?
• Are you noticing bony bumps on your index fingers? Or bony spurs on other joints?
• Are you anemic? Is your complexion very pale? Have you recently lost weight but weren't on a diet?
• Are you more than 20 pounds overweight and starting to feel the extra weight in your knees and hips?
• Do you have long-standing lung and bronchial congestion?
• Are you usually constipated? Do you suffer from ulcerative colitis?
• Do you take more than 6 aspirin a day? Are you on a long-term prescription of corticosteroid drugs?
  (Either of these may eventually impair the body's own healing powers.)

3-Day Arthritis Cleansing Diet

Does your body need an arthritis detox?

An arthritis detox diet helps dissolve and flush out inorganic mineral deposits, replacing them with healing nutrients. For best results, use Vitamin C powder with bioflavonoids, ½ tsp. at a time, in juice or water 4 to 6 times daily, and omega-3 flax oil, 3 tsp. daily in juice or water.

Lack of water is linked to arthritis pain and stiffness.

Chondroitin sulfate, a specific nutrient for arthritis, is the molecule in cartilage that attracts and holds water. Healthy joints are 85 to 90% water, but since cartilage doesn't have its own blood supply, chondroitin sulfate aids the chondroitin "molecular sponge" in providing joint nourishment, waste removal and lubrication. In fact, water often helps restore healthy cartilage as it relieves osteoarthritis symptoms. Include eight 8 oz. glasses of water daily in your arthritis healing diet. Limit your alcoholic beverages since they are especially dehydrating.

On rising: take a glass of lemon juice and water; or a glass of fresh grapefruit juice (Acidic citrus fruits help enzymes alkalize the body); or Crystal Star® Green Tea Cleanser™.

Breakfast: take a Potassium broth (pg. 16); or a glass of carrot/beet/cucumber juice.

Mid-morning: have black cherry juice; Green Foods Barley Essence; or Crystal Star® Energy Green Renewal™.

Lunch: have miso soup with snipped sea greens, and a glass of carrot juice with Bragg's Liquid Aminos.

Mid-afternoon: have a green drink, or alfalfa/mint tea, or Crystal Star® Cleansing & Purifying™ Tea.

Dinner: have a glass of cranberry/apple, or papaya juice, or another glass of black cherry juice.

Before Bed: take a glass of celery juice, or a cup of miso soup with 1 tbsp. of nutritional yeast.

Maintenance Recipes For Your Arthritis Detox

Use these recipes on an ongoing basis once your initial healing diet is producing good results.

Purifying Mineral Broth

2 tbsp. grapeseed oil	½ cup broccoli, chopped	2 tsp. Bragg's Liquid Aminos
¼ cup celery, chopped	½ cup carrots, grated	¼ cup parsley, chopped
¼ cup daikon radish, chopped	6 cups Potassium Essence Broth (pg.16)	
¼ cup leeks, chopped	2 tbsp. lemon peel, minced	

In the grapeseed oil, sauté briefly the celery, daikon radish, leeks, broccoli and carrots.

Add the Potassium Essence Broth, lemon peel, Bragg's Liquid Aminos and parsley. Heat for 1 minute, and serve hot. Makes about 8 cups.

Spring Cleanse Salad

1 peach   1 apricot   12 cherries, pitted
1 nectarine

Chop all ingredients, mix together in a bowl. Makes 2 servings.

Sprouts Plus

1 tub alfalfa sprouts   1 cup celery, minced   3 pinches lemon zest
2 cups carrot, grated

Mix all ingredients together in a bowl. Makes 2 servings.

Diet to Control Arthritis Symptoms

This alkalizing, anti-inflammatory diet can change your body chemistry and the way your body uses the nutrients you give it. It is particularly useful for gland nourishment where extreme inflammation shows that your body is not producing enough natural cortisone from adrenal cortex. It is free of nightshade plants, like potatoes, tomatoes, chilies, peppers, eggplant, etc. that impair calcium absorption. The diet is rich in vitamin C for connective tissue, full of fiber for regularity, and free of alcohol, caffeine and sugar that aggravate acidity. It is low in fat and meats to reduce pain, and high in whole grains and vegetables for better-formed bone and cartilage.

Note: In addition to arthritis itself, the diets in this chapter improve the following arthritis associated problems: rheumatism, bursitis, bone spurs, corns and carbuncles, chronic constipation, gout, shingles, lupus, prostate inflammation, post-menopausal bone loss and gum diseases.

On rising: take a glass of grapefruit juice; or a glass of apple cider vinegar in water with honey.

Breakfast: Bioflavonoids help connective tissue. Eat and drink cranberries, cherries (10 times stronger anti-inflammatory than aspirin!), papayas and citrus fruits, or JARROW GENTLE FIBERS drink. Mix 1 tbsp. each: sunflower seeds, lecithin granules, nutritional yeast and toasted wheat germ. Add 2 tsp. into yogurt, or sprinkle on fresh fruit or greens, but have some every day.

Mid-morning: take a POTASSIUM JUICE (pg. 16); or, if you have osteoarthritis, an Arthritis V-8 Special: add to a bottle of KNUDSEN'S VERY VEGGIE JUICE, 4 tbsp. each: wheat germ, lecithin granules and nutritional yeast flakes. Take 8 oz. twice daily. If you have rheumatoid arthritis, add 1 tsp. BRAGG'S LIQUID AMINOS to a green drink like SUN WELLNESS CHLORELLA or WAKUNAGA HARVEST GREENS.

Lunch: have a green leafy salad with lemon/oil dressing; and a hot miso broth or onion soup (there's a link between sulfur deficiency and arthritis). Eat sulfur-containing veggies like broccoli, onions, cabbage and garlic.

Mid-afternoon: a cup of miso soup with sea greens on top, alfalfa/mint tea, or Oregon grape/ginger tea.

Dinner: have a Chinese greens salad with sesame dressing; or a large dinner salad with soy cheese, nuts, tamari dressing, and a cup of black bean soup; or steamed vegetables with nutritional yeast sprinkled on top and brown rice for absorbable B vitamins. Have fish like salmon or tuna for high omega-3 oils twice a week.

Before bed: cranberry, black cherry juice, or celery juice; or a cup of miso soup with chopped sea greens.

Pointers for best results from your arthritis control diet:

- Avoid arthritis trigger foods: corn, wheat and rye breads; bacon and pork; beef; eggs; coffee; oranges; milk; nightshade foods like peppers, eggplant, tomatoes and potatoes; mustard; colas; chocolate.
- Cut down on: alcohol, fried foods, dairy foods, salty foods.

- Add balancing foods: green tea, artichokes, cherries, cabbages, brown rice, oats (not for rheumatoid arthritis), shiitake mushrooms, cold water fish, sea greens, fresh fruits, vegetables, leafy greens, garlic, onions, olive oil, flax seed oil, sweet potatoes. Note: Add ginger and parsley daily (almost immediate results).

Choose 2 or 3 supplements to enhance and accelerate your program:

- **Repair joints, protect cartilage:** Glucosamine-Chondroitin 4 daily (not if you have prostate cancer); Shark cartilage (natural chondroitin sulfates). Use with CMO (cetyl-myristoleate) 500 mg., like JARROW TRUE CMO for EFAs; LANE LABS ADVACAL ULTRA for calcium balance; Omega-3 flax or fish oil 3x daily—expect less pain in about 3 months.
- **Effective COX-2 inhibitors and anti-inflammatories:** DLPA 1000 mg.; NEW CHAPTER ZYFLAMEND AM & PM; SOURCE NATURALS MINOR PAIN COMFORT; Quercetin 1000 mg. w. Bromelain 1500 mg. daily; MSM 1000 mg.; Herbal anti-inflammatories: CRYSTAL STAR® ANTI-FLAM™ caps; cat's claw caps.
- **Antioxidants help regenerate cartilage:** SAMe protects cushioning sinovial fluid and blocks enzymes that degrade cartilage (can be as effective as ibuprofen); CoQ_{10} 300 mg. daily; Carnitine 2000 mg. daily for 3 months; LANE LABS NATURE'S LINING to strengthen the stomach wall (highly recommended for damage caused by Non-Steroidal Anti-Inflammatory Drugs (NSAIDs)).
- **Chlorophyll sources stimulate cortisone:** Alfalfa tabs 10 daily; SOLARAY ALFA JUICE caps; CRYSTAL STAR® ENERGY GREEN™ RENEWAL DRINK MIX; NUTRICOLOGY PRO-GREENS; WAKUNAGA KYO-GREEN; BARLEANS GREENS.
- **Enzymes help normalize body chemistry:** CRYSTAL STAR® DR. ENZYME™ WITH PROTEASE & BROMELAIN; TRANSFORMATION REPAIRZYME; CRYSTAL STAR® BITTERS & LEMON™ extract.
- **Nettles therapy:** nettles extract suppresses pro inflammatory proteins—their sting on affected joints can *dramatically* reduce symptoms. Use with guidance from an herbalist or holistic professional.
- **Stimulate natural cortisone production:** CRYSTAL STAR® ADRENAL ENERGY BOOST™ daily with Evening Primrose Oil 3000 mg. daily; PRINCE OF PEACE ROYAL JELLY/GINSENG vials, one daily; NUTRICOLOGY ADRENAL CORTEX caps.

Bodywork techniques relieve pain, improve circulation, hasten elimination of harmful deposits.

- **An arthritis sweat bath releases a surprising amount of toxic material.** Improvement after an arthritic sweat bath experience is notable.
- **How to take the arthritis bath:** For best results, take this bath at night before retiring. Note: Protect your mattress with a sheet of plastic. Make a tea of elder flowers, peppermint and yarrow. Drink it hot before the bath. Pour 3 pounds Epsom Salts or enough Dead Sea salts for 1 bath into very hot bath water. In the bath, rub arthritic joints with a stiff brush for 5 – 10 minutes—stay in the bath for 20 – 25 minutes. On emerging, do not dry yourself. Wrap up immediately in a clean sheet and go straight to bed, covering yourself with several blankets. The osmotic pressure of the Epsom salt solution absorbed by the sheet will draw off heavy perspiration. The next morning the sheet will be stained with wastes excreted through your skin—sometimes the color of egg yolk. Note: This is a strong detox procedure and it happens relatively quickly. Take extra care if you have a weak heart or high blood pressure. Repeat the bath once every two weeks until sheet is no longer stained, a sign that the body is cleansed. Drink water throughout the procedure to prevent dehydration and loss of body salts.
- **Another choice?** CRYSTAL STAR® HOT SEAWEED BATH™ normalizes body pH almost immediately.
- **To relieve pain:** Press the highest spot of the muscle between thumb and index finger. Press in the webbing between the two fingers, closer toward the bone that attaches to the index finger. Press for 10 seconds at a time into the web muscle, angling the pressure toward the bone of the index finger.
- **Exercise:** Lack of exercise weakens muscles putting more stress on joints. A daily stretching program and yoga are my favorites for keeping skeletal muscles strong.
- **Bodywork treatments:** Massage therapy, acupuncture, epsom salts baths, chiropractic treatments
- **Healing applications:** BAYWOOD TOPICAL SUPER COOL RELIEF; WAKUNAGA GLUCOSAMINE SOOTHING CREAM; NATURE'S WAY CAYENNE PAIN RELIEVING OINTMENT; BOERICKE & TAFEL TRIFLORA ARTHRITIS GEL; Emu oil (with omega-3, omega-6 EFAs.); Ayurvedic Boswellin creme; CRYSTAL STAR® ANTI-BIO™ GEL with una de gato; Cayenne/ginger compresses on affected areas; DMSO on clean skin.

Maintenance Recipes
For Your Arthritis Diet

Use these recipes on an ongoing basis once your initial healing diet is producing good results.

Breakfast

Raisin and Oat Muffins

1 cup unbleached flour	1 cup rolled oats	¼ cup grapeseed oil
½ cup whole wheat pastry flour	1½ tsp. baking soda	½ cup raisins
1 cup GRAPENUTS or raisin bran cereal	1 cup plain yogurt	
	½ cup honey	
	1 egg	

Oil 6 Pyrex custard cups. Preheat oven to 375°F. Combine dry ingredients: unbleached flour, whole wheat pastry flour, cereal, rolled oats, baking soda. Form a well in the center, and pour in yogurt, honey, egg, grapeseed oil and raisins. Stir until lumpy, and bake 25 minutes at 375° or until a toothpick comes out clean. Makes 6 big deli-style muffins.

Nutrition per serving:	Vitamin E --------- 5 IU	Cholesterol-------- 30 mg.	Potassium --------- 379 mg.
Calories ----------- 431	Carbohydrates ---- 75 g.	Calcium ----------- 110 mg.	Sodium------------ 168 mg.
Protein ----------- 11 g.	Fiber ------------- 6 g.	Iron -------------- 4 mg.	
Vitamin C--------- 2 mg.	Fat---------------- 12 g.	Magnesium ------- 76 mg.	

Ginger Grapefruit with Toasty Meringue Top

4 grapefruit halves	¼ cup honey
2 egg whites	¼ tsp. powdered ginger

Preheat oven to 300°F. Whip 2 egg whites to soft peaks. Add ¼ cup honey and ¼ tsp. powdered ginger and whip to meringue consistency. Spread meringue on grapefruit halves, and bake at 300° for 15 – 20 minutes. Makes 4 servings.

Nutrition per serving:	Vitamin E -- trace quantities	Cholesterol-------- 0	Potassium --------- 195 mg.
Calories ----------- 109	Carbohydrates ---- 27 g.	Calcium ----------- 16 mg.	Sodium------------ 24 mg.
Protein ----------- 2 g.	Fiber ------------- 2 g.	Iron -------------- 0	
Vitamin C--------- 47 mg.	Fat---------------- 0	Magnesium ------- 12 mg.	

New England Cranberry-Honey Compote

4 cups apple juice	½ cup raisins	½ cup cranberries (fresh or frozen)
½ cup honey	2 cinnamon sticks	walnuts, chopped and toasted
1 pound dried mixed fruit	6 thin lemon slices	
1 cup cranberry-apple juice	6 thin orange slices	

In a saucepan over medium-low heat, combine: apple juice, honey, dried fruit, cranberry-apple juice, raisins, cinnamon sticks, lemon slices and orange slices. Simmer until tender, about 25 minutes. Add cranberries, simmer for another 5 minutes and remove from heat. Cover, chill; top with toasted chopped walnuts. Makes about 6 cups.

Healing drinks

Arthritis Relief Detox

large handful spinach	large handful watercress	3 radishes
large handful parsley	5 carrots (with tops)	1 tbsp. BRAGG'S LIQUID AMINOS

Juice the spinach, parsley, watercress, carrots, and radishes. Add the BRAGG'S LIQUID AMINOS. Makes 1 large serving.

Nutrition per serving:	Vitamin E --------- 7 IU	Cholesterol-------- 0	Potassium --------- 4937 mg.
Calories ----------- 270	Carbohydrates ---- 44 g.	Calcium ----------- 279 mg.	Sodium------------ 879 mg.
Protein ----------- 10 g.	Fiber ------------- 14 g.	Iron -------------- 7 mg.	
Vitamin C--------- 147 mg.	Fat-------trace amounts	Magnesium ------- 137 mg.	

Apricot Orange Cream

4 fresh apricots, halved	1 frozen banana, in chunks	orange juice to taste
1 orange, peeled and sectioned	1 tbsp. almonds, chopped	
	1 tbsp. shredded coconut	

Blend smooth: apricots, orange, banana, almonds, coconut, orange juice. Makes 1 large serving.

Arthritis/Bursitis Relief

3 oranges, peeled	¼ pineapple or mango	½ apple, cored

Juice all ingredients. Makes 1 large serving.

Soups, Salads, Appetizers

Famous Soup
Achieved its fame through many years of requests.

½ cup sliced almonds	¼ cup red onion, diced	1 tbsp. tamari
1 tbsp. sesame seeds	¼ cup celery, diced	3 oz. pkg. ramen noodles
4 cups organic chicken broth or light miso soup	¼ cup carrot, diced	4 oz. shrimp, diced
6 dry shiitake mushrooms	¼ cup jicama, diced	1 pinch stevia leaves
½ cup water	2 tbsp. sake or sherry	1 cup shaved iceberg lettuce or shredded Belgian endive
	1 tbsp. brown rice vinegar	

Toast almonds and sesame seeds in a 350°F oven until golden. In a soup pot, bring chicken broth (or miso) to a boil. Soak the shiitake mushrooms in ½ cup water until soft; then sliver and discard stems. Add mushrooms and soaking water to broth and simmer 15 minutes. Add red onion, celery, carrot and jicama. Simmer gently for 5 minutes until tender yet crisp. Add sake, rice vinegar, tamari, ramen noodles, shrimp and stevia leaves. Simmer for 2 minutes and remove from heat. Top with iceberg lettuce, the toasted almonds and sesame seeds. Serve immediately. Makes about 6 cups.

Autumn Sweet Potato Spread for Pita Chips

2 sweet potatoes	1 tbsp. maple syrup	½ tsp. lemon-pepper seasoning
2 tsp. grapeseed oil	2 tbsp. sesame tahini	baked pita chips
1 yellow onion, minced		

Bake sweet potatoes at 350° until soft, 40 – 60 minutes. Let cool. Peel potatoes and drop into a blender. Heat grapeseed oil in a saucepan, add the onion and sauté until dark gold, about 20 minutes. Add onions to the blender. Add maple syrup, tahini and lemon-pepper. Blend until smooth. Serve warm or chilled with a big bowl of baked pita chips. Makes about 12 servings.

Sweet Waldorf Salad

2 Fuji apples, diced	½ cup oven-toasted walnuts	½ tsp. sweet-hot mustard
1 cup celery, diced	¼ cup lemon yogurt	2 tbsp. lemon juice
1 cup red seedless grapes, halved	2 tbsp. low-fat mayonnaise	½ tsp. honey

Toss together all ingredients. Serve on chilled plates. Makes 4 salads.

Nutrition per serving:	Vitamin C --------- 16 mg.	Fat ---------------- 11 g.	Magnesium ------- 44 mg.
Calories ----------- 218	Vitamin E --------- 3 IU	Cholesterol -------- 0	Potassium --------- 394 mg.
Protein ------------ 5 g.	Carbohydrates ---- 29 g.	Calcium ----------- 58 mg.	Sodium ------------ 50 mg.
Vitamin A --------- 19 IU	Fiber ------------- 3 g.	Iron -------------- 1 mg.	

Asparagus Soup

1 tbsp. olive oil	1 lb. fresh asparagus (cut in 1" pieces)	1 handful fresh parsley, with the stems removed
1 onion, chopped finely	1 stalk lemongrass	¼ cup white wine
1 clove garlic, minced	1 tsp. chervil	lemon-pepper seasoning
2 cups water		

In a pan, sauté the olive oil, onion, and garlic for 5 minutes. Add 2 cups water, asparagus, lemongrass, chervil, and parsley. Simmer 5 minutes only. Remove lemon grass stalk and discard. Pour mixture into blender or food processor and blend smooth. Add white wine and season with lemon-pepper to taste. Serve hot. Makes 4 servings.

White Gazpacho

1 long European cucumber, peeled and diced	2 cups plain low-fat yogurt	½ cup water
¼ tsp. garlic-lemon seasoning	2 cups onion broth	2 tbsp. fresh cilantro leaves, chopped
	2 tbsp. lemon juice	2 tbsp. green onions, chopped
	½ cup white wine	1 tbsp. fresh basil, chopped

In a blender, blend the cucumber, garlic-lemon seasoning, yogurt, ½ cup of the onion broth and the lemon juice. Pour into a large soup pot with: the remainder of the onion broth, white wine, and ½ cup water. Stir and heat gently until smooth. Remove from heat. Top with cilantro leaves, green onions, basil. Chill in the fridge for 1 – 2 hours before serving. Makes 6 servings.

Nutrition per serving:	Vitamin C --------- 8 mg.	Fat ---------------- 1 g.	Magnesium ------- 26 mg.
Calories ----------- 74	Vitamin E --------- 1 IU	Cholesterol -------- 4 mg.	Potassium --------- 332 mg.
Protein ------------ 5 g.	Carbohydrates ---- 9 g.	Calcium ----------- 158 mg.	Sodium ------------ 81 mg.
Vitamin A --------- 18 IU	Fiber ------------- 1 g.	Iron ----------- trace amounts	

Zucchini Carpaccio

An authentic Italian appetizer salad. Use a food processor to get the zucchini paper-thin.

tart garden greens, like arugula, endive or radicchio	4 small zucchini	lemon-pepper seasoning
sunflower sprouts or watercress leaves	olive oil	
	1 lemon	
	reggio-parmesan cheese	

Cover small, chilled salad plates with greens. Pile on sunflower sprouts (or watercress leaves) to cover. Slice zucchini paper-thin and divide between salad plates. Sprinkle a few drops of olive oil and squeeze a bit of fresh lemon juice over each salad, top with some grated reggio-parmesan cheese and sprinkle with lemon-pepper seasoning. Makes 4 servings.

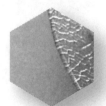 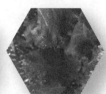 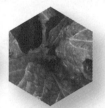 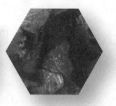 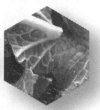 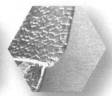

Sultan's Purses

6 dried shiitake mushrooms	1½ tsp. fructose	¼ cup green peas
large bunch of scallions	1 tsp. sesame salt (gomashio)	
1 egg	1 egg white	60 won ton wrappers
2 cups water	1½ tsp. toasted sesame oil	spinach leaves
¼ tsp. baking soda	1½ tsp. grated ginger	Boston lettuce leaves
8 oz. tiny cooked salad shrimp	½ tsp. grapeseed oil	
1 tsp. tamari	1 tbsp. sake	3 tbsp. dry mustard or Chinese hot mustard powder
2 tbsp. arrowroot powder	¼ tsp. black pepper	
	¼ cup water chestnuts, diced	1½ tsp. hot pepper sauce

Soak shiitake mushrooms to soften. Sliver and set aside. Separate white and green parts from the scallions. Sliver ¼ cup green slices for topping and set aside. Separate the white and yolk of 1 egg. Bring 2 cups water to a rapid boil. Add baking soda and the remainder of the scallions and blanch until bright green, about 2 minutes. Rinse under cold water and sliver.

In a blender, create the savory filling: shrimp, tamari, arrowroot, fructose, sesame salt, egg white, sesame oil, grated ginger, grapeseed oil, Sake and black pepper. Blend, then turn into a bowl, add water chestnuts and green peas. Mix lightly, and chill.

Separate 60 skins from a package of won ton wrappers. Put about 1 teaspoon of filling in the center of each. Draw the four points of the sides together, seal edges with egg yolk, and twist the top to form a drawstring "purse." Chill in the refrigerator until ready to steam.

Use a large steamer or wok with a steaming rack, and bring an inch of water to a boil. Cover with spinach leaves, and put purses in a single layer on the leaves. Steam for 10 minutes. Transfer purses to a serving plate lined with Boston lettuce leaves. Sprinkle with reserved scallions.

Make the dipping sauce: Mix mustard powder in a bowl with hot pepper sauce and enough water to make a dip. Makes 60 steamed pouches.

Nutrition per serving:	Vitamin C --------- 1 mg.	Fat ---------------- 1 g.	Magnesium ------- 14 mg.
Calories ---------- 20	Vitamin E ---- trace amounts	Cholesterol------- 10 mg.	Potassium -------- 42 mg.
Protein ----------- 1 g.	Carbohydrates ---- 2 g.	Calcium ---------- 6 mg.	Sodium----------- 30 mg.
Vitamin A --------- 10 IU	Fiber---------- trace amounts	Iron -------------- 1 mg.	

Entrées

Baked Turkey Sandwiches

4 cups herb stuffing cubes	½ tsp. sea salt	1 can cream of mushroom soup
4 cups cooked turkey, diced	¼ tsp. pepper	1 cup mozzarella cheese, shredded
½ cup onion, diced	1½ cups plain almond milk	2 eggs
½ cup celery, diced		1 tbsp. yellow mustard

Preheat oven to 350°F. Scatter herb stuffing over a large rectangular baking dish. In a skillet, sauté turkey, diced onion, celery, sea salt and pepper. Distribute mixture over top of stuffing. In a bowl, mix almond milk, cream of mushroom soup, mozzarella cheese, eggs and mustard. Pour over turkey and bake 40 minutes or until a knife inserted in the center comes out clean. Make 6 servings.

Trade Winds Tuna Casserole

½ cup onion, diced	1 (7 oz.) can water-packed white tuna	1 small package crispy chow mein noodles
1 tbsp. olive oil		
8 oz. can water chestnuts, sliced	4 tbsp. low-fat cream cheese	2 tbsp. fresh parsley, chopped
	½ tsp. curry powder	
1 (14 oz.) can cream of celery or cream of mushroom soup		

Preheat oven to 350°F. Sauté onion in olive oil for 10 minutes. Remove from heat; add water chestnuts, cream of celery or cream of mushroom soup, tuna, cream cheese, curry powder, 2 cups of the chow mein noodles and the fresh parsley. Pour into a lecithin-sprayed, 1 qt. covered casserole dish. Top with remaining chow mein noodles; cover and bake 35 minutes or until light brown. Serves 4.

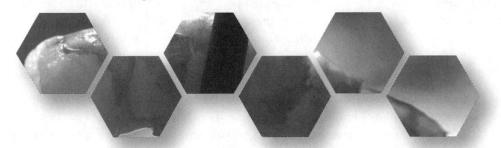

Grilled Prawns with Veggies and Sesame Sauce

½ cup sesame seeds	1 lb. prawns, shelled and butterflied	3 tbsp. olive oil
		4 tbsp. white wine
½ cup sake or sherry	8 green onions, sliced	1 tbsp. honey
2 tbsp. tamari	4 small zucchini, sliced	juice of 1 lemon
1 tbsp. toasted sesame oil	8 fresh shiitake mushrooms	2 tbsp. fresh ginger, minced
		pinch paprika
		pinch garlic powder

Dry roast sesame seeds in a pan until golden. Set aside.

Make the marinade: combine the sake, tamari and sesame oil. Use half to marinate the prawns, and the other half to marinate the onions, zucchini and mushrooms. Allow to marinate for at least an hour in the refrigerator.

Grill prawns over high heat until just opaque but still tender. Then grill vegetables until seared and tender. Baste twice. Remove from heat immediately. Put prawns and veggies on a platter and keep warm.

Make the Sesame Sauce: in a blender, combine the toasted sesame seeds, olive oil, white wine, honey, lemon juice, ginger, paprika, garlic powder. Drizzle over prawns and veggies. Makes 4 servings.

White Sea Bass with Braised Spinach

Loaded with EFAs

½ cup miso broth	6 tbsp. tamari	1 bunch scallions, thinly sliced
1 tbsp. fresh, grated ginger	2 tbsp. honey	
½ cup sherry	4 boned, skinned white sea	
1 tsp. Chinese five-spice	bass fillets	
powder	1 large package baby spinach	
2 tbsp. sesame seed	1" piece of fresh ginger	

Use a wok steamer for best results. Mix the miso marinade: miso broth, ginger, sherry, five-spice seasoning, sesame seed, tamari, honey. Pour over sea bass fillets; cover and let marinate overnight.

Thinly slice baby spinach and pile onto wok steamer tray. Place tray in wok filled with 2 cups boiling water and a 1" piece of fresh ginger. Cover spinach with marinated fish. Sprinkle scallions over fish, cover and steam 10 minutes or until fish flakes easily with fork. Makes 4 servings.

Healthy dessert options

Double Ginger Dessert

5 cups VANILLA RICE DREAM frozen dessert	¼ cup diced crystallized ginger	½ tsp. cinnamon ginger ale
	¾ tsp. cardamom	

Slightly soften the VANILLA RICE DREAM by letting it stand at room temperature about 10 minutes. Scoop into a large bowl. Add crystallized ginger, cardamom, and cinnamon; swirl ingredients together. Place bowl in freezer until dessert is firm enough to scoop… about 1½ hours; if storing up to 1 week, cover air-tight. Divide into 4 large water goblets. Slowly fill glasses with icy ginger ale, and serve immediately. Makes 4 servings.

Nutrition per serving:	Vitamin C ---- 1 mg.	Fat ---- 6 g.	Magnesium ---- 60 mg.
Calories ---- 147	Vitamin E ---- trace amounts	Cholesterol ---- 0	Potassium ---- 438 mg.
Protein ---- 9 g.	Carbohydrates ---- 17 g.	Calcium ---- 21 mg.	Sodium ---- 44 mg.
Vitamin A ---- 48 IU	Fiber ---- 1 g.	Iron ---- 2 mg.	

Baked Apples with Lemon and Tofu

4 granny smith apples	dried cranberries	2 tbsp. fresh lemon zest, finely
raisins	8 oz. soft silken tofu	minced
walnuts, finely chopped	1½ tbsp. maple syrup	½ tsp. cinnamon

Preheat oven to 375°F. Partially core the apples: remove the top ¾ of the core but leave the base intact. Drop into cavity of each apple: 1 tsp. raisins, 1 tsp. minced walnuts and 1 tsp. dried cranberries. Fill cavities to the top with water. Pour boiling water into a glass baking dish, and put the apples in. Bake uncovered for 35 minutes rotating the apples after 20 minutes to expose each inner half to the heat. While apples bake, whisk tofu in a bowl with maple syrup, lemon zest, and cinnamon. When the apples are done (they'll turn yellow), cut each in half vertically and top each half with tofu mixture. Sprinkle with lemon peel, raisins and dried cranberries. Makes 8 servings.

Nutrition per serving:	Vitamin C ---- 9 mg.	Fat ---- 3 g.	Magnesium ---- 41 mg.
Calories ---- 105	Vitamin E ---- 1 IU	Cholesterol ---- 0	Potassium ---- 201 mg.
Protein ---- 3 g.	Carbohydrates ---- 18 g.	Calcium ---- 47 mg.	Sodium ---- 4 mg.
Vitamin A ---- 21 IU	Fiber ---- 3 g.	Iron ---- 2 mg.	

Blood Sugar Imbalances:
Diabetes and Hypoglycemia

It's the bittersweet truth: Even after decades of warnings about their dangers we are a nation addicted to sugar and artificial sweeteners like aspartame. Over 60% of the U.S. population suffers from some degree of the "blood sugar blues." Twenty million Americans suffer from diabetes (high blood sugar) or hypoglycemia (low blood sugar).

Sugar has become an entire food group, counting for an astounding 20% of total daily calories for adult Americans. U.S. kids eat enough sugar to account for half of their daily calories! Sugar has so infiltrated our food supply that most of us hardly notice it's there. In August 1999, the Center For Science in the Public Interest filed a petition to the FDA to require more explicit labeling of added sugar in foods. Almost all snack foods and pre-prepared foods have added sugar in their ingredients to enhance their flavor.

Are you confused about sugar?

We need sugar, in the form of glucose or blood sugar, to live. But, our bodies get enough glucose from eating complex carbohydrates like vegetables, whole grains and legumes. We don't need it from simple carbohydrates like sugar or corn syrup. What we know as sugar today is actually a heavily refined substance that qualifies more as a drug than a food! Just two teaspoons of refined sugar is enough to throw off your body chemistry.

A high sugar intake heavily stresses your pancreas, causing abnormal insulin production, and inviting health problems like diabetes and hypoglycemia, high triglycerides and high blood pressure. Other research shows sugar causes changes in cellular proteins and nucleic acids related to premature aging. A sugar heavy diet suppresses immune response because refined sugar destroys the ability of white blood cells to kill germs for up to 5 hours after consumption! Sugar also disrupts hormonal health, and feeds candida yeast and some cancers.

Too much sugar leads to nutrition deficiencies, because sugar robs your body of B vitamins, minerals like magnesium and zinc, and trace minerals like copper and chromium. High sugar consumption is directly related to obesity, coronary thrombosis and periodontal disease. Hyperactivity and Attention Deficit Disorder (ADD) are aggravated by sugar. Sugar even affects energy and mood. Most of us know that our energy drops after a sugar binge, but did you know that too much sugar can cause depression? One recent study finds people with major depression clearly benefit when they eliminate refined sugar from their diet.

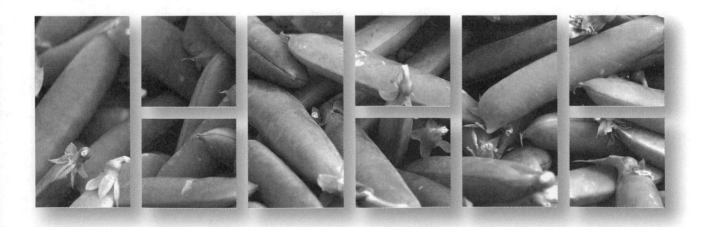

High fructose corn syrup, in almost all commercial sodas and juices today, isn't good for health either. Studies from Israel reveal that rats fed a high fructose diet age faster because changes in their collagen result in premature skin wrinkling and sagging. Studies also show that sodas sweetened with high fructose corn syrup cause mineral losses of phosphorous and calcium, which may contribute to osteoporosis.

Sugar-free artificial sweeteners, once thought to be healthier than sugar, are not foods you should include in your regular diet. New reports suggest they are setting up an environment where illnesses like lupus, multiple sclerosis and Alzheimer's disease may take hold.

The leader of today's artificial sweeteners is aspartame, a substance that has received more complaints about adverse reactions than any other food ingredient in FDA history. Fully 75% of the complaints reported to the FDA's Adverse Reaction Monitoring System are for aspartame-related symptoms. Aspartame's major brand names, NutraSweet and Equal, are everywhere… over 5,000 food products contain aspartame. Some people have immediate, serious reactions from aspartame—dizziness, attention problems, memory loss, slurred speech, headaches, throat swelling, allergic reactions and retina deterioration are just a few documented side effects. The American College of Physicians says aspartame is causing a plague of neurological diseases in the U.S. Pregnant and lactating women, toddlers or allergy-prone children, and those with PKU, should avoid aspartame products. One study shows that the more NutraSweet consumed, the more likely tumors are to develop. Aspartame is also associated with brain damage in fetuses, and ovarian tumors.

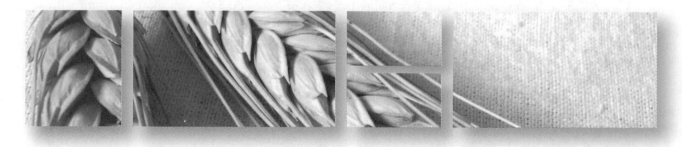

Aspartame's side effects can be serious…

Aspartame can affect your eyesight and memory. Formaldehyde builds up in the retina from aspartame causing blurred or tunnel vision, visual disturbances like bright flashes or black spots, and may even cause retinal detachment. Aspartame alters delicate brain chemistry, aggravating Parkinson's disease and increasing Alzheimer's risk. Without the other balancing amino acids found in protein, aspartame's ingredients, aspartic acid and phenylalanine, deteriorate brain cells, leading to memory loss, especially significant for the elderly who consume chemically sweetened beverages at record levels.

Aspartame can be dangerous for people with blood sugar problems like diabetes and hypoglycemia. Aspartame is 200 times sweeter than sugar, so it keeps blood sugar levels out of control by disrupting the way your body uses insulin. Diabetes and hypoglycemia may progress and worsen. Eyes diagnosed with diabetic retinopathy may be the result of aspartame toxicity instead. Neurological damage, memory loss and confusion, and dramatic changes in appetite and weight are frequently a problem for diabetic and hypoglycemic patients who use aspartame sweeteners.

What about Splenda and Acesulfame K? Are they safer sweeteners?

The public outcry about aspartame's side effects has resulted in the meteoric rise in sucralose, chlorinated sucrose (Splenda) as a commercial sweetener, especially in drinks and baked goods. Splenda is 400 to 800 times sweeter than sugar. Sucralose is seen as a chemical by your body, not as a carbohydrate, so it has no effect on insulin secretion or carbohydrate metabolism. But recent evidence suggests sucralose may impair glucose levels for diabetics. While the manufacturer says the absorption of sucralose is very limited, research from the Japanese Food Sanitation Council shows that up to 40% of sucralose is in fact absorbed, and may concentrate in the liver, kidneys and gastrointestinal tract.

Original FDA studies concluded sucralose is not carcinogenic and does not cause significant genetic change, birth defects, brain or nerve damage, or other health risks. Forty studies determined it was biodegradable, safe for plant and aquatic life. However, some experts feel the original data was flawed, and that sucralose may pose hazards to both health and to the environment. In animal tests, sucralose is linked to a variety of problems: up to 40% shrinkage of the thymus gland, atrophy of the lymph follicles in the spleen and thymus, enlarged liver and kidneys, decreased red blood cell count, and aborted pregnancy.

Acesulfame K, *(acesulfame potassium)*, a non-caloric organic salt, sold in the U.S. as Sunette, Sweet One and Swiss Sweet, is 200 times sweeter than sugar and boosts the sweetening effect of other sweeteners. It passes through the human digestive system unchanged. Yet, even after 90 safety studies, the Center for Science in the Public Interest has petitioned the FDA for a stay of approval because of "significant doubt" about acesulfame potassium. Newer animal tests show it aggravates hypoglycemia, produces lung tumors, breast tumors, thymus tumors, some forms of leukemia, and respiratory disease even when less-than-maximum doses were given.

Do you have the blood sugar blues? There are body signs to watch for.

Taking your blood sugar when you get up in the morning can give you some helpful clues. For a non-diabetic, blood sugar should be below 150 in the morning before eating and below 150 two hours after a meal.

For a diabetic, blood sugar should be between 80 – 120 in the morning before a meal and less than 180 two hours after a meal. If your blood sugar gets higher than 230 or lower than 70, you should consult with your physician about treatment for possible diabetes or hypoglycemia. Regular hypoglycemic blood sugar swings may be a sign that you're at risk for adult onset diabetes. Home blood glucose monitoring kits such as Stay Healthy U-Detect Glucose Test and Johnson & Johnson One Touch Profile are reliable.

What can you do to help yourself?

Blood sugar problems are one of America's biggest health threats.
• Read labels especially on the drinks you consume.
• The herb stevia, is a healthy drink sweetening choice, even for people with blood sugar problems.
• If you eat lots of sugary foods, look for healthier sweeteners like honey, molasses, rice syrup and fruit juice concentrates.

Have you heard about Stevia?

Stevia is a natural sweetener, safe even for diabetics. Yet it's been the source of controversy for years. I remember well when stevia was literally ripped off health food store shelves, its makers dragged to jail, their offices ransacked and computers confiscated. Stevia, or "sweet herb," native to Paraguay, is an herb with a turbulent history, not because it is unsafe or has rampant side effects, but because it is big competition for the billion dollar U. S. commercial sweeteners, especially aspartame.

Stevia has a centuries' long history of safe use as a natural, herbal sweetener. In South America, it's been used since the 16th century to sweeten foods and as a key ingredient in medicinal teas. Stevia has been grown in England since World War II as an inexpensive sugar substitute. The Japanese widely embraced stevia as a natural sweetener. Stevia holds almost 50% of the Japanese sweetener marketplace and has been enjoyed for over 25 years as a regular part of their diet. U.S. distribution began in the late seventies, as Americans demanded healthier alternatives to refined sugar and chemical sweeteners. Stevia immediately became a formidable rival to saccharin and aspartame sweeteners in the U.S. marketplace, widely used throughout the '80s. It wasn't long before the backlash began. The FDA admits it received trade complaints (not safety complaints) from sweetener companies about stevia in the early '80s.

In 1991, the FDA put an import ban on all stevia products to stop any "unapproved" use of the herb in the U.S., saying stevia was a food additive and should not be declared safe unless proven safe by U.S. (not foreign) research. Yet stevia, in its whole, unadulterated form, is a food, NOT a food additive, that meets the GRAS (generally recognized as safe) food criteria. Extensive modern research and experience with stevia in Japan and Brazil has proved stevia to be safe and non-toxic.

The truth: stevia was literally run out of the marketplace by a money driven conspiracy of manufacturers of other sweeteners like NUTRASWEET (aspartame) and saccharin to maintain control of the U.S. market. Stevia is still the target of FDA attack. In 1997, the FDA prepared a document with 19 "unresolved concerns" on stevia's safety. According to the FDA, certain studies indicated that stevia might contribute to hypoglycemia. Researcher, Mauro Alvarez Ph.D., whose work was cited in the document, disagrees with the FDA conclusions.

Can Americans enjoy the benefits of this "good for you" sweetener?

Stevia is a low-calorie, non-toxic sweetener even for people with blood sugar problems like diabetes and hypoglycemia for whom refined sugar and chemical sweeteners can be problematic. Today, in South America, stevia is recommended to diabetic and hypoglycemic patients as a healthy sweetener and blood sugar regulator.

Unlike sugar, stevia does not cause tooth cavities. Instead, stevia is a potent herbal antibiotic, actually helping to *prevent* tooth decay and gum disease. Regular stevia users report fewer colds and flu. Other studies find stevia lowers high blood pressure. (Stevia does not seem to affect normal blood pressure indicating that your body uses it as a balancer, instead of a drug.) Stevia can even be used as a weight management aid because it contains no calories, while significantly increasing glucose tolerance and inhibiting glucose absorption. People whose weight loss problems stem from a craving for sweets report that it decreases their desire for sugary foods. Many users report that stevia tea reduces desire for tobacco and alcoholic beverages. A facial mask of water-based stevia extract (full of AHA's) effectively smooths out skin wrinkles while healing skin blemishes, including acne. A drop of the extract may be applied directly on a blemish outbreak for fast results, sometimes within 24 hours.

For Americans, the FDA allows stevia to be sold as a dietary supplement. Even though it is not labeled a sweetener, once you buy it, you can use it any way you like. It has a slight licorice flavor that most people find pleasant. But, remember... stevia is 200 times sweeter than sugar. Just one teaspoon of dried leaves is sweeter than 1 full cup of sugar! A tiny pinch of dried leaves is all you need to sweeten a drink or cooking liquid. Liquid extracts and powders are recommended for cooking and as tabletop sweeteners. The powdered extract should be mixed with water and used by the drop according to directions. BODY ECOLOGY STEVIA LIQUID (liquid concentrate) and NOW STEVIA BALANCE (packets with chromium and inulin) are both quality stevia products.

Resources for those interested in cooking with stevia: Baking with Stevia: Recipes for the Sweet Leaf by Rita DePuydt and Stevia Sweet Recipes: Sugar Free Naturally by Jeffrey Goettemoeller.

Controlling Diabetes Naturally

New Center for Disease Control statistics show diabetes reaching epidemic proportions, doubling between 1999 to 2000. Today, 17 million people have diabetes. One million more are diagnosed each year. With its complications, diabetes is now the 7th leading cause of death in the U. S. It's a vicious circle disease, in which poor fat and sugar metabolism lead to obesity... which then leads to diabetes. The cycle keeps going. Diabetes makes you want to eat more, so symptoms are aggravated as well as brought on by eating too much fat, too many sugary foods and too much fast food (especially caffeine and alcohol).

This type of diet overworks, then damages the pancreas, so your body can't produce or correctly use insulin (the hormone that helps convert food into energy). As simple carbohydrates and sugars cease to be metabolized, they accumulate in the body and are stored as fat. Excess body fat and lack of exercise bring on insulin resistance. Even though Type 2 diabetics produce insulin, it isn't used properly (insulin resistance).

The worst news is about kids who now suffer from both kinds of diabetes:

Type 1 diabetes, a juvenile condition, is more severe and almost entirely dependent on insulin to sustain life. Some research links type 1 diabetes to drinking cow's milk in the first three months of life.

Type 2 diabetes is increasingly being diagnosed in overweight children and adolescents who get little exercise and live on snack foods. Type 2 diabetes is a degenerative disease, strongly linked to long term diet overloads of highly processed carbohydrates and sugar, and lack of fiber.

Do you think you or your child might have diabetes? Here are the signs.

Type II/Adult-Onset Diabetes
• Are you always thirsty? Do you urinate very frequently?
• Do you get frequent infections? Do cuts and bruises heal slowly?
• Have you lost weight but weren't on a diet?
• Are you constantly tired or drowsy? Is your vision blurry from time to time?
• Do you get leg cramps, or prickling in your fingers or toes?
• Have you experienced episodes of impotence?

Juvenile Diabetes
• Is your child unusually thirsty? Does he or she urinate very frequently?
• Is your child extremely hungry?
• Is your child unusually irritable? Is he or she unusually tired or drowsy?

Diabetes Control Diet

Both types of diabetes benefit from diet improvement, exercise and natural supplements. Diet improvement is absolutely necessary to overcoming diabetes. High blood sugar is also an indication of high triglycerides, a risk factor for heart disease. The following diet, in addition to reducing insulin requirements and balancing blood sugar, has the nice "side effects" of healthy weight loss and better heart protection.

This diet supplies slow-burning, complex carbohydrate fuels that do not need much insulin for metabolism. Meals are small, largely vegetarian, and low in fats of all kinds. Proteins come from soy foods and whole grains that are rich in lecithin and chromium. Fifty percent of the diet is based in fresh or simply cooked vegetables for low calories and high digestibility. Avoid caffeine and caffeine foods, hard liquor, food coloring and sodas. Even "diet" sodas have phenylalanine that can affect blood sugar levels.

Note: Don't skip meals. Most diabetics should eat 6 mini meals a day, especially if they're on insulin therapy.

Check your blood sugar regularly to monitor high and low swings that may require medical attention!

On rising: take the juice of two lemons in a glass of water with 2 tsp. Sun Wellness Chlorella granules.

Breakfast: have aloe vera juice; or All One Vitamin-Mineral drink in apple juice or water to balance sugar curve. Make a mix of 2 tbsp. each: nutritional yeast, toasted wheat germ, lecithin granules and rice or oat bran. Sprinkle into yogurt with fresh fruit and grated almonds on top; or have a poached egg on whole grain toast; or granola with apple juice or vanilla rice milk; or buckwheat pancakes with apple juice or molasses.

Mid-morning: have a green drink like Crystal Star® Energy Green Renewal™ or Fit for You, International Miracle Greens; or green tea. Recent USDA research shows green tea's catechins enhance insulin activity.

Lunch: have a green salad, with celery and sprouts, marinated tofu and mushroom soup; or tofu burgers or turkey with steamed veggies and rice or cornbread; or a baked potato with yogurt or kefir cheese, and miso soup with sea greens; or a whole grain sandwich, with avocado, rice cheese, a low fat spread and watercress.

Mid-afternoon: have a glass of carrot juice; and/or fruit juice sweetened cookies with a bottle of mineral water or and a sugar balancing herb tea, such as licorice, dandelion, or pau d'arco tea; or watercress-cucumber sandwiches with a kefir cheese sandwich spread; or a hard boiled egg with sesame salt, or a veggie dip.

Dinner: Keep it light—have baked or broiled seafood with brown rice and peas; or a Chinese stir-fry with rice, veggies and miso soup; or Spanish beans and rice with onions and peppers; or a light Italian polenta with a hearty vegetable soup, or whole grain or veggie pasta salad; or a mushroom quiche with whole grain crust and yogurt/wine sauce, and a green salad. Beware! Consuming any alcohol can cause blood sugar to soar.

Before bed: take a cup of miso soup, or mix 1 tsp. Red Star nutritional yeast in 1 tsp. warm water.

Choose 2 or 3 supplements to help normalize your high blood sugar:

- **Stabilize blood sugar:** CRYSTAL STAR® SUGAR CONTROL HIGH™ capsules help insulin balance; Bitter Melon capsules help both high and low blood sugar attacks; NUTRICOLOGY GLUCOSOL WITH BANABA is clinically proven to activate cellular glucose transport. Adapters like GTF CHROMIUM or chromium picolinate 200 mcg. daily and Vanadium 25 mcg. daily (diabetics usually make enough insulin, chromium and vanadium help them use it). Siberian eleuthero extract or GRIFRON MAITAKE SX FRACTION caps to enhance insulin sensitivity. Vitamin E 800 IU daily; fenugreek seed, or rosemary tea balance blood sugar. Neem and turmeric powders (¼ tsp. each in 1 tsp. honey before a meal).
- **Lower blood sugar levels:** Alpha Lipoic acid 600 mg. daily lowers glucose levels up to 30%; CRYSTAL STAR® FEEL GREAT NOW™ caps (with ginseng, a proven aid to blood sugar control), or Olive Leaf extract; high dose biotin - 3000 mcg. daily; Vitamin C 3000 mg. daily with magnesium 400 mg. daily combats insulin resistance; ALL ONE TOTALLY FIBER COMPLEX helps insure a low-glycemic diet; HERBCARE CHARANTIA tea.
- **Normalize pancreas activity and insulin function:** Take gymnema sylvestre extract before meals to help repair damage; Ester C 3000 mg. daily increases insulin tolerance, normalizes pancreatic activity. Glutamine 1000 mg. with carnitine 1000 mg.; NUTRICOLOGY PRO-LIVE olive leaf extract as directed; DHEA 25 mg. daily increases cell sensitivity to insulin. Burdock, Pau d'arco or Astragalus tea, 2 cups daily for 3 months; raw pancreas glandular or PREMIER VANADIUM 25 mcg. daily.
- **Prevent nerve damage with EFAs:** Evening Primrose Oil capsules 1000 – 2000 mg. daily, Omega-3 flax or fish oil (for DHA) 3000 mg. daily.
- **Raise antioxidants:** Pycnogenol or grapeseed PCOs 200 mg. daily.
- **Boost energy:** CRYSTAL STAR® ADRENAL ENERGY BOOST™ caps for cortex support with ENERGY GREEN RENEWAL™ caps for stable energy. Spirulina tablets 6 daily to elevate mood.

Bodywork and lifestyle techniques are critical to success in overcoming blood sugar irregularities.

- **Don't smoke.** Nicotine increases the desire for sugar and sugary foods.
- **Hot tub therapy:** A study reported in the New England Journal of Medicine shows soaking in a hot tub for 30 minutes a day for three weeks lowers blood sugar levels 13%!
- **Walking is good exercise for diabetics** to increase metabolic processes and reduce need for insulin. Insulin resistance drops by nearly 2% for every 200 calories burned through exercise.
- **Lose excess weight.** A fiber weight loss drink, like ALOELIFE FIBER-MATE is effective.
- **A regular deep therapy massage is effective** in regulating sugar use through the body.
- **Strive for eight hours of sleep a night.** Sleep deprivation increases diabetes risk and complications.

Hypoglycemia Control Plan

Hypoglycemia and diabetes stem from the same causes. Hypoglycemia is also an epidemic in America today. Like diabetes, hypoglycemia is caused by sugar overload, but a hypoglycemic body reacts to the sugar in the opposite way. The pancreas produces *too much* insulin rather than too little. The blood sugar swings are just as wild, though. In fact, regular hypoglycemic episodes can be a marker that your body is on the pathway to diabetes.

If your adrenals are exhausted (they sit atop your kidneys and they hurt when pressed if they're exhausted), if you diet excessively, or if you abuse drugs or alcohol, you're on a road to hypoglycemia. Hypoglycemia can also result from prolonged, strenuous exercise, fasting, and in early pregnancy.

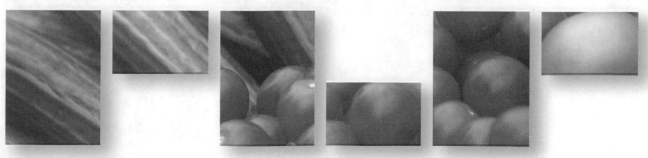

There are two types of hypoglycemia:

1.   Endogenous hypoglycemia, related to a serious medical condition like liver disease, is the most severe and needs immediate medical supervision.

2.   Reactive hypoglycemia, which happens a few hours after a meal, is the type we're talking about in this section. Reactive hypoglycemia occurs when the excess insulin secreted by the pancreas lowers blood sugar to the point of body disruption. This form of hypoglycemia is an internal body condition, not a disease. It is less severe than endogenous hypoglycemia, but symptoms become apparent swiftly. Your decision making and thinking abilities are affected first, because your brain requires 50% of all blood glucose as an energy source to think clearly.

Hypoglycemia in children is widely seen as a cause of hyperactivity and learning disorders. If your child has mood swings, aggressive behavior, is always negative with obstinate resentment to all discipline, take the self-test below, as well as a Glucose Tolerance Test from a physician. I find that for children, hypoglycemia can only be managed by a diet with all forms of concentrated sugars removed, including fruit juices.

Do you think you have low blood sugar?

The importance of correct diagnosis and treatment of sugar instabilities is essential. Hypoglycemia symptoms are often mistaken for other problems. Low blood sugar is the biological equivalent of a race car running on empty. It is not so much a disease as a symptom of other disorders. The human body possesses a complex set of checks and balances to maintain blood glucose levels within a narrow range. Some of the symptoms can be improved right away by eating something, but this does not address the cause.

Here are signs to watch for:

- severe fatigue, memory lapses and mental dullness
- dizziness, confusion
- mood swings, especially aggressive behavior
- depression and anxiety
- insomnia
- blurry vision that goes to frequent headaches or migraines
- periodic ravenous hunger, especially cravings for sweets
- shakiness, racing heartbeat resulting in temporary incoordination
- severe PMS

If you have any of these symptoms regularly for two weeks or more, consult with a physician to determine whether you have hypoglycemia. Hypothyroidism or chronic stress can mimic hypoglycemia symptoms. A blood test is a quick way to determine whether hypoglycemia is causing your symptoms. Home blood glucose monitoring kits are also available from your pharmacist.

Natural therapies can help you reduce blood sugar swings

Natural therapies for hypoglycemia are much the same as those for diabetes because the conditions are so closely related and their underlying causes are similar. Like diabetes, hypoglycemia responds quickly to natural therapies. The rewards of a commitment to a diet change are well worth it.

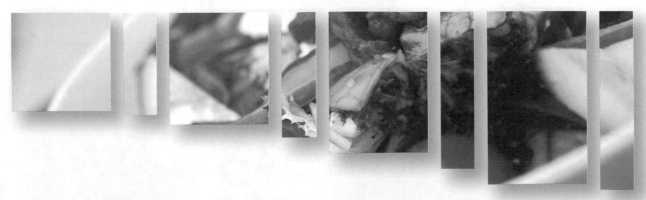

- **Eat small, frequent, low-glycemic meals**, with plenty of fresh foods to keep sugar levels in balance.
- **Avoid "trigger" foods** like refined carbohydrates and sugary foods, alcohol, cheese, vinegar, condiments like ketchup and mayonnaise, and salad dressing. Hypoglycemics get a double whammy if they have food allergies, because the pancreas often over-secretes insulin in response to an allergen food in addition to its sugar response. Drinking alcohol on an empty stomach is especially dangerous.
- **Keep a sugar-free, high protein drink on hand** for acute reactions. Try CRYSTAL STAR® RESTORE YOUR STRENGTH™ drink mix, (excellent results) or METABOLIC RESPONSE MODIFIERS WHEY PUMPED drink (high quality).
- **Boost brain power.** Lack of protein, potassium or other minerals can cause mental burnout and sugar swings. Make a brain booster: mix 2 tbsp. each: lecithin for phosphatides and memory lapses, nutritional yeast for chromium. Take 1 – 2 tbsp. of the mix daily in juice.
- **Take plant enzymes to enhance sugar absorption.** Try CRYSTAL STAR® DR. ENZYME II: FAT & STARCH BUSTER™ or TRANSFORMATION DIGESTZYME.
- **Address hypothyroidism regularly involved with hypoglycemia.** Iodine and potassium rich sea greens like dulse, wakame and sea palm can reactivate the thyroid and increase body energy.

Diet for Hypoglycemia Control

The key factors in hypoglycemia are stress and poor diet… both a result of too much sugar and refined carbohydrates, like pastries and desserts. These foods quickly raise glucose levels, causing the pancreas to over-compensate and produce too much insulin, which then lowers body glucose levels too far and too fast. This diet supplies your body with fiber, complex carbohydrates and protein—slow even-burning fuel that prevents sudden sugar swings. I recommend a diet like this for 2 – 3 months until blood sugar levels are regularly stable.

Diet watchwords:
- Eat potassium-rich foods: oranges, broccoli, bananas, and tomatoes.
- Eat chromium-rich foods: nutritional yeast, mushrooms, seafood and sea greens, beans and peas.
- Eat high quality vegetable protein at every meal.

On rising: take a "hypoglycemia cocktail:" 1 tsp. each in apple or orange juice to control morning sugar drop: glycine powder, powdered milk, protein powder, and nutritional yeast; or a protein/amino drink, like WAKUNAGA HARVEST BLEND, or CRYSTAL STAR® RESTORE YOUR STRENGTH™.

Breakfast: the most important meal of the day for hypoglycemia. Include ⅓ of daily nutrients; have oatmeal with yogurt and fresh fruit; or poached or baked eggs on whole grain toast with butter or kefir cheese; or whole grain cereal or pancakes with apple juice, soy milk, fruit, yogurt, nuts or fruit sauce; or tofu scrambled "eggs" with bran muffins, whole grain toast and a little butter; or my favorite: brown rice with tofu and tamari sauce and steamed veggies for breakfast.

Mid-morning: have a Stress Cleanse juice (page 18), GREEN FOODS GREEN MAGMA with 1 tsp. BRAGG'S LIQUID AMINOS, or CRYSTAL STAR® ENERGY GREEN RENEWAL™ drink ; or a sugar balancing herb tea, such as licorice, dandelion, or CRYSTAL STAR® DR. VITALITY™ tea; and some crisp, crunchy vegetables with kefir or yogurt cheese.

Lunch: have a fresh salad, with cottage cheese or soy cheese, nuts, noodle or seed toppings, and lemon oil dressing; or a seafood or chicken sandwich on whole grain bread, with avocados and low-fat cheese; or a bean or lentil soup with tofu or shrimp salad or sandwich; or a seafood and whole grain pasta salad; or a vegetarian pizza on a chapati crust with low fat cheese.

Mid-afternoon: have a hard boiled egg with sesame salt, and whole grain crackers with yogurt dip; or a licorice herb or dandelion root tea, or another green drink; or yogurt with fruit, nuts and seeds.

Dinner: have some steamed veggies with tofu, or baked or broiled fish and brown rice; or an Asian stir fry with seafood, rice and vegetables; or a vegetable pasta dish with verde sauce and hearty soup (add green beans for pancreatic support); or a Spanish beans and rice dish, or paella with seafood and rice.

Before bed: have a cup of RED STAR nutritional yeast or miso broth; or papaya juice with a little yogurt.

Choose 2 or 3 supplements to help normalize your low blood sugar:

- **Normalize blood sugar swings with herbs and nutrients.** CRYSTAL STAR® SUGAR CONTROL LOW™ is designed to balance blood sugar levels, support stressed adrenals and encourage a feeling of well-being; or SOURCE NATURALS GLUCO SCIENCE (highly effective nutrient support); CRYSTAL STAR® FEEL GREAT NOW™ with ginseng helps remove excess sugar from the blood; ALL ONE TOTALLY FIBER COMPLEX helps insure a low-glycemic diet to balance sugar curve.
- **Supercharge adrenals for long-term recovery:** When blood glucose is low, the adrenals compensate by secreting extra adrenaline which brings sugar levels back up. Eventually, the adrenals become exhausted by repeated attempts to normalize your blood sugar. Consider vitamin C with bioflavonoids 3000 mg. or PURE PLANET AMLA C PLUS tabs with spirulina to revitalize the adrenal glands. (Take vitamin C immediately during an attack). CRYSTAL STAR® ADRENAL ENERGY BOOST also provides adrenal support and helps stabilize blood sugar levels. NUTRICOLOGY ADRENAL CORTEX extract and PLANETARY SCHIZANDRA ADRENAL COMPLEX nourish exhausted adrenals. Gentle whole herbs like kava kava, passionflowers, scullcap and gotu kola caps fight stress linked to hypoglycemia; Evening Primrose Oil caps 2000 mg.; B Complex 100 mg. 2x daily with extra PABA 100 mg., and pantothenic acid 500 mg.
- **Boost energy:** Glutamine 500 mg. daily; 1 tsp. each: spirulina granules and bee pollen granules in apple juice, or RAINBOW LIGHT HAWAIIAN SPIRULINA between meals. BEEHIVE BOTANICALS ROYAL JELLY caps or PRINCE OF PEACE RED GINSENG-ROYAL JELLY VIALS for a noticeable energy boost. Take aloe vera juice concentrate before meals (add pinches of cinnamon, ginger and nutmeg to help control cravings—good results).
- **Enzyme therapy for glucose homeostasis:** CoQ-10 60 mg. 3x daily for 3-6 weeks; Pancreatin 1200 mg. with meals; CRYSTAL STAR® DR. ENZYME™ WITH PROTEASE AND BROMELAIN; TRANSFORMATION BALANCEZYME with MASTERZYME; PURE ESSENCE LABS CANDEX before meals, especially if candida yeast is also a problem.
- **Chromium may be critical:** GTF Chromium 200 mcg.; SOLARAY CHROMIACIN; Chromium picolinate 200 mcg.

Bodywork and lifestyle changes for hypoglycemia pay off for total health, too

- Eat 6 – 8 mini-meals throughout the day to keep blood sugar levels up. Large meals throw sugar balance way off, especially at night.
- Eat relaxed, never under stress. Regular massage therapy treatments can do wonders.
- Get some exercise everyday to work off unmetabolized acid wastes.
- Some oral contraceptives can cause glucose intolerance and poor sugar metabolism. Ask your doctor.

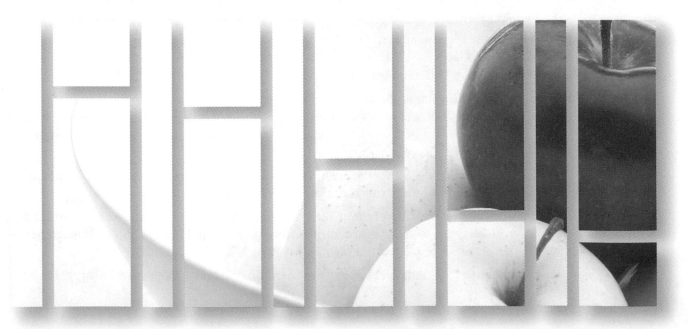

Maintenance Recipes for Your Sugar Control Diet

Note: The same diets that will benefit diabetes will, generally, benefit hypoglycemia. Check with your physician and monitor blood sugar fluctuations for the best results.

Breakfast

Basic Breakfast Grains

1 cup apple juice	½ cup toasted, sliced	cinnamon
1 cup whole grains (oats,	almonds	1 – 2 tsp. honey
brown rice, millet,	sunflower seeds	yogurt to taste
couscous)	½ cup raisins	

Combine apple juice and 1 cup water in a pot, heat to a low boil. Add your choice of whole grains (see above for suggestions). Reduce heat to medium, cover and cook until liquid is absorbed, about 25 minutes. May be served hot with almonds and sunflower seeds, raisins and a dash of cinnamon. To serve cold, add honey and fruit yogurt to taste. Makes 4 servings.

Nutrition per serving:	Vitamin E --------- 2 IU	Cholesterol-------- 0	Potassium --------- 439 mg.
Calories ----------- 301	Carbohydrates ---- 46 g.	Calcium ----------- 58 mg.	Sodium----------- 8 mg.
Protein ----------- 10 g.	Fiber ------------- 6 g.	Iron -------------- 3 mg.	
Vitamin C--------- 23 mg.	Fat---------------- 9 g.	Magnesium ------- 103 mg.	

Green Tea Fruit Bowl

1 cup granola	½ cup apples, sliced	¼ cup slivered almonds, toasted
1 cup vanilla yogurt	½ pint raspberries	
½ cup sunflower seeds, toasted	½ cup green tea	

Cover bottom of a bowl with granola. Gently spread on vanilla yogurt, and smooth it with the back of a spoon. Cover with toasted sunflower seeds. Top with apple slices, then smooth on another thin coat of yogurt. Mix raspberries with the green tea in a blender. Pour in the bowl and sprinkle with almonds. Makes 2 servings.

Healing Drinks

Honey-Almond Protein Drink

½ cup almonds	2 drops almond extract	1 tsp. spirulina powder
⅓ cup honey	¼ tsp. vanilla extract	
1 cup apple juice	1 tbsp. toasted wheat germ	

Combine all ingredients in a blender and blend until smooth. Makes 2 drinks.

Nutrition per serving:	Vitamin E --------- 13 IU	Cholesterol-------- 0	Potassium --------- 482 mg.
Calories ----------- 442	Carbohydrates ---- 70 g.	Calcium ----------- 106 mg.	Sodium----------- 35 mg.
Protein ----------- 9 g.	Fiber ------------- 4 g.	Iron -------------- 3 mg.	
Vitamin C--------- 3 mg.	Fat---------------- 116 g.	Magnesium ------- 117 mg.	

Homemade Root Beer

Buy the herb ingredients at a health food store. Great energy booster.

3 oz. sassafras bark pieces   3 oz. fennel/anise seed   ½ oz. ginger root pieces
3 oz. sarsaparilla root pieces   1 oz. roasted dandelion root   ½ oz. Chinese star anise
3 oz. licorice root pieces   1 oz. burdock root   ¼ oz. lemon peel pieces

Steep all ingredients in 1 quart steaming water for 20 – 30 minutes. Use about 4 tbsp. of the resulting liquid for 1 – 2 glasses of root beer, mixed with chilled sparkling water.

Soups, salads, sandwiches, appetizers

Hot Potato Salad

3 large red potatoes   ¼ cup soy bacon bits   2 cups dark greens (spinach,
4 eggs   1 tsp. sea salt   arugula)
2 tbsp. grapeseed oil   ½ tsp. pepper   nutmeg
1 onion, chopped   ½ cup low-fat cheddar
           cheese, shredded

Cut potatoes in bite-size pieces and steam until tender. Put into a large salad bowl. Hard-boil 4 eggs. Cool under running water and peel. Sauté the onion, bacon bits, salt and pepper in grapeseed oil until aromatic. Remove from heat; put into a salad bowl and toss with potatoes. Add cheddar and toss. Place dark greens like spinach or arugula on individual salad plates. Divide potato mixture among plates. Chop hard boiled eggs and sprinkle over top. Sprinkle each salad with nutmeg. Serve right away. Makes 6 salads.

Nutrition per serving:	Vitamin C	13 mg.	Fat	8 g.	Magnesium	54 mg.
Calories	181	Vitamin E	1 IU	Cholesterol	152	Potassium	501 mg.
Protein	14 g.	Carbohydrates	14 g.	Calcium	196 mg.	Sodium	537 mg.
Vitamin A	295 IU	Fiber	3 g.	Iron	3 mg.		

Black Bean Tortilla Wrap

Rich in protein and chlorophyll

2 cups short-grain brown   1 red bell pepper, diced   1 tbsp. olive oil
    rice, cooked   1 tomato, diced   1 tsp. garlic-lemon seasoning
4 large wheat tortillas   2 tbsp. fresh cilantro leaves,   plain yogurt
15 oz. can black beans, rinsed   minced
    and drained

In a bowl, combine the black beans, bell pepper, tomato, cilantro, olive oil and garlic-lemon seasoning. Warm each tortilla in a dry skillet until soft. Lay flat and spread ½ cup of the brown rice down the center. Cover rice with bean filling. Roll up, tucking sides toward the center to form a bundle. Slice each in half and serve with several tablespoons of plain yogurt. Makes 4 wraps.

Nutrition per serving:	Vitamin C	24 mg.	Fat	6 g.	Magnesium	75 mg.
Calories	321	Vitamin E	1 IU	Cholesterol	0	Potassium	269 mg.
Protein	12 g.	Carbohydrates	61 g.	Calcium	87 mg.	Sodium	616 mg.
Vitamin A	23 IU	Fiber	10 g.	Iron	5 mg.		

Classic Avo-Jack Sandwich

¼ tsp. herbal seasoning salt
2 tbsp. low fat mayonnaise
2 slices whole grain bread,
    toasted

several leaves romaine
    lettuce, thinly sliced
3 thin slices of avocado
1 slice of cheese (jack,
    cheddar or rice cheddar)

alfalfa sprouts to taste
1 small cucumber, thinly sliced
toasted sunflower seeds
soy bacon bits

Mix seasoning salt with the mayonnaise. Spread on toast. Thinly slice several leaves romaine lettuce and cover toast slices. On one of the slices, layer the avocado, cheese, alfalfa sprouts, cucumber. Sprinkle with sunflower seeds and soy bacon bits. Top with the other toast slice. Makes 1 sandwich.

Nutrition per serving:
Calories ----------- 420
Protein ----------- 17 g.
Vitamin A --------- 108 IU

Vitamin C--------- 6 mg.
Vitamin E --------- 8 IU
Carbohydrates ---- 34 g.
Fiber ------------- 8 g.

Fat----------------- 25 g.
Cholesterol-------- 31 mg.
Calcium ----------- 278 mg.
Iron -------------- 3 mg.

Magnesium ------- 110 mg.
Potassium --------- 434 mg.
Sodium----------- 657 mg.

High Energy Sprout & Seed Salad

½ cup Asian snack mix (or
    use your favorite crunchy
    snack mix)
2 tbsp. toasted sesame seeds
2 tbsp. sunflower seeds
2 tbsp. almond granola

1 carrot, cut into sticks
3 tbsp. fresh cilantro leaves,
    chopped
8 oz. carton lemon-lime
    yogurt
¼ tsp. pepper

Boston lettuce leaves
1 hard-boiled egg, chopped
grated parmesan cheese to taste
½ cup alfalfa sprouts

In a bowl, mix the snack mix, sesame seeds, sunflower seeds, almond granola, carrot, cilantro leaves, yogurt and pepper, until just moistened. Place onto Boston lettuce leaves and top with the egg, parmesan and alfalfa sprouts. Makes 3 salads.

Spinach-Shrimp Salad with Mustard Dressing

2 (12 oz.) packages baby
    spinach leaves
1 lb. salad shrimp, cooked

1 tbsp. honey
1 tsp. arrowroot powder
⅓ cup Dijon mustard
2 tbsp. white wine

1 tbsp. balsamic vinegar
2 tbsp. fresh dill, minced
    (or 1½ tsp. dried dill)

Place the spinach in a large bowl and toss with the shrimp. Make the dressing in a saucepan over medium heat. Mix in the honey and arrowroot. Whisk in the mustard, 2 tbsp. water, white wine and balsamic vinegar. Cook, stirring constantly, until dressing comes to a low simmer. Stir in the dill and remove from heat. Pour dressing over salad. Mix well and serve at once. Makes 6 servings.

Egg Salad Light

An excellent protein source and very nutritious food, egg yolk cholesterol (which got such a bad "rap" for years) is balanced by the egg white lecithin phosphatides.

6 eggs, hard-boiled and
    peeled
2 tbsp. low-fat mayonnaise
2 stalks celery, minced

2 tsp. Dijon mustard
2 tbsp. parsely, chopped
2 tbsp. low-fat plain yogurt
¼ tsp. curry powder

juice of 1 lemon
¼ tsp. lemon-pepper
Boston lettuce leaves
paprika

Mash the eggs in a bowl together with the mayonnaise, celery, Dijon mustard, parsley, yogurt, curry powder, lemon juice, and lemon-pepper seasoning. Place scoops of the mixture in individual Boston lettuce leaves and top with a dash of paprika. Makes 4 servings.

Entrées

Veggies, Kasha & Cheese
Full of minerals as well as protein.

¾ cup bulgur or kasha
2 cups onions, diced
2 cloves garlic, minced
2 tbsp. olive oil
3 cups zucchini
3 cups fresh spinach
1½ tsp. Italian herbs

¼ tsp. lemon-pepper
   seasoning
1 cup feta cheese,(about 5
   oz.) crumbled
1 cup low fat cottage cheese
¾ cup fresh parsely, chopped
2 eggs

2 tbsp. tomato paste
¼ cup green onions, chopped
2 tomatoes, sliced
1 cup low-fat cheddar cheese, grated
1½ tbsp. sesame seeds

Preheat oven to 350°. Prepare a 9" x 9" baking dish. Place bulgur into a bowl and cover with ¾ cup boiling water and set aside. In a large frying pan, sauté onions and garlic cloves in the olive oil for 10 minutes. In a food processor, shred the zucchini. With a knife, thinly slice the fresh spinach and add to the frying pan along with the Italian herbs, lemon-pepper seasoning and zucchini, and sauté for an additional 3 minutes. In a bowl, mix the feta, cottage cheese, parsley, eggs, tomato paste, and green onions. Stir into the bulgur. To assemble casserole, layer bulgur mix on bottom of the baking dish. Cover with vegetable mixture, then the cheese mix. Cover with the sliced tomatoes and sprinkle with the cheddar cheese. Top with sesame seeds and bake covered for 45 minutes; then uncover and bake an additional 15 minutes. Let stand for 10 minutes before serving. Makes 8 servings.

Chicken & Vegetables
High in protein and minerals, low in fat.

2 cups low-fat organic
   chicken broth
1½ cups mixed whole grains
4 organic chicken breasts,
   skinned, boned and sliced
   into strips

2 tbsp. grapeseed oil
1 tbsp. grapeseed oil
1 red onion, diced
2 shallots, diced
1 red bell pepper, sliced
3 large tomatoes, diced

½ tsp. dried basil
1 tsp. cumin
½ tsp. oregano
½ tsp. black pepper
2 cups fresh pea pods, trimmed

Preheat oven to 350°. In a soup pot, bring the chicken broth to a boil and stir in the whole grains. Reduce heat, cover and simmer for 10 minutes. Fluff, turn into a large grapeseed oil-sprayed casserole dish. In a large skillet, brown the chicken strips in the grapeseed oil until opaque, firm and tender. Arrange on top of the grain in the casserole dish. Add 1 tbsp. grapeseed oil to the skillet and sauté the onion, shallots, and bell pepper for 5 minutes. Add the tomatoes, basil, cumin, oregano, and black pepper and sauté for 5 minutes more. Arrange vegetable mixture over the chicken, cover and bake for 30 minutes. Uncover, and stir in the pea pods. Cover again, turn off oven, and let peas steam until green, about 10 minutes. Delicious and fragrant with herbs. Makes enough for 8 people.

Nutrition per serving:			
Calories ----------- 227	Vitamin C--------- 43 mg.	Fat ---------------- 3 g.	Magnesium ------- 89 mg.
Protein ------------ 20 g.	Vitamin E --------- 2 IU	Cholesterol-------- 34 mg.	Potassium --------- 562 mg.
Vitamin A--------- 121 IU	Carbohydrates ---- 37 g.	Calcium ----------- 67 mg.	Sodium------------ 57 mg.
	Fiber ------------- 4 g.	Iron -------------- 2 mg.	

Paella

6 tbsp. olive oil	3 tsp. saffron threads	2½ cups arborio rice
1 lb. large shrimp, shelled and deveined	½ cup fresh cilantro, chopped	4 cups fish stock or vegetable broth
24 mussels	2 tbsp. lemon juice	1 cup white wine
1 lb. sea bass or monkfish fillets, cut into pieces	2 cups yellow onion, diced	1 can garbanzo beans
1 tbsp. sweet paprika	5 cloves garlic, minced	1 jar artichoke hearts, quartered
	3 cups tomatoes, chopped	lemon wedges
		cracked black pepper

Heat the olive oil in a paella pan or your widest heavy skillet and sauté the shrimp for a few minutes. Remove with a slotted spoon to a large bowl and set aside. Add the mussels and cook 3 minutes until shells open (discard any that don't open). Remove to the bowl with the slotted spoon. Add the sea bass and sauté 5 minutes and remove to bowl. Combine the paprika, saffron, cilantro and lemon juice in a small bowl and mix well. Sprinkle over the seafood and let the flavors blend. Sauté the onions, garlic and tomatoes in the pan for 10 minutes. Add the rice, fish stock, white wine, garbanzo beans and artichoke hearts. Reduce heat, cover and simmer untouched for 15 minutes until rice is done but still chewy. You'll have a rich, crusty brown layer on the bottom of the pan. Turn off heat. Add entire contents of seafood bowl to paella. Cover and let stand for 10 minutes. Serve with lots of lemon wedges and cracked black pepper. Makes 9 servings.

Lemon Mushrooms

These mushrooms are absolutely delectable.

20 – 24 gourmet mushrooms (a blend of chanterelles, shiitakes, enokis, buttons), brushed clean and halved or sliced	1 small red onion, sliced	½ cup white wine
	1 cup olive oil	¼ cup lemon juice
	1 shallot, minced	½ tsp. lemon-pepper seasoning
	1 tbsp. fresh oregano or 1 tsp. dry oregano	⅓ cup watercress leaves or sunflower sprouts

Combine the mushrooms and onion in a bowl. To create the marinade, combine the olive oil, shallot, oregano, white wine, lemon juice, lemon-pepper. Toss marinade with mushroom mix. Chill, covered, overnight. Top with the watercress and serve. Makes 4 salads.

Very Low-Fat Chinese Chicken Salad

2 whole organic chicken breasts	1 tbsp. soy bacon bits	1 bunch broccoli
3 – 4 cups organic vegetable broth	1 tbsp. RED STAR nutritional yeast	3 cups mixed baby Asian greens
	½ tsp. black pepper	½ cup celery, diced
2 tbsp. brown rice vinegar	¼ tsp. dry mustard	2 tbsp. white daikon radish, thinly sliced
2 tbsp. soy sauce	1 tsp. grated orange zest	2 scallions, thinly sliced
2 tbsp. green onions, sliced	½ cup olive oil	1 hard boiled egg, crumbled

Simmer the chicken breasts in the broth for 1 hour until tender. Skin, bone, and cut into bite-size pieces. To create the marinade, combine the vinegar, soy sauce, green onions, bacon bits, yeast, black pepper, mustard, orange zest, olive oil. Pour over chicken pieces. Chop the broccoli Chinese restaurant style. (To do this, cut off ends of each stalk to make 5" stems and slit lengthwise.) Cook in boiling salted water until broccoli turns bright green. Drain, add to chicken pieces and chill. In a salad serving bowl, mix the Asian greens, celery, daikon radish and scallions. Remove chicken and broccoli from the marinade with a slotted spoon, and pour remaining liquid over greens. Toss to mix. Arrange broccoli with stems to the center in a ring over the top of the greens. Fill the ring with the chicken. Sprinkle with crumbled hard boiled egg. Makes 6 servings.

Nutrition per serving:	Vitamin C --------- 42 mg.	Fat ---------------- 12 g.	Magnesium ------- 54 mg.
Calories ----------- 227	Vitamin E --------- 3 IU	Cholesterol -------- 117 mg.	Potassium --------- 571 mg.
Protein ----------- 25 g.	Carbohydrates ---- 6 g.	Calcium ----------- 71 mg.	Sodium------------ 190 mg.
Vitamin A --------- 128 IU	Fiber ------------- 3 g.	Iron -------------- 2 mg.	

Healthy dessert options

Double Ginger Molasses Cookies

½ cup granulated maple sugar

4 tbsp. butter

4 tbsp. grapeseed oil

½ cup molasses

2 tbsp. lemon juice

2 tbsp. honey crystallized ginger

2 cups whole wheat pastry flour

1 tsp. ground ginger

1 tsp. baking powder

½ tsp. baking soda

1 tsp. allspice

1 tsp. cinnamon

1 tsp. ground cloves

½ tsp. sea salt.

raisins

chopped nuts

nutmeg

Preheat oven to 350°F. Combine the following ingredients in a saucepan until melted: the maple sugar, butter, grapeseed oil, molasses, lemon juice and crystallized ginger. In a separate bowl, stir together the flour, ground ginger, baking powder, baking soda, allspice, cinnamon, cloves and sea salt. Combine mixtures together and roll out into a dough; decorate with raisins, chopped nuts and sprinkles of nutmeg. Cover with plastic wrap and chill. Then cut with a cookie cutter, saving and reworking in scraps. Use a grapeseed oil-sprayed baking sheet. Bake for 15 minutes and cool on racks. Makes 24 cookies.

Lemon-Lime Pie

¾ cup honey-sweetened graham cracker crumbs

2 tbsp. melted butter

½ tsp. allspice

1 packet gelatin

2 tbsp. apple juice concentrate

1 cup low-fat cream cheese

1 cup kefir cheese

1 cup lemon-lime yogurt

4 tbsp. granulated maple sugar

2 pinches stevia powder (or 6 drops stevia extract)

2 tsp. grated lemon zest

2 tsp. grated lime zest

4 tbsp. lemon juice

4 tbsp. lime juice

½ cup lemon-lime yogurt

1 pinch stevia powder (or 2 drops stevia extract)

Preheat oven to 325°F. Use a 9" pie pan. To make the crust, mix the graham cracker crumbs with the butter and allspice, press into the bottom the pie pan and bake for 10 – 12 minutes. Remove and cool. To make the filling, sprinkle the gelatin over apple juice concentrate in a sauce pan. Let sit 5 minutes to soften, then heat gently until gelatin dissolves. Remove from heat. Put in a blender and blend until smooth, adding the cream cheese, kefir cheese and ½ of the yogurt. Add the maple sugar granules, stevia, lemon zest, lime zest, lemon juice and lime juice. Pour into crust. Chill until somewhat set. For the topping, mix the rest of the yogurt with the stevia and spread on top. Serves 12.

Pears in Raspberry Sauce

3 pears, sliced

¼ cup honey-sweetened raspberry jelly

½ cup orange juice

½ cup fresh raspberries

chopped, toasted almonds

Preheat oven to 350°F. Place the pears in a baking dish. In a blender, combine the raspberry jelly, orange juice and fresh raspberries. Pour over pears. Cover with foil; bake for 30 minutes. Place in a serving dish and spoon sauce over top. Sprinkle on more fresh raspberries and the toasted almonds. Makes 4 – 6 servings.

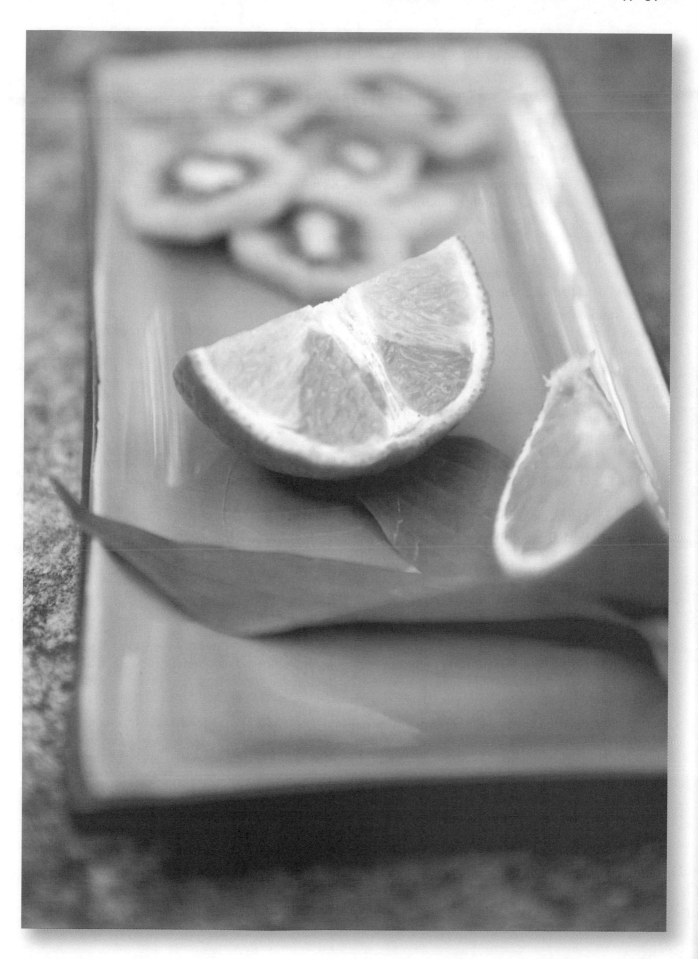

Cancer: Controlling and Rebuilding Health

What do we know about cancer development today?

Cancer is reaching epidemic proportions in the U.S.: it's now overtaking heart disease as the leading cause of death in the United States. Despite billions of dollars in research, and decades of studies, sad statistics show that now more than one in three Americans will eventually get cancer. Cancer used to be extremely rare. In 1971, when the highly publicized National War on Cancer was declared, the chances of falling victim to cancer were one in six. By 1983, those chances doubled to one in three. Today, the incidence of cancer is rising almost exponentially. More than 3 million Americans are being treated for cancer. 1.3 million are newly diagnosed each year. Cancer treatment costs the economy $172 billion *every year*, our most expensive disease by far.

Yet, studies show that conventional therapies fail 50% of the time. The percentage is even higher for lung and advanced breast cancer, and pancreatic, liver, bone, ovary and colon cancers. The traditional medical community recognizes the downsides of current treatments and aims its new drugs and technologies at killing cancer, but not patients. Even so, the newest research shows that if we spent more time on cancer prevention rather than treatment, the number of cancer deaths in the U.S. could drop by nearly a third. That translates into 100,000 fewer cancer cases and 60,000 prevented cancer deaths by 2015!

Is our lifestyle really that bad?

The dramatic, late 20th century increase is only minimally due to new diagnostic tests, or to calling old diseases, like consumption, cancers. The devastating disease we know as cancer today appears to have emerged gradually and then started rising at extraordinary rates as industrial societies became more and more dependent on technology instead of nature. Over 200 different diseases are now classified as cancer. Chasing every cancer with a drug for its different requirements and ramifications is futile. Evidence from a rising group of cancer survivors shows us that using our lifestyle to normalize cells that are out of control offers the best chance for success.

Is the cure worse than the disease?

More than $30 billion has been invested in cancer research since 1971, yet chemotherapy drugs, radiation and surgery are the main "approved" cancer therapies, and these treatments come at great cost. Cancer experts at Duke University estimate that 40% of cancer patients actually die from malnutrition, largely as a result of the severe nausea, vomiting, lack of appetite and poor nutrient intake that follows chemotherapy treatment. The Surgical Forum analyzed 100 clinical studies where chemotherapy was the sole treatment for breast cancer patients. Their report showed no benefits, but did show significant damage.

Chemo drugs don't distinguish between healthy cells and cancer cells, so many healthy cells are damaged during chemo treatments. Immunity is greatly compromised, leaving many patients wide open to supergerm infections that can be contracted in today's hospitals. One of my research assistants lost a friend suffering from leukemia not to his cancer, but to a virulent lung fungus he caught in the hospital while in chemotherapy treatment.

Anemia, hair loss and severe weakness are common side effects of chemo drugs. Still, chemotherapy is the treatment of choice for an astounding 75% of all cancer patients.

Radiation treatment, given to about 60% of cancer patients, has debilitating side effects, too. Painful swallowing, great fatigue and skin reactions are acute. Long-lasting ulcers, painful sores, reproductive malfunction and chronic diarrhea are frequently reported. Many patients actually develop other cancers because the risk for leukemia and internal scarring is so greatly increased. (For more, see page 74.)

Where do we go from here?

In May 2002, the National Cancer Institute and American Cancer Society acknowledged that the medical community is not winning the war on cancer at all. Overall, cancer survival rates have risen from 38% in 1971 to 50% today. Deaths for ovarian cancer and cancers of the liver and pancreas are still as high as 1 in 20. And, the five-year survival rates for all cancers have remained virtually static since 1970. Cancer incidence is expected to double by 2050 due to aging population.

There are a few bright spots. Testicular cancer, Hodgkin's disease and childhood leukemia are now treatable. Women with breast cancer may now choose a breast-sparing lumpectomy, followed by radiation, instead of a radical mastectomy. Colon cancer treatments, that almost always required a colostomy in times past, now allow most patients to keep significant amounts of colon structure.

A new class of drugs, angiogenesis inhibitors, in early testing stages, starve the blood vessels that feed oxygen and nutrients to cancerous tumors. Some of the angiogenesis inhibitors do arrest tumor growth. Some tumors actually shrivel up and disappear. Human testing of two angiogenesis inhibitors, angiostatin and endostatin, is now underway. Side effects appear to be minimal, but data on tumor response has not been yet released.

Cancer vaccines are being designed to stop cancer recurrence for non-Hodgkin's lymphoma which kills 25,000 patients each year. The vaccines work by fusing tumor cells to antibody-producing cells, while boosting the immune system's ability to fight cancer growth. The vaccines will not be available for another 2 or 3 years.

Herceptin, a new breast cancer drug, targets cancer genes to stop tumor growth. Specifically, it pinpoints the gene HER2, which appears to fuel aggressive tumor growth. Unlike chemo drugs and radiation, Herceptin attacks only the tumor while leaving healthy cells intact. Studies show it can extend lifespan for women with the gene who have advanced breast cancer. But Herceptin is useless for the 70% of cases that don't involve this gene, and it may weaken the heart muscle, leading to congestive heart failure.

Some surgeons are experimenting with "cryotherapy" to freeze tumors of the breast and prostate, and then surgically remove them, a process which experts say is less harmful and more effective than other therapies.

Molecular biologists have spent the past 25 years trying to pry the lid off the "black-box" of the cancer cell. Scientists are re-designing cells to contain cancer-killing properties that nature doesn't provide, such as an immune cell with a gene for TNF (tumor necrosis factor).

What about stem cell research and cancer?

Molecular research convinces most scientists that cancer is a genetic disease where mutations damage the genes that control cell division. I believe that while respecting all ways of healing, we should also be quite careful about the wider consequences of genetic engineering. The world is already crowded with drugs that increase the risk of cancer, drugs that work at far less elemental body levels than our genes. The human body is incredibly complex. I don't believe we can ever fathom or take into account all of the ramifications of "playing God" through genetic construction. Fantasy and science fiction films like "Jurassic Park" depict some of the problems of science trying hopelessly to control and predict nature, which is fundamentally illogical, uncontrollable and unpredictable.

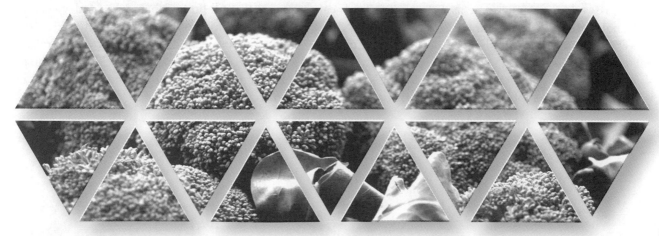

Do we know more today about what causes cancer to develop?

Diet: The foods you're eating (or not eating) could be skyrocketing your cancer risk. 40 to 60% of cancer risk is determined by your diet choices. Studies show a lack of fruits, veggies and fiber is the biggest link to cancer. A high fat diet is another offender. Naturopaths know that harmful genetic mutations can result from a diet with excess fat, because fat is involved in gland and hormone activity. Trans fatty acids from fried fast foods and commercial snack foods are especially dangerous; European studies show breast cancer risk is 40% higher in women who have high body levels of trans fatty acids! New studies reveal a diet high in protein (especially from animal sources, like the popular "Zone" and low carb diets) may increase cancer risk. Alcohol abuse, too much sugar and red meat (barbecue-charred meat is the most carcinogenic) can also be traced to cancer development.

Lifestyle: Up to 90% of cancer risk is determined by lifestyle factors like smoking, inactivity, and a fatty diet. If you live on your couch, you're boosting your cancer risk. While one out of three Americans falls victim to cancer, only one out of seven active Americans does. Exercise acts as an antioxidant to enhance body oxygen use, alters body chemistry to control fat retention, and accelerates passage of cancer-causing waste out of the body.

We all know tobacco smoke is a carcinogen. The American Cancer Society estimates that in 2004, more than 180,000 cancer deaths will be caused by tobacco use. Don't smoke! Protect yourself from second hand smoke by asking smokers to smoke away from you.

Environment: Clinical studies show that environmental toxins can damage cell DNA, which leads to cell mutation and tumor development. Factors like overexposure to the sun's UV rays, air pollution, estrogen-containing pesticides play a significant role in cancer development. The chemical link to cancer is becoming undeniable. 20,000 of the 70,000 chemicals people come in contact with regularly are toxic. After World War II, America's use of synthetic chemicals exploded. Billions of tons of new chemicals were dumped into our water and onto our land. Only a meager 3% were ever tested for safety. A 1979 confidential report to the chemical industry trade association conceded that exposures to occupational carcinogens were responsible for at least 20% of all cancers. Moreover, many chemicals have hormone-mimicking effects—a primary reason they're implicated in hormone-driven breast and prostate cancers.

Women, in particular, have been hit hard. Human breast milk contains more dioxin, PCBs, DDT and other pesticides than any other food on the planet! A study in the International Journal of Epidemiology shows breast cancer mortality rates rise the closer women live to toxic waste dumps. Until about 20 years ago, both breast cancer rates and contamination levels of PCB pesticides in Israel were among the highest in the world. An aggressive phase-out of these pesticides has led to a sharp reduction in contamination levels, followed by a dramatic drop in breast cancer death rates for Israeli women. Here in the U.S., breast cancer rates have more than doubled since 1950. Today, one in eight American women will develop breast cancer in their lifetime.

Men are getting a cancer wake-up call of their own. Testicular cancer is on the rise in young men. The rate of prostate cancer has doubled since the WWII chemical era.

The dental chemical link to cancer has been vastly understated. Hydrogen peroxide used in teeth whitening toothpastes and dental bleaches may accelerate mouth cancer. Research from University of Buffalo shows hydrogen peroxide may turn pre-cancerous cells into full-blown cancer; lesions already present grow even larger!

EMFs (electromagnetic fields): Do electric fields cause cancer? It's still hotly debated, but today even the National Institute of Environment Health Sciences (NIEHS) says exposure to strong electromagnetic fields from power lines and electric appliances may be a cause of cancer. Most notable are studies which show high rates of leukemia in children living near high voltage power lines. Electric-utility workers exposed to EMFs on the job show increases in lymphoma. Exposure to EMFs may cause enzyme, and cell behavior changes. There are some who say that EMFs suppress the hormone melatonin, a cancer protector.

Do you know the early detection signs of cancer?

• a change in bowel or bladder habits, especially blood in the stool.
• chronic indigestion, bloating and heartburn, especially difficulty swallowing.
• unusual bleeding or discharge from the vagina.
• lumps or thickening of the breasts or testicles.
• a chronic cough or constant voice hoarseness; bloody sputum.
• inflamed warts or moles, or scaly skin patches that won't go away, especially if they ulcerate.
• unexplained weight loss usually accompanied by anemia or great fatigue.

Can diet and alternative therapies really help you cut your risk?

While it seems like we're assaulted from all sides by cancer activators that we can't control, lifestyle causes mean that we can positively affect most cancer sources ourselves - both to prevent cancer from occurring and helping ourselves when it has. Diet is the first place to look. Improving your diet directly improves your defenses against cancer. The latest estimates show that good food choices could have helped prevent 395,000 to 750,000 new cancer cases, and between 180,000 to 350,000 cancer deaths in 1996 in the United States alone.

Cancer treatment is a place where conventional treatments and alternative therapies can come together for the good of the patient. More and more physicians and patients are embracing a complementary approach—using both today's technologies and natural healing therapies like biofeedback, imagery, acupuncture and nutrition in the battle against cancer. The use of supplements and herbs to beat cancer is exploding. Research reveals 80% of cancer patients are using some type of unconventional cancer therapy, but 50% don't tell their doctors!

(See my book HEALTHY HEALING, 12th Edition for the latest information, or visit www.healthyhealing.com)

Eight ways to cut your cancer risk. Watchwords for cancer prevention:

Your diet is the place to start.

Your diet is your major weapon against cancer. Whole food nutrition allows the body to use its built-in restorative and repair abilities. A healthy diet can intervene in the cancer process at many stages, from its conception to its growth and spread. Even if your genetics and lifestyle are against you, your diet may still make a tremendous difference in your cancer odds. For example, certain body chemicals must be "activated" before they can initiate cancer. Antioxidant foods can block the activation process, snuff out carcinogens, nip free radical cascades in the bud, even repair some cellular damage.

Certain foods help your body detoxify, and prevent the genetic ruin of cells, a prelude to cancer (one of the reasons I emphasize a detoxification diet as part of cancer control). Healthy food elements can determine whether a cancer-causing virus, or a cancer promoter like too much estrogen will turn tissue cancerous. Even after cells have massed into structures that may grow into tumors, food compounds can intervene to stop more growth. Some actually shrink the patches of precancerous cells.

Although far less powerful at later stages, diet can still influence the metastasis or spread of cancer, and help prolong your life. Wandering cancer cells need the right conditions in which to attach and grow. Food agents can foster a hostile or a favorable environment. Massive new research is validating what naturopaths have known for decades. The more fruits and vegetables you eat, the less your cancer risk.

Even small to moderate amounts of fruits and vegetables make a big difference. Two fruits and three vegetable servings a day have shown amazing anti-cancer results. Eating fruit twice a day, instead of twice a week, can cut the risk of lung cancer by 75%, even in smokers. One National Cancer Institute spokesman said it is almost mind-boggling, that ordinary fruits and vegetables could be so effective against such a potent carcinogen as nicotine. The evidence is so overwhelming that some researchers view fruits and vegetables as powerful preventive drugs that could substantially wipe out cancer. What an about-face for cancer study!

1.   **Reduce your intake of fat,** especially animal fats and trans fats. Environmental toxins lodge in the fatty tissue of animals in our food chain, and in tissue of humans who eat them. Protect yourself from chemical overload by eating organic foods and integrating a detoxification program in your life at least twice a year.

2.   **Reduce your intake of red meats.** Cancer is closely related to the protein and fat, in red meats, fast foods and fried foods, and sometimes the added hormones injected into red meats.

3.   **Eat fruits and vegetables every day.** People who eat plenty of fruits and vegetables have half the risk of people who eat few fruits and vegetables. Berries, citrus fruits and cruciferous veggies are among the most potent cancer fighters. Try a green drink like FIT FOR YOU MIRACLE GREENS or CRYSTAL STAR® ENERGY GREEN RENEWAL™.

4.   **Use enzyme therapy.** High enzymes are essential to protect against cancer protection and to fight cancer. Have a fresh green salad every day; use a supplemental proteolytic enzyme like CRYSTAL STAR® DR. ENZYME WITH PROTEASE & BROMELAIN to stimulate immune response.

5.   **Use free radical-neutralizing antioxidants.** Free radical damage to cellular DNA and RNA causes the loss of normal cell regulatory control, allowing cells to multiply at a much faster rate contributing to cancer.

6.   **Detoxify and cleanse your body at least twice a year to defend against chemical overload.** Superfoods like barley grass and chlorella, and vegetable juices accelerate natural body detox activity. (See the special STRESS DETOX DIET on page 14 for details.)

7.   **Keep your immune system strong with minerals.** Minerals set the baseline for your immune system. They're the foundation your body works with to build everything else. Minerals increase enzyme production and help establish normal pH levels, vital for immune maintenance. Electrolyte minerals offer maximum absorption. Try ALACER EMERGEN-C drink mix.

8.   **Develop your own spirituality.** The newest research shows that prayer really works for healing. It's a sad but well-established fact among healers that one major commonality between cancer patients is a traumatic event like divorce, or loss of a loved one that occurs in the year or two before their diagnosis. Reducing stress through relaxation therapies like yoga, massage and meditation can be invaluable.

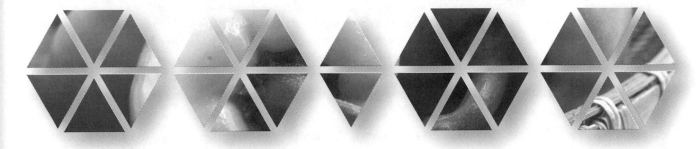

The foods that provide prime cancer-fighting nutrition:

• Vitamin C-rich, antioxidant-rich fruits and vegetables—citrus fruits, tomatoes, peppers and broccoli, reinforce a strong immune system to prevent wandering cancer cells from attaching to new tissue.
• Yogurt cultures help neutralize carcinogens and de-activate enzymes that allow body substances to turn into cancer.
• Antioxidant foods, like wheat germ, soy foods, yellow, orange and green vegetables, green tea, citrus fruits, and olive oil help normalize pre-cancerous cells, and neutralize cancer-causing free radicals. The darker green the vegetables, like kale, dandelion, arugula and spinach, the more cancer-inhibiting carotenoids they have.
• Fiber-rich foods like whole grains, fruits and vegetables absorb excess bile, increase elimination of toxins and improve healthy intestinal bacteria.
• Phytochemical food compounds like indole 3 carbinole in cruciferous vegetables and algin in sea greens break down carcinogens and remove them from the body. These same vegetable compounds also break down excess estrogens that are responsible for some types of breast cancer.
• Folic acid foods—whole wheat and wheat germ, leafy vegetables, beets, asparagus, fish, sunflower seeds, and citrus fruits, are critical to normal DNA synthesis so healthy cells do not mutate and turn cancerous.

Can a macrobiotic diet control cancer?

The greatest benefit of a macrobiotic diet is that it is cleansing and strengthening at the same time. This balanced way of eating is non-mucous forming, high in vegetable fiber and protein, low in fats that can alter body chemistry. It stimulates heart and circulatory systems with Asian foods like miso, green tea, and shiitake mushrooms. It alkalizes with umeboshi plums, sea greens and soy foods. It is high in potassium, natural iodine and other minerals. It is easily individualized for one's environment, the seasons, and the constitution of the person using it. The form recommended here for an intensive healing program can be followed for three to six months.

Twenty minutes before each meal, and before bed: take a glass of aloe vera juice (detoxifies and eases nausea if you are undergoing chemotherapy or radiation).

On rising: take a potassium broth (page 16); or carrot-beet-cucumber juice to clean liver and kidneys; or cranberry concentrate (2 tsp. in water) or red grape juice; or a ginseng restorative tea like Yogi Ginseng NRG Tea; or Crystal Star® Restore Your Strength™ drink; or a superfood drink like Green Foods Carrot Essence.

Breakfast: take this Pulsating Parsley Juice for vitamin A and carotenes: juice 6 carrots, 1 beet with top, a large handful of spinach leaves and ¼ cup fresh parsley; then, make a mix of: Red Star nutritional yeast, wheat germ, lecithin granules, CC Pollen High Desert Bee Pollen granules. Sprinkle some daily on granola, or mix with yogurt and fruit, or on fresh fruit like strawberries or apples with kefir or kefir cheese; or have a breakfast pilaf like brown rice or Kashi, with apple juice or kefir cheese topping.

Mid-morning: take a cup of Crystal Star® Cleansing & Purifying™ Tea; or a mixed vegetable juice; or Sun Wellness Chlorella, Green Foods Green Magma, or fresh wheat grass juice. Or take an herb tea, like pau d'arco, Natural Energy Plus Caisse's Tea, Essiac Tea, or a glass of fresh carrot juice; or a cup of miso soup with fresh ginger and sea greens snipped on top. (Have 2 tbsp. dry sea greens daily.)

Lunch: have Super V-7 veggie juice : juice 2 carrots, 2 tomatoes, 1 handful each spinach and parsley, 2 celery ribs, ½ cucumber, ½ bell pepper. Add 1 tbsp. green superfood: like Crystal Star® Energy Green Renewal™, Nutri-Cology Pro-Greens, or Fit For You, Inc. Miracle Greens. Have steamed broccoli with brown rice, or an Asian stir fry with brown rice and miso sauce; or a green salad; or a black bean, onion or lentil soup, or a 3 bean salad.

Mid-afternoon: a cup of green tea, or Crystal Star® Green Tea Cleanser™ for chemoprotective effects, and some whole grain crackers with kefir cheese.

Dinner: mix brown rice and steamed veggies with maitake or shiitake mushrooms. Maitake's unique natural killer cells are powerful against tumors. Add 1 tbsp. flax oil, nutritional yeast and snipped dry sea greens; or have a whole grain casserole with tofu and steamed vegetables, or a big salad with sea greens, nuts and seeds; or baked or broiled fish or seafood with veggies, or rice-stuffed cabbage rolls and baked carrots with ginger syrup.

Before bed: have a cup of shiitake mushroom or ginger broth, or apple juice; or papaya-pineapple juice to enhance enzyme activity; or a cup of green tea (anticancer and cancer chemoprotective effects).

Note: In order for the macrobiotic balance to work correctly with your body, avoid the following foods: Red meat, poultry, preserved, smoked, cured meats of all kinds, and dairy foods except occasional eggs. Coffee and carbonated drinks. All refined, frozen, canned, processed foods; white vinegar, and table salt. Nightshade plants: tomatoes, potatoes, peppers, eggplant; and hot spices. (Modified macrobiotic diets may use these foods sparingly.)

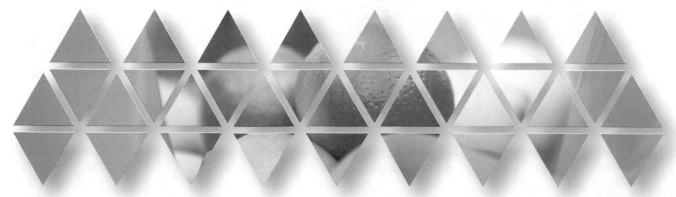

Choose 2 or 3 supplements to enhance your immune response against cancer:

- **Macrobiotic cleansing support:** CRYSTAL STAR® LIVER CLEANSE FLUSHING™ TEA; DAILY DETOX BY M.D.; ARISE & SHINE CLEANSE THYSELF PROGRAM - a specific for cancer patients, with many reports of success.
- **Enzyme support:** CRYSTAL STAR® DR. ENZYME WITH PROTEASE & BROMELAIN™ or TRANSFORMATION PUREZYME (proteolytic enzymes) dissolves fibrin coating on cancer cells so immune defenses can work. Purifies by breaking down protein invaders. DOUGLAS LABS COQMELT (fast acting, high potency); HERBAL ANSWERS HERBAL ALOE FORCE.
- **Immune support:** Herbs: CRYSTAL STAR® ENERGY GREEN RENEWAL™; NUTRICOLOGY PRO-GREENS; VIBRANT HEALTH GREEN VIBRANCE; PLANETARY FORMULAS SHIITAKE MUSHROOM SUPREME. Supplements: ALLERGY RESEARCH GLUTATHIONE with vitamin C; NUTRICOLOGY LAKTOFERRIN with colostrum (not for leukemia); GRIFRON MAITAKE D-FRACTION extract; EIDON SILICA MINERAL; ALPHA LIPOIC ACID 600 mg. daily; BIOTEC CELL GUARD.

Bodywork techniques are a key to establishing an anti-cancer body environment

- **Sunlight:** Get some sunlight on the body every day possible (esp. for organ cancers).
- **Guided imagery:** effective in helping immune response, balancing hormones, and reducing production of abnormal cells. I have personally seen results with several people. See a good practitioner for real help.
- **Enemas:** Enemas (especially coffee enemas) are a specific for cancer detoxification: Take an enema the first, second and the last day of your cleansing program to help release toxins out of the body.
- **Exercise:** Regular exercise is almost a "cancer defense" in itself, acting as an antioxidant to boost immune response, accelerating waste passage out of the body, altering body chemistry to control fat retention.
- **Overheating therapy:** highly effective against cancer (see my book *Healthy Healing* for technique).
- **Deep breathing:** Deep, relaxed breathing removes stress, composes the mind, increases energy levels. 1. Shift focus away from your racing mind to focus attention on your breath. 2. Take slow, deep, regular breaths to calm the mind. 3. Recall a pleasant experience. 4. Physically feel thankfulness or love about the good people you have in your life. 5. Question your inner intuition to help find a health solution, or a better response to the situation.

Maintenance Recipes for a Macrobiotic Diet
Appetizers

Macrobiotic Mushroom Pâté

1 tbsp. grapeseed oil
6 scallions, chopped
1 rib celery, chopped
1 cup whole grain bread crumbs
1 cup walnuts, chopped
1 cake tofu, cubed

5 cups mixed mushrooms, sliced (try button, cremini, and shiitake)
½ tsp. dry basil (or 1 tbsp. fresh)
¼ tsp. dry thyme
½ tsp. dry tarragon
¼ tsp. rosemary

¼ tsp. paprika
¼ cup sesame tahini
2 tbsp. soy sauce
2 tbsp. white wine
black pepper
baby salad greens
rice crackers

Preheat oven to 400°. Sauté grapeseed oil, scallions and celery in a hot skillet. Add bread crumbs, walnuts, tofu. Toss to coat and remove from heat. Add mushrooms; sauté until fragrant. Season with basil, thyme, tarragon, rosemary, paprika. Mix in the tahini, soy sauce and white wine. Add black pepper to taste.

Mix ingredients. Oil a loaf pan with lecithin spray, and line it with oiled waxed paper. Spoon in pâté, and fold extra waxed paper over top. Bake 1 hour and 15 minutes until a toothpick comes out clean. Cool in pan. Invert on a plate, peel off paper and surround with greens. Serve with rice crackers. Makes 16 appetizer servings.

Famous Soy Bean Spread

Use for raw veggies, crackers, chips or dip up with Belgian endive leaves.

1 lb. soy beans (2½ cups dry)	½ cup tamari	½ tsp. garlic powder
½ cup olive oil	2 tbsp. minced fresh parsley	½ tsp. paprika
½ cup lemon juice	½ tsp. onion powder	¼ tsp. cumin powder

Cook soy beans well until <u>very</u> soft; mash. To create the sauce, blend the olive oil, lemon juice, tamari, parsley, onion powder, garlic powder, paprika, cumin powder. Mix the sauce with the cooked beans and chill until flavors bloom. Enough for 12 people.

Macrobiotic soup

Green Ginger Soup

Making this delicate healing broth from scratch takes a little time, but it makes all the difference, and the soup is so delicious.

2 tbsp. grapeseed oil	8 dry shiitake mushroom	4 oz. snow peas, trimmed
6 cloves garlic, minced	caps (discard woody stems)	1 cup frozen peas
1 large onion, chopped	1 small can water chestnuts, sliced	brown rice vinegar
6 slices fresh ginger, minced	8 oz. firm tofu, in cubes	toasted sesame oil
1 tsp. sesame salt	2 tbsp. soy sauce	green onion, diced
7 cups water	1 bunch baby bok choy, sliced	
2 – 3 tbsp. miso paste	4 scallions, chopped	

In a large soup pot, make the ginger broth. In the grapeseed oil, sauté the garlic, chopped onion, fresh ginger, and sesame salt. Add 7 cups water, the miso paste and shiitake mushrooms. Partially cover and simmer 45 minutes until aromatic. Add water chestnuts, tofu, soy sauce and bok choy. Partially cover and simmer 5 minutes. Add scallions, snow peas, and frozen peas. Simmer briefly until everything is hot and fragrant. Serve in individual soup bowls. Drizzle drops of brown rice vinegar and toasted sesame oil over top of each bowl, and top with a bit of green onion. Makes 10 bowls.

Nutrition per serving:	Vitamin C --------- 15 mg.	Fat ----------------- 6 g.	Magnesium ------- 40 mg.
Calories ----------- 125	Vitamin E --------- 1 IU	Cholesterol-------- 0	Potassium --------- 281 mg.
Protein ------------ 7 g.	Carbohydrates ---- 12 g.	Calcium ----------- 93 mg.	Sodium------------ 323 mg.
Vitamin A --------- 370 IU	Fiber -------------- 3 g.	Iron --------------- 3 mg.	

Macrobiotic dessert

Icy Granita

Perfect over plain fruit for a fat-free healthy dessert that works with macrobiotics.

3 tbsp. honey	12 fresh mint leaves	7 tsp. green tea

Simply mix the honey and mint leaves in a bowl; lightly crush leaves with a wooden spoon. Pour 3 cups boiling water over 6 tsp. of the green tea in a warm teapot or pitcher, add mint leaves and honey; allow to steep about 4 – 5 minutes. Strain. Freeze in ice trays 2 – 3 hours.
Grind 1 tsp. green tea leaves to a powder in a food processor. Add a few tea ice cubes at a time and process on high until broken into granules. Spoon over fruit, garnish with a sprig of mint. 6 servings.

Cancer Control and Prevention Diet

Naturopaths believe that a healthy body with strong immune response does not develop cancer, and that cancer is a reflection of the body as a whole rather than a disease in one part. Alternative therapists seek to strengthen immune response, using a multifaceted, non-toxic approach, incorporating treatments which rely on bio-chemistry, metabolic, nutritional and herbal therapies, and immune enhancement.

Watchwords:

- Boost your intake of veggie juices, citrus juice and green tea. Add a glass of red wine a day.
- Have miso, shiitake mushrooms, sea greens and nutritional yeast 3 times a week.
- Reduce red meat, dairy foods, fat. Watch your BBQ, blackened meat has carcinogenic hydrocarbons.
- Drink 8 glasses of water daily. Avoid excessive alcohol (especially beer) and caffeine.
- Have a fresh green or seaweed salad every day!

Dramatic diet changes can mean dramatic results. The best (organic) cancer-fighting foods:

- **carotene-rich foods:** all red, orange and yellow fruits and veggies; tomatoes; green vegetables.
- **antioxidant foods soak up free radicals:** garlic, onions, broccoli, wheat germ, sea greens, leafy veggies, chili peppers, grapes, berries, carrots, turmeric, green tea, rooibos (red) tea, citrus fruits.
- **steamed cruciferous vegetables:** broccoli, cabbage, brussels sprouts, cauliflower, all dark greens.
- **protease inhibitors:** beans (esp. soy), potatoes, corn, hibiscus tea, brown rice.
- **high fiber foods:** whole grains, especially brown rice, apples, fruits and vegetables.
- **enzyme-rich foods and herbs:** pineapple, papaya, mangoes, miso, sprouts, ginger, fresh fruits and veggies.
- **lignan foods:** fish, flax oil, walnuts, berries.

On rising: take 2 tbsp. ALOELIFE ALOE GOLD drink, in orange juice.

Breakfast: make a mix of 2 tbsp. each RED STAR nutritional yeast, lecithin granules, toasted wheat germ, CC POLLEN HIGH DESERT BEE POLLEN granules and flax seeds. Sprinkle some on your choice of fresh fruits, plain or with yogurt; or a whole grain granola with apple juice, yogurt, or rice milk topping; or whole grain toast or muffins with a little kefir cheese; or a baked or poached egg or omelet.

Mid-morning: a Personal Best V-8 (pg. 18) or SUN WELLNESS CHLORELLA, (high beta carotene fights tumor formation); WAKUNAGA GREEN HARVEST, GREEN KAMUT JUST BARLEY, or CRYSTAL STAR® ENERGY GREEN RENEWAL™ drink in apple juice; or a tonifying herb tea, such as Siberian eleuthero, red clover, NATURAL ENERGY PLUS CAISSE'S TEA.

Lunch: have a leafy green salad with a cup of miso or ramen noodle soup; or a cup of black bean, lentil, or other protein soup with baked potato and kefir cheese or yogurt sauce; or a fresh organic fruit salad with cottage cheese or yogurt cheese, and whole grain baked chips or crackers; or a light seafood or organic turkey salad; or a hot spinach pasta salad.

Mid-afternoon: have whole grain crackers, rice cakes or crunchy raw veggies with a vegetable, soy or kefir spread, and a cup of light broth; or a cup of ginseng tea, or add 1 PRINCE OF PEACE ROYAL JELLY-GINSENG vial to hot water, or peppermint tea, or CRYSTAL STAR® DR. VITALITY™ TEA.

Dinner: a high protein vegetable, nut and seed salad with soup and whole grain muffins or cornbread; or a stir-fry with brown rice and miso soup with sea greens; or a baked veggie, tofu and rice casserole; or baked or broiled fish or seafood with a green salad, brown rice or steamed veggies. Relax with a glass of white wine.

Before Bed: have a cup of chamomile tea, apple or papaya juice, or a cup of miso soup.

Choose 2 or 3 supplements to enhance your immune response against cancer:

- **Detoxification support:** CRYSTAL STAR® DETOX BLOOD PURIFIER™ capsules as directed, and GREEN TEA CLEANSER™ every morning. Give yourself a weekly vitamin C flush (also relieves pain) – up to 10 g. daily (or until stool turns soupy). Una da gato capsules, especially if liver fluke parasites are involved (many cancers).
- **Ginseng reinforces tumor immunity:** IMPERIAL ELIXIR SIBERIAN GINSENG-ROYAL JELLY, or Eleuthero extract.
- **Protect against free radical damage:** Glutathione 150 mg.; Lipoic acid, or JARROW ALPHA LIPOIC ACID 600 mg.
- **Discourage tumor growth:** DR. RATH'S VITACOR PLUS; Ginger extract; European mistletoe helps repair damaged DNA (ask your health practitioner); NUTRICOLOGY MODIFIED CITRUS PECTIN for metastasis; CARNIVORA RESEARCH CARNIVORA® IMMUNE ENHANCER; CRYSTAL STAR® RESTORE YOUR STRENGTH™ drink; probiotics, like UAS LABS DDS-PLUS WITH FOS; JARROW IP-6; FLORA FLOR-ESSSENCE.
- **Protease enzymes have remarkable activity against cancer:** CRYSTAL STAR® DR. ENZYME WITH PROTEASE & BROMELAIN™; TRANSFORMATION PUREZYME; Bromelain 1500 mg. with Quercetin 1000 mg. daily; CoQ_{10} 200 mg. 3x daily.
- **Boost anti-angiogenesis to block tumor nourishment:** NUTRICOLOGY ANGIOBLOCK (bindweed extract); PHOENIX BIOLOGICS VITACARTE BOVINE TRACHEAL CARTILAGE; Garlic 10 tabs daily; Pau d'arco tea, 4 cups daily.
- **Polyphenol compounds:** red wine, green tea, aloe vera juice, maitake mushroom, GRIFRON PRO MAITAKE D-FRACTION; NUTRICOLOGY IMMUBLAST.
- **Natural anti-neoplaston substances reduce tumors:** Green tea; folic acid 800 mcg. Evening Primrose oil 3000 mg. daily; fish or flaxseed oil, 1 oz daily; selenium 400 mg. daily with vitamin E 800 IU.

Bodywork techniques are a key to establishing an anti-cancer body environment

- **Exercise regularly:** Morning sunlight (esp. for organ cancers), and regular exercise accelerate the passage of toxins. Yoga is especially good.
- **Guided imagery:** effective in helping the immune system work better, and the hormone system to stop producing abnormal cells.
- **Enemas can clean out putrefaction fast:** Take a coffee enema once a week for a month (1 cup strong brewed in a qt. of water) or chlorella implants, or a wheat grass retention enema.
- **Reduce external growths:**
  - HERBAL ANSWER'S HERBAL ANSWER ALOE GEL.
  - Effective poultices: Garlic/onion poultice; comfrey leaf poultice; green clay poultice.
  - CRYSTAL STAR® ANTI-BIO™ gel with una da gato.
  - PHYCOTENE CREME (contains a complex of 17 carotenoids) available from royalbodycare.com.
  - DR. CHRISTOPHER'S BLACK DRAWING ointment (very strong)

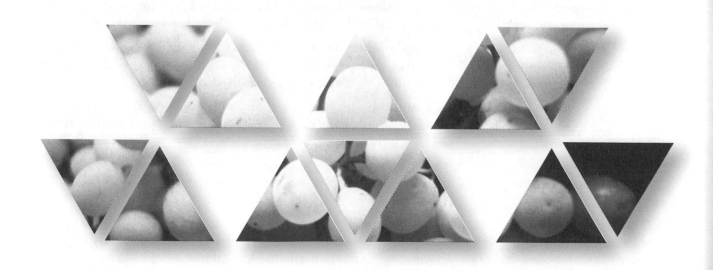

Normalize after Chemotherapy and Radiation

Chemotherapy and radiation treatments are widely used by orthodox medicine for most types, stages and degrees of cancer. While some partial successes have been proven, the effects of both treatments are often worse than the disease in terms of healthy cell damage, body imbalance, and reduced immunity. Doctors and therapists recognize the drawbacks to chemotherapy and radiation, but under current government and insurance restrictions, neither they nor their patients have alternatives. Even when a new treatment is substantiated, there is no reasonable investment certainty that government (and therefore health insurance) approval can be obtained through the maze of red tape and politics.

Amazingly, even with all the new information on alternative methods, new procedures, and even new drugs, surgery, chemotherapy, radiation and a few extremely strong drugs are still the only protocols approved by the FDA for malignant disease. Medical insurance will not reimburse doctors or hospitals if they use other healing methods. Thus, exorbitant medical costs and special interest regulations have bound medical professionals, hospitals, and insurance companies in a vicious circle where no alternative measures may be used to control cancer. Scientists admit that current treatments are pushed to their limits. Yet, even today, the vast majority of funds provided by the National Cancer Act support research to improve the effectiveness of existing therapies — radiation, surgery and chemotherapy— leaving patients with the same three therapies, just a more precise use of them.

Some of this is changing as cancer patients refuse to become victims of their medical system as well as the disease. The American people are demanding access, funding and insurance approval for alternative health techniques and medicines. Slowly, state by state, legislators and regulators are listening, health care parameters are expanding, and insurance limitations are lessening.

A Healing Diet after Chemotherapy

You can help your body clean out drug residues, get over treatment side effects, and rebuild strength after chemotherapy and radiation with the following healing diet. You can live with this diet for health on a lifetime basis, for cancer resistance to disease recurrence, and for good immune strength. It is high in absorbable vitamins and minerals, oxygenating foods, and immune and liver stimulating nutrients. Keep your diet about 60% fresh foods for the first month after chemotherapy.

On rising: take ALL 1 vitamin/mineral drink; GARDEN OF LIFE GOATEIN, or NATURE'S PLUS SPIRUTEIN in orange juice; or make your own fresh V- 8 juice (page 18) and add 1 tbsp. BRAGG'S LIQUID AMINOS.

Breakfast: have a high fiber, whole grain cereal with yogurt, kefir or soy milk, and add some nuts, seeds and dried fruit. Make a mix of 2 tbsp. each: RED STAR nutritional yeast, lecithin granules, and toasted wheat germ, and sprinkle it each morning over your breakfast - some fresh fruit, or yogurt, or a baked or poached egg.

Mid-morning: have some raw crunchy veggies with kefir or yogurt cheese or a veggie/soy spread; or a glass of carrot juice (at least once a week). Have a green supplement drink like SUN WELLNESS WAKASA GOLD (chlorella's high beta carotene content fights tumor formation). Take aloe vera juice as needed for nausea.

Lunch: have a seafood salad, or a large green salad with cucumbers, kiwi, and peas, and yogurt or lemon-flax oil dressing; or a cabbage coleslaw salad with yogurt or lemon dressing; or a quiche with asparagus, broccoli, or artichokes and a whole grain crust; or ahi tuna salad, or a tofu burger on a whole grain bun; or a baked potato with a little butter and a mushroom salad side dish.

Mid-afternoon: a cup of green tea or CRYSTAL STAR® DR. VITALITY™ TEA; or miso soup with sea greens snipped on top; or baked tofu chunks with low-fat dressing.

Dinner: have a light whole grain pasta meal, with fresh mozzarella cheese or soy mozzarella; or a sweet potato pie, or baked yams and carrots with a little butter and brown rice; or a broccoli-Chinese cabbage stir-fry with miso soup; or steamed broccoli, cauliflower, green beans or zucchini with toasted walnuts and dressing; or a salmon, rice and green bean casserole; or fresh grilled or baked fish with peas and rice; or a zucchini and rice frittata.

For 3 months after chemo or radiation, take these supplements to enhance your immune response:

CRYSTAL STAR® RESTORE YOUR STRENGTH™ broth daily.

Maitake mushroom has a powerful anti-cancer punch to shrink tumors. In combination with the chemotherapy drug mitomycin-C (Mit C), it may produce an amazing 99% tumor reduction. Side effects from chemo like nausea, vomiting and hair loss are reduced by maitake. GRIFRON MAITAKE D-FRACTION.

CoQ_{10} capsules, 360 mg.; in combination with germanium 150 mg. daily, and beta carotene 50,000 IU daily, and Vitamin C crystals with bioflavonoids, ¼ tsp. in liquid every hour, about 5 to 10,000 mg. daily. An adjunct to chemotherapy treatment as a heart protector.

800 mcg. folic acid to normalize DNA synthesis, especially if methotrexate was used in your treatment.

FLORADIX HERBAL IRON, 1 tsp. 3x daily, or CRYSTAL STAR ENERGY GREEN RENEWAL™ drink to counteract the anemia that causes such extreme fatigue after chemo treatments.

Protease enzymes have remarkable activity against cancer; CRYSTAL STAR DR. ENZYME WITH PROTEASE & BROMELAIN™; TRANSFORMATION PUREZYME. Co-enzymate B complex sublingual, for hair regrowth.

NUTRICOLOGY LAKTOFERRIN blocks cancer angiogenesis and boosts strength against infection from chemotherapy. Caution: Lactoferrin is contraindicated during pregnancy as high of levels of lactoferrin may cause rejection of the fetus. Also contraindicated for leukemia.

Medicinal mushrooms rebuild immunity, and may help prevent cancer reoccurrence—Royal Agaricus, Reishi, Cordyceps and Turkey Tail, available through MAITAKE PRODUCTS, INC.

For chemo-induced stomatitis, consider BHI's TRAUMEEL (found effective by injection in recent studies. Injectable TRAUMEEL is available by prescription).

Chamomile tea or liquid for inflammation of mucous membranes.

For chronic dry mouth, add flax seed oil to the diet.

Bodywork techniques are a key to establishing an anti-cancer body environment.

- Regular exercise is a healing nutrient in itself. Exercise can actually change body chemistry. Exercise with regular, moderate sunshine is the best choice of all.
- Avoid tobacco in all forms. Curtail caffeine intake. Avoid alcohol except for moderate wine.
- Even small amounts of radiation are sometimes proving to engender cancer growth in delicate tissue. Be extremely cautious of having X-rays, mammograms, etc. If you feel you are at risk for breast, uterine, ovarian, cervical or prostate cancer, avoid hormone replacement therapy; consciously avoid meats and dairy products that are regularly injected with hormones.
- Reduce the effects of chemotherapy and radiation: Reishi or Maitake mushroom extract; Astragalus extract; Nettles tea to dissolve adhesions. Apply kukui nut oil for chemotherapy or radiation burning.

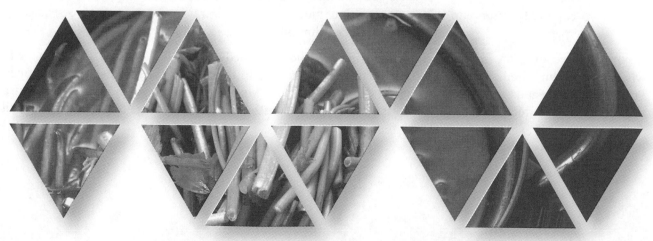

Maintenance Recipes for a Cancer Control Diet

Use these recipes on an ongoing basis once your initial healing diet is producing good results.

Research links good nutrition to the prevention of 40 – 60% of all cancers. Further, a nutritious diet can dramatically improve your survival odds if you have the disease.

Breakfast

Beta-Carotene Shake

10 – 12 fresh apricots, pitted	½ large papaya, peeled and seeded	4 ice cubes
		10 – 12 fresh mint leaves
		1 tsp. spirulina powder

In a blender, combine all ingredients and blend until smooth. Makes 2 drinks.

High Mineral Fruit Shake

1 cup vanilla lowfat soy or rice milk	1 frozen banana	2 kiwi fruit, diced
	4 tbsp. plain low-fat yogurt	2 tbsp. soy protein powder

In a blender, combine all ingredients and blend until smooth. Makes 2 drinks.

Nutrition per serving:

Calories ----------- 210	Vitamin C--------- 80 mg.	Fat ----------------- 1 g.	Magnesium ------- 59 mg.
Protein ------------ 12 g.	Vitamin E --------- 2 IU	Cholesterol-------- 1 mg.	Potassium --------- 598 mg.
Vitamin A--------- 23 IU	Carbohydrates ---- 38 g.	Calcium ----------- 320 mg.	Sodium------------ 99 mg.
	Fiber ------------- 3 g.	Iron -------------- 7 mg.	

Original Old-Fashioned Granola

6 cups rolled oats	2 cups toasted wheat germ	½ cup grapeseed oil
2½ cups toasted sunflower seeds	¼ cup sesame seeds	1½ cups honey
	½ cup shredded coconut	4 cups dried chopped fruits, like
1 cup toasted pumpkin seeds (pepitas)	1 cup walnut pieces	raisins, currants, apricots, dates
	2 cups sliced almonds	and pitted prunes

Preheat oven to 250°. In an extra large bowl, mix together the rolled oats, sunflower seeds, pumpkin seeds, wheat germ, sesame seeds, shredded coconut, walnuts and almonds. In a pan, warm the grapeseed oil and honey. Pour over granola and toss. Spread on two 11" x 17" jelly roll pans; bake for 25 minutes. Remove and stir. Return to oven and reduce temperature to 150°. Stir every 10 minutes or so. Return to the large bowl. Add dried fruit and toss to blend. Let cool before storing. Enough for 20 servings.

Healing drinks

Blood Cleanser/Builder

2 bunches grapes	8 lemons, peeled	¼ cup honey
6 oranges	2 cups water	

In a juicer, juice the grapes, oranges and lemons, before stirring in the water and honey. If you don't have a juicer, or for convenience's sake, you can substitute 2 cups grape juice, 2 cups orange juice, and 1 cup lemon juice for the fresh fruit. Makes 4 large drinks.

Immune Enhancer

½ bunch parsley	2 tomatoes	a dash of hot pepper sauce (or
1 garlic clove	1 bell pepper	cayenne pepper)
6 carrots	4 romaine leaves	1 tsp. miso paste mixed with a
3 stalks celery with leaves	1 stalk broccoli	little water

Juice all of the vegetables in the juicer before adding the hot pepper sauce and miso. Makes 2 drinks.

Immune Protection Broth

1 oz. dry maitake mushrooms	4 tbsp. dry sea greens, chopped (any kind)	4 tbsp. pearled barley
1 oz. dry shiitake mushrooms	1 oz. astragalus bark	4 tbsp. organic brown rice
	1" piece ginger root	2 cups organic leafy greens, chopped

Soak the maitake mushrooms, shiitake mushrooms, sea greens, astragalus bark and ginger root in just enough water to cover them. Sliver mushrooms; discard astragalus and ginger. Save soaking water. Simmer 8 cups water and add soaking water, barley, brown rice and greens. Simmer 30 minutes. Drink hot. Store in fridge and reheat. Makes 6 large servings (a week's supply).

Nutrition per serving:			
Calories ----------- 103	Vitamin E ---- trace quantities	Cholesterol -------- 0	Potassium --------- 334 mg.
Protein ----------- 12 g.	Carbohydrates ---- 22 g.	Calcium ----------- 34 mg.	Sodium ----------- 19 mg.
Vitamin C --------- 35 mg.	Fiber ------------- 3 g.	Iron -------------- 1 mg.	
	Fat --------------- 2 g.	Magnesium ------- 49 mg.	

Mineral-Rich Aminos Drink

A complete, balanced vitamin/mineral electrolyte drink—rich in greens, amino acids and enzymes.

4 – 6 packets miso soup powder	1 tbsp. RED STAR nutritional yeast	2 tbsp. bee pollen granules
1 tbsp. dry sea greens (any type), crumbled	½ cup soy protein powder	1 tsp. spirulina granules
	1 packet instant ginseng tea	1 tsp. acidophilus powder
		2 tbsp. fresh parsley leaf

Powder dry ingredients in the blender, then mix about 2 tbsp. powder into 2 cups of hot water for 1 drink. Let flavors bloom for 5 minutes before drinking. Sip over a half hour period for best assimilation. Enough powder for 8 drinks. Note: Add 1 tsp. BRAGG'S LIQUID AMINOS to each drink if desired.

Nutrition per serving:			
Calories ----------- 60	Vitamin E --------- 3 IU	Cholesterol -------- 0	Potassium --------- 915 mg.
Protein ----------- 6 g.	Carbohydrates ---- 17 g.	Calcium ----------- 41 mg.	Sodium ----------- 143 mg.
Vitamin C --------- 86 mg.	Fiber ------------- 3 g.	Iron -------------- 1 mg.	
	Fat ---- trace quantities	Magnesium ------- 25 mg.	

Green Broth with Echinacea and Astragalus

2 tbsp. olive oil
6 minced cloves garlic
1 diced leek (white and light green parts only)
5 sliced scallions
1 diced fennel bulb

6 cups vegetable or organic chicken stock
1 cup chopped green cabbage
1 cup sliced broccoli
2 cups frozen peas
4 cups sliced spinach leaves

1 handful chopped fresh parsley
1 tsp. astragalus extract
1 tsp. echinacea extract
1 tsp. lemon-pepper seasoning

Heat the olive oil in a soup pot. Add the garlic, leek, scallions, and fennel and sauté for few minutes. Add 6 cups vegetable or organic chicken stock, 1 cup chopped green cabbage, 1 cup sliced broccoli. Simmer 10 minutes. Add frozen peas, spinach leaves (for EFAs), parsley, astragalus extract, echinacea extract, and lemon-pepper seasoning. Serve immediately. Makes 8 cups.

Nutrition per serving:
Calories ----------- 144
Protein ------------ 8 g.
Vitamin C--------- 55 mg.

Vitamin E --------- 3 IU
Carbohydrates ---- 24 g.
Fiber ------------- 6 g.
Fat---------------- 3 g.

Cholesterol-------- 0
Calcium ----------- 93 mg.
Iron -------------- 3 mg.
Magnesium ------- 80 mg.

Potassium --------- 773 mg.
Sodium------------ 154 mg.

Soups, salads, appetizers

Healing Shiitake Broth

1 tsp. grapeseed oil
1 piece ginger root, peeled and slivered
¼ tsp. ground tumeric
½ tsp. Chinese five-spice powder
6 cups organic, low-fat chicken broth

1 tbsp. tamari
1 small carrot, diced
1 small daikon radish, cut in matchsticks
4 oz. fresh shiitake mushrooms, stemmed and sliced

4 oz. thin wheat noodles (somen), cooked and cooled
¼ cup cilantro leaves
1 tsp. toasted sesame oil
garlic-lemon seasoning

In a soup pot, heat the grapeseed oil. Add the ginger root, tumeric and five-spice. Cook and stir until fragrant, about 3 minutes. Add chicken broth, tamari, carrot, daikon radish, and the mushrooms. Simmer until mushrooms are very tender, about 15 minutes. Add noodles and cilantro, and warm through, 2 minutes more. Season with sesame oil, and garlic-lemon seasoning to taste. Serve immediately in warmed soup bowls. Makes 4 servings.

Nutrition per serving:
Calories ----------- 141
Protein ------------ 6 g.
Vitamin C--------- 18 mg.

Vitamin E --------- 1 IU
Carbohydrates ---- 18 g.
Fiber ------------- 3 g.
Fat---------------- 4 g.

Cholesterol-------- 0
Calcium ----------- 28 mg.
Iron -------------- 1 mg.
Magnesium ------- 19 mg.

Potassium --------- 251 mg.
Sodium------------ 968 mg.

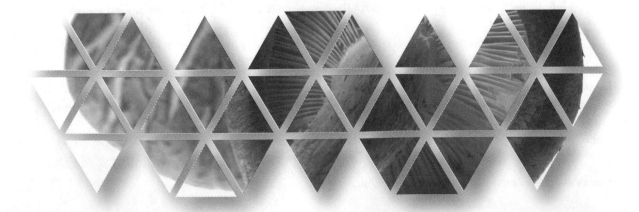

Chinese Stuffed Mushrooms

20 large fresh shiitake mushrooms, stemmed and cleaned
arrowroot powder
1 tbsp. seasoned rice vinegar

1 tsp. arrowroot powder
1 tbsp. sherry
½ tsp. fructose
8 water chestnuts, minced
¼ cup scallions, minced

¼ cup bok choy, chopped
¼ cup bean sprouts, diced
¼ cup cilantro, chopped
¼ cup onion stock
2 tbsp. oyster sauce

Preheat oven to 350°F. Sprinkle a little arrowroot powder on the open side of each mushroom cap.

Mix filling in a bowl: combine the rice vinegar, 1 tsp. arrowroot powder, sherry, fructose, water chestnuts, scallions, bok choy, bean sprouts and cilantro. Fill caps. Press a cilantro or watercress leaf on top. Coat a round baking pan with lecithin spray and arrange mushrooms in a layer. Mix onion stock with oyster sauce and pour around mushrooms. Cover with foil and bake 15 – 20 minutes. Remove foil. Baste and heat again briefly. Remove with slotted spoon to serving plate. Makes 20 appetizers.

Nutrition per serving:			
Calories ----------- 22	Vitamin C--------- 1 mg.	Fat---------------- 0	Magnesium ------- 4 mg.
Protein ----------- 1 g.	Vitamin E ---- trace quantities	Cholesterol------- 0	Potassium --------- 49 mg.
Vitamin A --------- 30 mg.	Carbohydrates ---- 4 g.	Calcium ----------- 5 mg.	Sodium------------ 12 mg.
	Fiber ------------- 1 g.	Iron -------------- 1 mg.	

Macrobiotic Purifying Soup

May be used for the start of almost any healing diet.

⅔ cup lentils
⅔ cup split peas
⅔ cup brown rice
2 cloves garlic, minced

1 onion, chopped
1 chopped carrot
1 rib celery, chopped
3 cups onion or veggie broth

3 cups water
1 tsp. turmeric powder
½ tsp. lemon-pepper seasoning
½ tsp. ginger powder

In a large pan, toast lentils, peas, rice and garlic until aromatic (about 5 minutes). Add onion, carrot, celery, broth, 3 cups water, turmeric powder, lemon-pepper and ginger powder. Simmer gently 1 hour, stirring occasionally. Makes about 6 cups.

Nutrition per serving:			
Calories ----------- 341	Vitamin E --------- 1 IU	Cholesterol------- 0	Potassium --------- 446 mg.
Protein ----------- 13 g.	Carbohydrates ---- 4 g.	Calcium ----------- 24 mg.	Sodium------------ 88 mg.
Vitamin C--------- 1 mg.	Fiber ------------- 14 g.	Iron -------------- 1 mg.	
	Fat---------------- 1 mg.	Magnesium ------- 71 mg.	

Cancer-Fighting Soup

Especially good after chemotherapy.

10 astragalus sticks
¼ cup pearl barley
10 dry shiitake mushrooms
1 cup carrots, diced
1 cup beets, diced

1 cup yams, diced
1 cup broccoli stems, diced
1 dropperful reishi mushroom extract

1 dropperful Siberian eleuthero extract
1 tbsp. barley grass powder

Fill a large soup pot with 4 qts. water, the astragalus sticks and barley. Soak mushrooms in ½ cup water until soft; then sliver and discard stems. Add mushrooms and soaking water to soup. Simmer 15 minutes. Add carrots, beets, yams and broccoli. Simmer for 30 minutes. Remove from heat. Discard astragalus pieces. Stir in reishi mushroom extract, Siberian eleuthero extract, and barley grass powder. Eat hot. Store in the fridge for easy re-use. Makes 12 servings.

Firebird

1 cup fresh alfalfa sprouts or sunflower sprouts	2 tbsp. grapeseed oil	1 tsp. sesame salt (gomashio)
2 cups carrots, grated	3 tbsp. tomato juice blend (like KNUDSEN'S VERY VEGGIE)	
1 cup celery, minced	2 tbsp. lime juice	

Toss alfalfa sprouts, carrots, celery. Make the dressing: Mix the grapeseed oil, tomato juice, 2 tbsp. lime juice, sesame salt. Pour over salad just before eating. Makes 2 appetizer salads.

Nutrition per serving:	Vitamin C -------- 25 mg.	Fat ---------------- 14 g.	Magnesium ------- 31 mg.
Calories ----------- 190	Vitamin E --------- 6 IU	Cholesterol -------- 0	Potassium --------- 608 mg.
Protein ----------- 3 g.	Carbohydrates ---- 16 g.	Calcium ----------- 63 mg.	Sodium ------------ 305 mg.
Vitamin A --------- 15,590 IU	Fiber ------------- 5 g.	Iron -------------- 1 mg.	

Wakame Succotash

1 oz. dried wakame	1 cake tofu, cubed	2 tbsp. green onions, minced
10 oz. package of frozen succotash vegetables	1 red onion, thin-sliced	2 tbsp. seasoned brown rice vinegar
	2 tsp. grapeseed oil	

Soak dried wakame in water for 30 minutes. Drain and steam for 10 minutes until tender. Chop into 1" pieces, removing the tough stems. Cook succotash vegetables and tofu in a pan according to package directions. Sauté red onion in grapeseed oil until fragrant. Toss with vegetables and wakame. Add and toss green onions and rice vinegar, and let marinate for 3 – 4 hours before serving. For 4 servings.

Tofu Dumplings

A tasty addition, they add protein and make the soup a full meal.

1 lb. fresh tofu	1 tbsp. soy flour	1 tsp. arrowroot dissolved in 1 tsp. water
1 tbsp. light miso	½ tsp. toasted sesame oil	

Mash all ingredients together and form into balls. Drop balls into a simmering soup, and let cook for 15 minutes. For 4 – 6 dumplings.

Entrées

Thai Broccoli Pie

2 cups brown rice, cooked	2 tsp. wasabi paste	4 cups low-fat chicken broth
2 tbsp. brown rice vinegar	½ tsp. sea salt	¼ cup fresh cilantro, chopped
1 tbsp. olive oil	½ tsp. cracked black pepper	1 cup firm tofu, cubed
½ cup red onion, diced	½ tsp. cumin powder	2 cups broccoli florets, chopped
2 garlic cloves, minced	2 tbsp. whole wheat flour	1 yellow squash, diced

Preheat oven to 375°F. Use a deep ceramic baking dish. Make the crust by spreading the brown rice mixed with rice vinegar in the baking dish. Bake for 10 minutes until crusty.

Make the filling in a pot: Heat olive oil and sauté the onion, garlic, wasabi, salt, pepper and cumin. Stir in whole wheat flour. Stir until bubbly. Add chicken broth and blend until smooth. Add cilantro, tofu, broccoli and squash. Spoon on top of rice and bake covered for 35 – 40 minutes.

Five Minute Easy Chicken, Peas and Brown Rice

3 cups chicken breasts, diced
and cooked
2 cups basmati rice, cooked
2 tbsp. butter
10 oz. box of frozen green peas

4 oz. can sliced mushrooms
with juice
1 organic chicken bouillon
cube
1 cup plain yogurt

4 eggs
½ tsp. sea salt
2 tbsp. fresh parsley, chopped
3 tbsp. grated romano cheese

Preheat oven to 325°F. Use a 9" x 13" baking pan. Layer chicken in the oiled baking pan. Sprinkle with a layer of basmati rice. Dot with butter. Spread a layer of peas. Sprinkle on the mushrooms with juice. Whisk together 2 cups water, the chicken bouillon, yogurt, eggs, sea salt, and parsley. Pour over casserole. Sprinkle with romano cheese and bake 45 minutes until set. Makes 6 servings.

Fresh Seared Ahi

½ cup tamari
¼ cup sake
3 sprigs fresh basil, minced
1 tsp. fresh lemon zest
2 tsp. toasted sesame oil
1½ lbs. very fresh ahi tuna

2 carrots, diced
2 tbsp. crystallized ginger,
minced
½ tsp. olive oil
½ tsp. toasted sesame oil
½ cup white wine

½ tsp. lemon-pepper seasoning
¼ cup low-fat cream cheese
4 mint leaves, chopped
fresh cilantro

Mix a marinade in a bowl: tamari, sake, basil, lemon zest, sesame oil. Marinate ahi tuna for 1 hour. Sear ahi in a hot, heavy skillet about 10 seconds each side. Remove, chill as you make the salad. Sauté for 1 minute the carrots, ginger, olive oil, sesame oil. Add ½ cup water, the white wine and lemon-pepper; simmer 3 minutes. Remove from heat and blend in the cream cheese and mint. Divide sauce onto 6 salad plates; divide the tuna—sliced very thin—over the top of the sauce. Sprinkle fresh cilantro over the top. Serves 6.

Nutrition per serving:			
Calories ----------- 255	Vitamin C--------- 4 mg.	Fat---------------- 8 g.	Magnesium ------- 76 mg.
Protein ----------- 30 g.	Vitamin E --------- 4 IU	Cholesterol------- 48 mg.	Potassium --------- 463 mg.
Vitamin A--------- 1459 IU	Carbohydrates ---- 8 g.	Calcium ----------- 42 mg.	Sodium----------- 422 mg.
	Fiber ------------- 1 g.	Iron -------------- 2 mg.	

Snow Peas with Shiitake Mushrooms

15 dry shiitake mushrooms
2 tbsp. miso paste
1 tsp. arrowroot powder
½ tsp. sesame salt

2 tsp. soy sauce
peanut oil
2" slice fresh ginger, shredded
4 green onions, diced

3 tbsp. oyster sauce
8 oz. fresh snow peas, trimmed
½ tsp. sesame salt

Soak mushrooms in 1 cup water until soft; sliver and discard stems. Save soaking water. Mix miso paste with 1½ cups water and the mushroom soaking liquid. Set aside. Mix sauce ingredients in a bowl: arrowroot, sesame salt, fructose and soy sauce. Add slivered mushrooms; toss to coat, and set aside.

Heat wok for 1 minute over medium heat. Add 2 tbsp. peanut oil and sauté the ginger until aromatic, about 1 minute. Add mushrooms and green onions and simmer 1 minute. Add miso sauce and bring back to a boil, cover and simmer for 5 minutes. Add oyster sauce and arrowroot mixture. Stir to thicken and place on a serving platter. Add another 2 tsp. peanut oil to the wok, heat; then add the snow peas and sesame salt. Toss and sauté until color changes to bright green, about 2 minutes. Spoon over mushroom mix and serve. Makes 8 servings.

Healthy dessert options

Asian Rice Pudding

2 cups cooked jasmine rice
3 tbsp. raisins
1 pinch salt
2 pinches cinnamon

¾ cup apple juice
¾ cup water
2 tsp. sesame tahini
2 tsp. lemon juice

2 tbsp. rice syrup
1 tbsp. kuzu or arrowroot powder
toasted, slivered almonds

In a large saucepan, combine the rice, raisins, salt and cinnamon. Add the apple juice, water, sesame tahini, lemon juice and rice syrup. Simmer on low heat for 25 minutes. Dissolve arrowroot powder in 3 tbsp. cold water; add to other ingredients and stir so it will thicken the mixture—just a few minutes. Spoon into dessert dishes and let sit until ready to serve. Top with toasted, slivered almonds. Serves 4.

Nutrition per serving:	Vitamin E --------- 3 IU	Cholesterol-------- 0	Potassium --------- 201 mg.
Calories ----------- 262	Carbohydrates ---- 52 g.	Calcium ----------- 38 mg.	Sodium------------ 16 mg.
Protein ----------- 5 g.	Fiber ------------- 2 g.	Iron -------------- 2 mg.	
Vitamin C--------- 2 mg.	Fat--------------- 5 g.	Magnesium ------- 43 mg.	

Pineapple Enzyme Sundae

3 cups fresh pineapple, chopped

3 cups fresh apricots, chopped

12 fresh strawberries, chopped
6 tbsp. toasted almonds, chopped

Toss all ingredients in a bowl. Makes 6 servings.

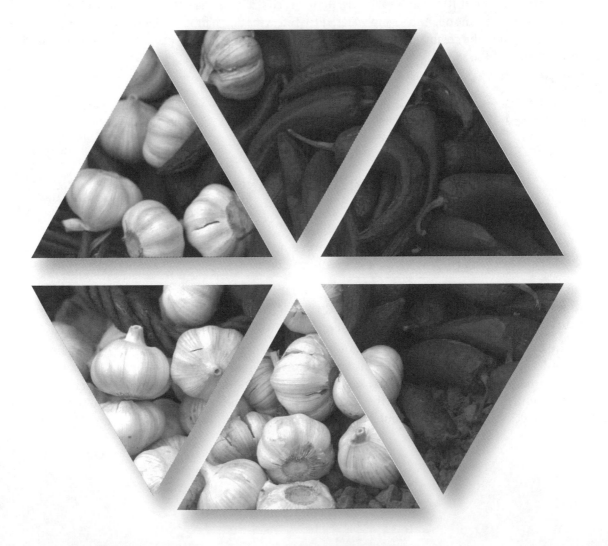

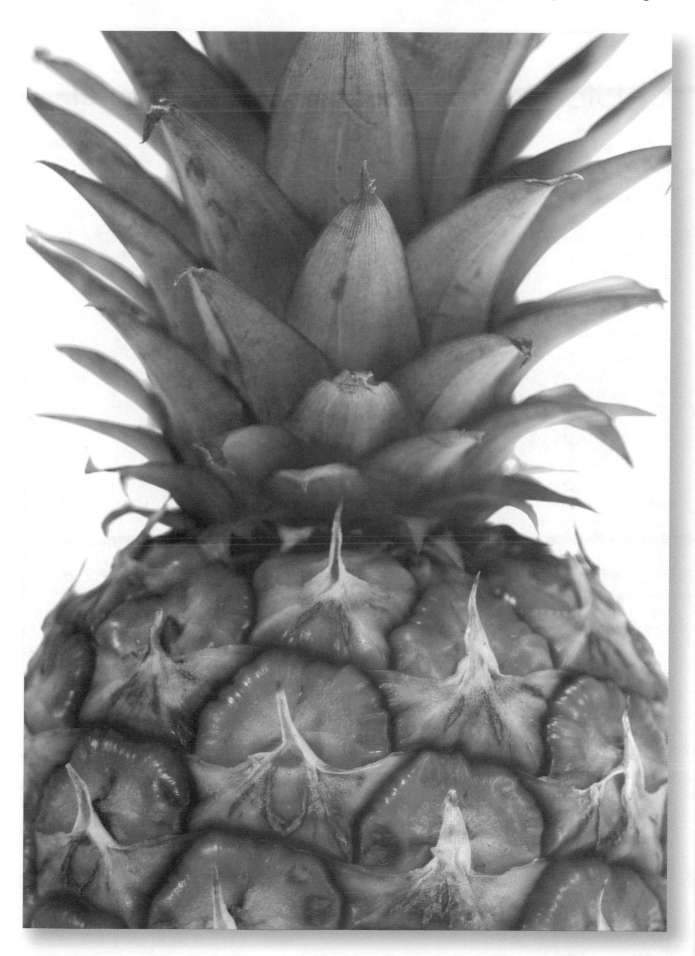

Digestive Disorders:
Ulcers, Heartburn, Irritable Bowel

Most digestive disorders are long standing, deeply ingrained from inherited eating habits and early lifestyle. Low enzyme activity plays a role in almost every digestive problem because enzymes are critical to proper metabolism. Poor metabolism is at the root of health problems from obesity to arthritis, even to some kinds of cancer. Low enzymes mean you have little protection from food allergens. Food allergies are also increasing in America as more chemicals are added to our food and soil, and as more foods are refined and genetically altered.

High fat foods with chemical additives cause the worst digestive problems. Too much meat, especially red meat which stays in the stomach too long, and too little fiber which favors constipation, are not far behind. Low stomach HCL and bile reduces digestion of acids and proteins, resulting in an over-acid system and fermentation. Many meals in today's busy lifestyles are hurried and eaten under stress, again leading to poor digestion.

It's never easy to change daily habits. But since life isn't going to slow down, a conscious effort must be made to break the vicious digestive circle. Keep remembering how much better you will feel.

Find a way to relax before you eat. Breathe deep. Do some mild stretches. Listen to calming music. Lighten up your meals. Simplify complex meals. Eat less concentrated foods. Take two capsules of acidophilus before each meal to build up your friendly bacteria.

5 Easy Steps to Less Indigestion, Heartburn and Gas

1. **Take ENZYMES.** America is an enzyme deficient nation. We eat on the run, under stress, out of boxes or cans. Many of the foods we eat are so processed they are completely devoid of nutrients. More importantly, they lack enzymes! Enzymes are the spark plugs for every body function. We are each born with a limited supply of enzymes which become depleted with age. But enzymes can be easily brought into your body through fresh foods. If your food is cooked, microwaved, or processed above 118° Fahrenheit, its enzymes are destroyed. If the foods you eat don't have enough enzymes for digestion, the body has to pull from reserves in your liver or pancreas, weakening enzyme-dependent processes like detoxification or hormone secretion. Without enough enzymes for digestion, bacteria feed off the undigested food in your GI tract, a process that generates gas, bloating, heartburn and constipation.

In almost every case, when someone with digestive disorders adds more plant enzymes either through fresh foods or enzyme supplements, digestive problems dramatically lessen. People carrying extra weight from body congestion can drop up to 10 lbs! People who are constipated become more regular. People with food allergies are often able to overcome them. Amylase, the plant enzyme which digests starches, can render gluten-rich grains like wheat and rye harmless to people with gluten enteropathy, a severe intestinal malabsorption syndrome caused by an allergy to gluten grains. Have a green salad every day! And consider CRYSTAL STAR® DR. ENZYME II: FAT & STARCH BUSTER™, for extra enzyme help in processing fats and starches (good results for weight loss).

2. **Take PROBIOTICS.** Meaning "for life", probiotics are friendly bacteria, like Lactobacillus acidophilus and Bifidobacteria bifidum, that inhabit your digestive tract and maintain the inner ecology critical to digestion. They keep out pathogens like viruses, yeasts and harmful microorganisms by competing with them for space in the gastrointestinal tract. Probiotics are a powerful preventive against digestive problems like diarrhea, constipation, more serious problems like inflamed bowel disease, even colon cancer. University of Delaware research finds that bifidobacteria can actually remove cancer cells or the enzymes which lead to their formation!

Your natural probiotics are depleted by: chemicals in your food or environment (like chlorine in drinking water), a stressful lifestyle, excessive alcohol, smoking, and some prescription drugs. Over-using antibiotics is the biggest offender in probiotic depletion. (In Japan and India, doctors routinely recommend acidophilus when they prescribe antibiotics.) Probiotics keep your digestion smooth. Eat cultured foods rich in these organisms, like yogurt, kefir or raw sauerkraut. Consider probiotic supplements like UAS Labs DDS-Plus with FOS or Jarrow Jarro-Dophilus.

Are PREBIOTICS the future of probiotic supplementation? Prebiotics are homeostatic soil organisms (HSOs), naturally present in the Earth's soil that protect plants from disease and help them absorb nutrients. Supplemental prebiotic HSOs help flush waste matter lodged in our intestines, improve our nutrient absorption, and produce lactoferrin, an immune stimulant. Some manufactures say HSOs are more effective than traditional probiotic products because they can withstand heat, cold, chlorine, fluorene, ascorbic acid, stomach acids, even pH changes. (Note: I myself have had the best results using probiotic supplements while adding cultured foods, like fermented soy foods, kefir and raw cultured vegetables.)

3. Begin good FOOD COMBINING. Sometimes, it's not *what* you eat that's making you sick, it's the way you eat it. Different foods need different enzymes to digest properly. Your intelligent body activates the proper enzyme when it detects a certain food in your mouth. (That's why digestion actually begins in your mouth.) When you eat foods that need widely different enzymes for digestion, the food tends to stay too long in your stomach waiting for digestion. It starts to ferment instead, leading to gas, constipation or diarrhea - clear signs that food is not being assimilated well. Proper food combining can make a lot of difference to your digestion.

Most experts think human digestion evolved very early, when our species ate almost all fresh or dried foods. Foods we ate together fell naturally into certain harvest times and seasons, and we developed the capacity to digest them at the same time. Today we eat any type of food we want when our taste-buds want it. Enzymes which digest one type of food but are incompatible with another type eaten in the same meal, get either blocked or confused, and we get the non-compatible food signs of gas and bloating.

Yet our digestive systems adapt somewhat to our eating habits. Unless your digestion is seriously compromised, you probably don't need to follow all the food combining rules. Sometimes we let these things control our lives and lose the pleasure of eating.

I follow just two principles: 1. I eat fruits alone and on an empty stomach in the morning. 2. I don't eat fruits and vegetables together. Check out page 89 in this chapter for a Good Food Combining Diet, and a Good Food Combining Chart.

4. Eat more FIBER. Why is fiber so good for us? Fiber from whole grains, fruits and vegetables lowers harmful LDL cholesterol levels linked to heart disease. It speeds weight loss by suppressing the appetite and reducing colon congestion. It improves glucose tolerance for people with diabetes. It provides protection against breast and colon cancer development, diverticulitis and irritable bowel. Fiber also keeps the digestive system running smoothly by decreasing the transit time of food in the intestines. Two types of fiber are important for digestive health: insoluble fiber and soluble fiber. **Insoluble fiber** is available in bran (wheat, oat, and rice); wheat germ; cauliflower; green beans; potatoes; and celery. Insoluble fiber passes through the intestines largely unchanged and is the main type of fiber that helps prevents constipation and adds bulk to the stool. **Soluble fiber** is available in peas; beans; oats; barley; some fruits and vegetables (apples, oranges, carrots); and psyllium. It helps slows digestion, allowing the body to better absorb nutrients. Many foods contain both types for digestion protection.

Today's statistics tell us that most Americans need to double their fiber intake to get the 30 to 35 grams a day recommended for digestive health. Six half-cup servings of whole grains, cereal or legumes and 4 servings of fresh fruits and vegetables each day give you the fiber you need. Fiber supplements are good as an addition, not a substitute. Try Nature's Secret Ultimate Fiber, or All One Totally Fiber Complex.

5.   **Eat more ALKALINE FOODS.** The typical American diet relies on too many acid-forming foods. They're the primary cause of GERD (Gastro-Esophageal Reflux Disorder), the most common cause of heartburn for 40 million Americans. By design, our bodies are slightly alkaline, with a pH of 7.4. When our systems become too acidic, alkaline minerals like sodium, calcium, potassium and magnesium are pulled from reserves to restore alkaline pH. But disrupting mineral balance becomes dangerous. Even small mineral deficiencies are linked to severe depression, osteoporosis and premature aging. Acidity is also implicated in chronic fatigue syndrome, arthritis, cancer, allergies and fungal infections. Bring more alkaline foods into your diet to ease indigestion and heartburn.

> ***Acid-forming foods to limit:** refined sugars, white flour, alcohol, sodas, coffee, red meat, fried, fatty foods.*

> ***Alkaline-forming foods to add:** mineral water, land and sea veggies, herb tea, miso, brown rice, honey, fruits.*

Do you rely on antacids for heartburn protection?

15 million Americans have heartburn daily. Another 50 million suffer heartburn at least once a week severe enough to disrupt their sleep. We spend $1.7 billion on indigestion remedies each year! But antacids are designed to provide only temporary relief. Evidence is piling up that excessive use of over-the-counter antacids may cause long term problems for digestive health. They may even become a health problem themselves because they radically change your digestive chemistry.

Do any of these problems pertain to you?

- **The tolerance effect:** The more you use antacids, the more you need them. Antacids neutralize stomach HCl (hydrochloric acid), needed for digestion, or they block it, confuse the body and disrupt its normal processes. If you take a lot of antacids, your body overcompensates, producing *excess* stomach acid.
- **Antacids disrupt your pH balance:** Optimum pH is between 7.35 and 7.45. If you take lots of antacids, your GI tract fluctuates between over alkaline and over acid, leading to problems like diarrhea or constipation, gallbladder disorders and hiatal hernia. A friend thought his heartburn symptoms would improve if he doubled his acid blocker dosage. He ended up in the bathroom all night, passing completely undigested food. Disrupting body pH alters bowel ecology, potentially causing dramatic growth of harmful organisms, like candida yeasts.
- **Pernicious ingredients:** Many antacids contain aluminum which causes constipation and bone pain. Others overdose you on magnesium causing diarrhea. Some contain both aluminum and magnesium, so you may get alternating constipation and diarrhea. Antacids full of sodium may cause water retention. Most are laden with chemical coloring agents that can cause allergic reactions in some people or lead to mood changes if taken regularly… the very way many people take them.
- **Some drugs interact with antacids:** People on drug therapy for HIV should know antacids can decrease their HIV drug absorption by up to 23%. Oral contraceptives like "the pill" may lose their effectiveness if taken with antacids. People using NSAIDS drugs for arthritis along with antacids suffer 2½ times more serious gastrointestinal complications than those taking a placebo! Antacids not only block drug absorption, they also block your food absorption of nutrients, especially B_{12}, necessary for virtually all immune responses.
- **Some antacids build up and impede body processes:** I know a woman who was hospitalized three times for kidney stones. Her physician advised her to stop taking her antacids because the unabsorbed calcium in them was causing her kidney stones.
- **By blocking critical stomach acid, your natural line of defense against germs,** proton pump inhibiting drugs can lead to serious disease. The newest research reveals PRILOSEC and PREVACID, now available over-the-counter, double the risk of pneumonia, especially dangerous for the elderly or those with weakened immune systems.

Is heartburn or GERD (gastroesophagael reflux disease) a daily problem for you?

GERD (Esophageal reflux disease) is due to leaking of stomach acid back into the esophagus and acid coming up into the throat. GERD also occurs in severe cases of osteoporosis, when the rib cage and upper body collapse to the point where normal food transit is impeded. (My Mother suffered from this; it was extremely painful.) People who suffer from acid reflux are far more likely to develop cancer of the esophagus, now the fastest growing type of cancer in the western world. Antacids do not reduce the cancer risk, only mask symptoms and often do more harm than good. They don't prevent or cure the underlying condition and can upset stomach pH causing it to produce even more harmful acids. Modern surgical procedures like Laparoscopic are minimally invasive and can greatly reduce GERD, but surgery side effects like diarrhea may be permanent.

What puts you at risk for GERD? Overeating and resulting obesity, enzyme deficiency, constipation from a low residue diet and too many fast foods, fried foods and dairy foods (all acid-forming), prescription drug side effects, and severe osteoporosis can all lead to GERD. A hiatal hernia is another common cause of GERD. A hiatal hernia occurs when a part of the stomach protrudes through the diaphragm wall, causing difficulty swallowing and breathing, burning and reflux in the throat, and great nervous anxiety. Today's American diet habits mean that a hiatal condition is common… and so is GERD.

Signs you may have GERD:

– Chest pains, heartburn and bloating after eating
– Belching, hiccups and regurgitation after eating
– Difficulty swallowing and a full feeling at the base of the throat, leading to chronic hoarseness
– Raised blood pressure usually accompanied by gastrointestinal bleeding, or a stomach ulcer

Nutritional plan for chronic heartburn or GERD:

Cleanse the digestive system and establish good enzymes:

1.   Start with a cleansing, pectin mono diet of apples and apple juice for 2 days. (For people that really suffer, this makes them feel better almost right away.) Then for 4 days, use a diet of 70% fresh foods and brown rice for B vitamins. Take 2 glasses of mineral water or aloe vera juice daily. Add fresh veggies and high fiber foods gradually if digestion is delicate. When digestion has normalized, follow a low fat, low salt, high fiber diet.

2.   Juices for stomach acid balance: Carrot juice, or GREEN FOODS CARROT ESSENCE for healing vitamin A; Carrot/cabbage, a stomach healer; Pineapple-papaya for extra enzymes; Liquid chlorophyll or SUN WELLNESS CHLORELLA, 1 tsp. in water before meals is also effective.

Follow with an alkalizing, plant-based diet:

1.   Eat plenty of cultured foods like yogurt, kefir and miso soup, fresh vegetables, fruits, and enzyme-rich foods like papaya and pineapple. Especially include lightly steamed vegetable fiber foods during healing.

2.   Eliminate fried and spicy foods—they slow the rate at which your stomach empties, allowing food to travel back to the esophagus. Eliminate refined carbohydrates and sugary foods—they boost gastric acidity.

3.   Omit red meats, fatty dairy foods, dried fruits, sodas and caffeine (coffee forms acid). Switch to herbal teas, like CRYSTAL STAR® DR. VITALITY™ green and white tea blend with ginger for better digestion.

4.   Foods that aggravate a hiatal hernia: coffee, chocolate, red meats, hard alcohol drinks, sodas.

5.   Frequent bouts of hiccups are very common today—try Wild Cherry tea (sometimes dramatic help).

Quick Tips:
- If 1 tsp. cider vinegar in water relieves your heartburn you need more stomach acid.
- If you are bloated, take ½ tsp. baking soda in water to ease distension.
- If you have flatulence, take a catnip or slippery elm enema for immediate relief.
- If your stomach is sour, settle it with lime juice and a pinch of ginger.
- If you absorb poorly, a glass of wine can offer better absorption.
- At first sign of heartburn, take 2 oz. aloe vera juice.
- What triggers indigestion: late night snacks, chocolates, fatty fried foods, rich desserts or sauces, alcohol, smoking, coffee, lots of sugar-free sorbitol candies (cramping and diarrhea).

Choose 2 or 3 supplements to help normalize digestion and smooth out heartburn:

- **Bitters herbs help the cause of heartburn:** CRYSTAL STAR® GERD GUARD™ caps before and after meals; CRYSTAL STAR® BITTERS & LEMON CLEANSE™ extract each morning as a preventive; FLORA GALLEXIER; GAIA HERBS SWEETISH BITTERS.
- **Get to the heart of heartburn:** L-glutamine 1500 mg. daily for long-term relief; LANE LABS NATURE'S LINING to strengthen the stomach wall (highly recommended); Betaine HCl capsules after meals.
- **Soothe the burn:** Slippery elm tea or lozenges; Marshmallow tea; HYLANDS HOMEOPATHIC INDIGESTION after meals; Umeboshi plum paste. Acute indigestion: NATURE'S HERBS DGL POWER; 2 tbsp. Aloe vera juice.
- **For belching and burping:** AKPHARMA BEANO drops; RAINBOW LIGHT ADVANCED ENZYME SYSTEM.
- **Good digestive teas:** Peppermint, spearmint or alfalfa-mint tea; ginger, dill, caraway ease digestion. Catnip-fennel-lemon peel tea; Chamomile tea; Wild Yam tea, especially if you have eaten too much refined sugar.
- **Enzyme therapy:** •Bromelain 1500 mg. daily; NATURE'S PLUS chewable bromelain; AMERICAN HEALTH PAPAYA CHEWABLES; CRYSTAL STAR® DR. ENZYME II: FAT & STARCH BUSTER™; TRANSFORMATION DIGESTZYME AND GASTROZYME.
- **Probiotics for friendly flora:** NUTRICOLOGY SYMBIOTICS + FOS, dairy free; UAS DDS-PLUS + FOS.

Bodywork and lifestyle changes do wonders for digestion

- **Avoid all tobacco.** Nicotine affects gastric functions.
- **Commercial antacids neutralize stomach acid,** inviting the stomach to produce even more acid, often making the condition worse in the long run. New tests even show that chronic use of aluminum-containing antacids causes bone loss. Avoid over-using antibiotics. They destroy friendly flora in the digestive tract, too, which you'll need to replace with probiotics.
- **Apply hot ginger compresses to abdomen** and over liver area (upper right abdomen).
- **Lie on your back and draw knees up to chest to relieve abdomen pressure.** To prevent night time reflux, elevate head off bed 6 – 8 inches. Don't eat within two hours of your bedtime.
- **Have a chiropractic adjustment** to the area or a massage therapy treatment at least once a month. (I have personally seen massage therapy work for many people.)
- **NAET** (Nambudripad Allergy Elimination Technique) helps eliminate food allergy reflux.
- **Try to eat when relaxed.** Eat smaller meals. Chew food very well. No liquids with meals. Eat slowly so that you are less likely to swallow air and belch. Don't lie down after eating.

About Food Combining

Keep it simple. The human digestive system works best when the number of different foods in a meal is small—about four or five. Each category of foods—fruits, starches, proteins, sweets, etc. requires different acid/alkaline mediums, different enzymes and different digestion times. Eating foods together that have drastically different digestive needs often results in poor assimilation. The body simply passes foods through with no digestion, or holds them back to wait for the proper enzyme medium. Sometimes the unassimilated food decomposes in the digestive tract and then ferments, producing gas along with resulting heartburn or elimination problems. People have known about good digestion and good food combining for centuries. In simpler times, when we ate with the harvests and seasons, food combinations almost fell into place by themselves. Things that were available at the same time were eaten at the same time… and so our digestive systems adapted. Today, we can have literally any food, any time, from any where, at any season. Food combinations come from all over the globe. We eat summer, winter, spring and autumn foods in any combo or all together.

America's "melting pot" of ethnic foods, fast foods and pre-prepared foods is one of the worst for good food combining or easy digestion. Most of us start off "not right" each morning because we eat citrus juice, coffee and bread or grain together. We continue through the day drinking milk with meals, eating fruits with meats, veggies and grains. At the end of the day we have a heavy, concentrated starch and protein meal that discourages enzyme activity. A lot of food is only partially digested, or not digested at all, left in the stomach, fermenting and causing gas. Undigested or poorly digested food is a primary cause of the epidemic food intolerances and sensitivities we experience today.

It can get very confusing. Yet, food combining is only one factor in healthy eating. It doesn't guarantee good digestion. Overeating, eating under stress or fatigue, eating before strenuous exercise, or during strong emotional experiences also reduces digestive capacity. Caffeine and alcohol retard digestion considerably. Fever and inflammatory illness may partially suspend digestion to conserve energy. As your diet incorporates more fresh, unprocessed foods, good food combining naturally becomes part of good eating habits. I have included a simple chart on the basics of good food combining. (See below.)

The bottom line:

1. Small amounts of poor combinations don't seem to cause problems, and sometimes really enhance taste and enjoyment, such as a handful of raisins in a cake, or a whole grain cereal with a little apple juice or yogurt.

2. Fruits of all kinds are better eaten fresh, by themselves, in the first half of the day.

3. Don't let food combining rule your life. Most natural food recipes work out as good combinations.

Good Enzyme-Rich, Food Combining Diet

Ease your new diet into your life. This diet improves faulty food combining gently and moderately by avoiding red meats, caffeine, sugary, fatty and fried foods. It keeps your system alkaline by avoiding dairy foods (except cultured dairy foods, like yogurt, cottage cheese, and kefir that offer "friendly flora"). It's full of enzyme-rich foods like fresh vegetables and fruits (like papaya and pineapple) to keep digestion strong.

You can use this diet for a lifetime. It is varied, yet observes good food combining for easiest digestion. It features simply cooked high mineral dishes. It emphasizes high fiber to give you a full feeling with little calorie expenditure. It maintains proper acid/alkaline balance, and stimulates and increases your own enzyme production.

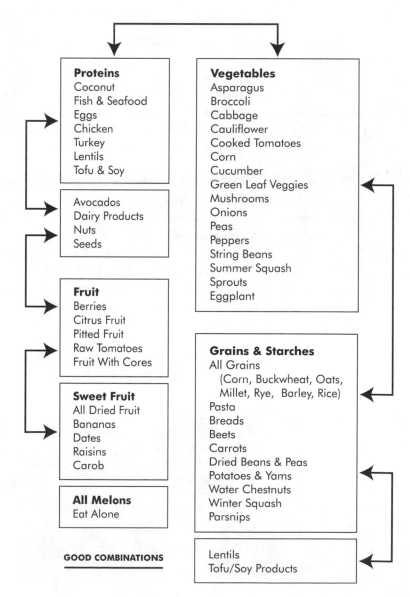

Proteins
Coconut
Fish & Seafood
Eggs
Chicken
Turkey
Lentils
Tofu & Soy

Avocados
Dairy Products
Nuts
Seeds

Fruit
Berries
Citrus Fruit
Pitted Fruit
Raw Tomatoes
Fruit With Cores

Sweet Fruit
All Dried Fruit
Bananas
Dates
Raisins
Carob

All Melons
Eat Alone

Vegetables
Asparagus
Broccoli
Cabbage
Cauliflower
Cooked Tomatoes
Corn
Cucumber
Green Leaf Veggies
Mushrooms
Onions
Peas
Peppers
String Beans
Summer Squash
Sprouts
Eggplant

Grains & Starches
All Grains
   (Corn, Buckwheat, Oats,
   Millet, Rye, Barley, Rice)
Pasta
Breads
Beets
Carrots
Dried Beans & Peas
Potatoes & Yams
Water Chestnuts
Winter Squash
Parsnips

Lentils
Tofu/Soy Products

GOOD COMBINATIONS

On rising: have grapefruit, papaya, or apple juice; or 2 tbsp. cider vinegar in water with 1 tsp. maple syrup and 1 tsp. acidophilus; or 10 drops CRYSTAL STAR® BITTERS & LEMON™ extract in water; or aloe vera juice with 1 tsp. chlorophyll liquid.

Breakfast: have a high fiber, whole grain cereal, with yogurt, apple juice or vanilla rice or almond drink; or fresh fruit with yogurt or kefir; or oatmeal or buckwheat pancakes with maple syrup or apple juice or kefir.

Mid-morning: have some whole grain muffins and a green drink; or carrot juice with 1 tsp. spirulina granules or chlorophyll liquid added, and some whole grain crackers with kefir cheese or a vegetable dip.

Lunch: before eating, have another glass of aloe vera juice with 1 tsp. acidophilus liquid; then have a green veggie salad, and a cup of miso soup with sea greens snipped on top; or a baked potato with yogurt cheese or non dairy topping, and a green salad; or cole slaw with yogurt dressing and cornbread.

Note: Follow any above choice with ginger extract or 1 tsp. New Chapter Ginger Wonder Syrup.

Mid-afternoon: have some crunchy raw veggies with kefir or yogurt cheese or a veggie dip, and a mineral drink, like CRYSTAL STAR® RESTORE YOUR STRENGTH™ drink; or an herb tea, like slippery elm or peppermint tea.

Dinner: take another lemon and water drink or aloe vera juice with acidophilus liquid before eating: then have some brown rice with tofu and veggies; or an Asian stir-fry with brown rice and miso soup; or grilled fish or seafood dinner with a light vegetable quiche with yogurt-wine sauce; or some millet or bulgar grains with steamed veggies and teriyaki sauce or light yogurt/chive dressing; or a hearty veggie stew with whole grain bread.

Note: A little white wine at dinner can often help digestion.

Before bed: have some pineapple/papaya juice, or apple juice; or make a broth with RED STAR NUTRITIONAL YEAST; or alfalfa/mint tea.

Choose 2 or 3 supplements to help normalize digestion and boost enzyme production:

• **Add enzymes:** CRYSTAL STAR DR. ENZYME WITH PROTEASE & BROMELAIN, between meals (to overcome food sensitivities); TRANSFORMATION DIGESTZYME; AMERICAN HEALTH PAPAYA CHEWABLES; CRYSTAL STAR RESTORE YOUR STRENGTH™ drink; PANCREATIN capsules 1400 mg.; HERBAL PRODUCTS AND DEVELOPMENT POWER PLUS ENZYMES; Garlic-parsley caps.

• **Add cultured foods:** like yogurt, kefir, miso; cultured vegetables like REJUVENATIVE FOODS RAW SAUERKRAUT.

• **Add green superfoods:** chlorella, spirulina, or liquid chlorophyll daily.

• **For heartburn:** Ginseng-licorice elixir; L-glutamine therapy 1500 mg. daily for long-term relief; PREVAIL ACID EASE or Betaine HCl caps after meals.

• **For gas and bloating:** Ginger capsules 2 – 4 as needed; Homeopathic remedies: BIOFORCE INDIGESTION RELIEF, or NUX VOMICA, or DIOSCOREA for bloating. Take 2 – 4 peppermint oil drops in water. (Also helpful for irritable bowel syndrome). CRYSTAL STAR® DR. ENZYME II: FAT & STARCH BUSTER™ after meals for weight loss help. Relieve gas quick: pinches of cinnamon, nutmeg, ginger, cloves in water and drink down.

• **For cramping and diarrhea:** Activated charcoal tabs (short term help); Apple pectin tabs (long term help); BODY ESSENTIALS SILICA GEL; NUTRICOLOGY PERM A VITE to reduce gut permeability; CRYSTAL STAR® STRESS OUT™ muscle relaxer drops (fast activity); CRYSTAL STAR® STRESS ARREST™ tea (gentle activity). Add probiotics: UAS LABS DDS-PLUS WITH FOS; GARDEN OF LIFE PRIMAL DEFENSE; JARROW FORMULAS JARRO-DOPHILUS; LANE LABS GI48.

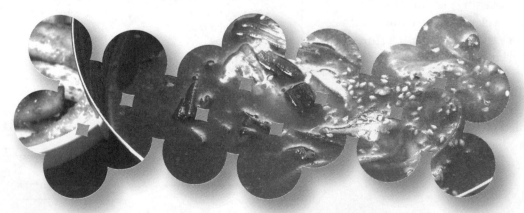

For more information on this topic, visit www.healthyhealing.com

Maintenance Recipes for a Digestive Disorder Diet

Use these recipes on an ongoing basis once your initial healing diet is producing good results.

Breakfast

Cinnamon Oatcakes with Mango Topping

12 oz. package frozen mango pieces	grated zest of 1 orange	1 tsp. baking powder
3 tbsp. brown sugar	1 egg	¼ tsp. baking soda
½ tsp. cinnamon	2 tbsp. brown sugar	2 pinches sea salt
2 cups low-fat buttermilk	1 tsp. grapeseed oil	1 tsp. grapeseed oil
1 cup instant oatmeal	½ cup oat flour	½ cup of water
	½ cup buckwheat flour	

To make the topping, place the frozen mango chunks in a saucepan with 3 tbps. brown sugar and the cinnamon; set aside to thaw.

To make the pancake batter: In a bowl, mix the buttermilk, oatmeal, orange zest and anise seed. Set aside for 15 minutes to soften the oatmeal. Beat in the egg, 2 tbsp. brown sugar, and 1 tsp. grapeseed oil. In a separate bowl, mix together the oat flour, buckwheat flour, baking powder, baking soda, sea salt and stir into the batter. In a nonstick skillet, heat 1 tsp. grapeseed oil over medium heat and spoon batter circles into the pan. Cook, flipping once when top becomes bubbly. While pancakes cook, add ½ cup of water to mango mixture; simmer just until the mango chunks and syrup are hot. Serve pancakes topped with mango sauce. Makes 4 servings (3 pancakes per serving).

Raisin GRAPENUTS Muffins

1 cup unbleached flour	1 cup rolled oats	1 egg
½ cup whole wheat pastry flour	1½ tsp. baking soda	¼ cup grapeseed oil
1 cup GRAPENUTS	1 cup plain yogurt	½ cup raisins
	½ cup honey	

Preheat oven to 375°F. Mix dry ingredients: the unbleached flour, whole wheat pastry flour, GRAPENUTS, rolled oats, and baking soda. Form a well in the center and pour in the plain yogurt, honey, egg, grapeseed oil, raisins. Stir until lumpy and bake in oiled custard cups for 30 minutes until springy when touched. For 6 big deli-style Sunday breakfast muffins.

Healing drinks

After Dinner Mint Tea for Good Digestion

1 tsp. peppermint	½ tsp. papaya leaf	½ tsp. rosemary
1 tsp. hibiscus		

In a tea pot, add all ingredients to 24 oz. of water. Add boiling water and let steep for 10 minutes. Makes 4 cups.

Cultured Fruit Shake

½ cup strawberry soy protein powder

½ cup pineapple juice

½ cup orange juice

1 cup brewed green tea

½ cup strawberries or orange segments

2 tbsp. lemon juice

2 tsp. acidophilus powder

½ cup vanilla yogurt (or 1 banana)

In a blender, mix the protein powder, pineapple juice, orange juice, green tea, strawberries, lemon juice, and acidophilus powder, and vanilla yogurt. Makes 2 servings.

Chai Tea

Like a spicy latte without quite as much caffeine. Good hot or iced.

2 rounded teaspoons of your favorite tea

6 oz. soy milk or rice milk

ground ginger

ground cinnamon

ground cardamom

vanilla extract

fructose

Steep the tea for 10 minutes in 2 cups of hot water. Steam the soy milk until hot and add to tea. Add small pinches of ground ginger, ground cinnamon, and ground cardamom. Add 2 – 3 drops vanilla and a pinch of fructose. Let sit 5 minutes. Makes 2 cups.

Soups, salads, appetizers

Orient Express Hot & Sour Soup

½ lb. firm tofu, frozen and thawed

1 tbsp. sesame oil

2 shallots, minced

½ cup scallions, diced

2 carrots, cut to matchsticks

½ cup fresh shiitake mushrooms, sliced

3 tbsp. miso paste

4 cups water

¼ cup brown rice vinegar

1 tbsp. honey

½ tsp. cracked black pepper

2 tbsp. finely grated ginger

1 tbsp. dried arame or sea palm, chopped

sesame seeds

2 cups cooked brown rice

Have the thawed tofu ready with excess water pressed out. In a wok, heat the sesame oil and sauté the shallots, scallions, carrots and shiitake mushrooms for 5 minutes. Crumble tofu and stir into vegetable mixture. Simmer for five minutes. In a bowl, mix the miso paste, water, brown rice vinegar, honey, cracked pepper, and finely grated ginger. Stir mixture into vegetables. Let simmer another 5 minutes. Divide among soup bowls. Sprinkle on the dried arame and sesame seeds. Serve hot with brown rice. Makes 4 servings.

Crunchy Top Tofu Salad

2 cakes extra-firm tofu, cubed

½ cup bottled natural French dressing

½ cup soy mayonnaise

½ cup yogurt sour cream (or kefir cheese)

1½ cups celery, diced

½ cup toasted sliced almonds

2 cups crisp Chinese noodles

1 cup low-fat cheddar cheese

Blanch the tofu in boiling salted water for 10 minutes. Drain. Pour the French dressing over the tofu. Chill in the fridge for 30 minutes. Assemble rest of the salad in a baking dish. Mix the mayonnaise, sour cream, celery, almonds and half of the Chinese noodles. Mix salad with the marinated tofu. Mix in the rest of the Chinese noodles and the cheddar cheese. Serve cold or run under a broiler for 30 seconds until the top is brown and crunchy. Serves 6 people.

Lemon Cucumber Pickles

8 lemon cucumbers	4 tbsp. fructose	½ tsp. celery seed
sea salt	1 tsp. stevia powder	cinnamon
1 cup tarragon vinegar	1 tsp. sea salt	dill weed
1 cup water	1 tsp. mustard seed	

Slice 8 lemon cucumbers in rounds; place in a colander. Sprinkle with sea salt; let drain 1 hour. In a saucepan, combine the tarragon vinegar, water, fructose, stevia powder, sea salt, mustard seed, celery seed, turmeric and a pinch of cinnamon. Bring to a simmer; taste. Add more sweetener or vinegar if needed. Remove from heat. Rinse and add cucumbers. Sprinkle with pinches of dill weed. Let stand until cool. Then, cover and chill 2 days before serving. Serves 6 people.

Spring Bitters Salad

a blend of organic fresh spring greens, young dandelion leaves, fresh parsley, fresh baby spinach, young violet leaves (use 2 cups greens per serving)	fennel	1 tbsp. scallions, minced
	lemon mint	1 tbsp. black sesame seeds
	tarragon	1 tbsp. white sesame seeds
	4 cups red leaf lettuce	salt and fresh ground pepper to taste
	2 tbsp. cold-pressed olive oil	lemon wedges
	1 clove garlic, pressed	young nasturtium flowers
chives, diced tips	2 tsp. fresh lemon juice	

Rinse greens, then gently tear them into bite-size pieces and place in a salad bowl with the red leaf lettuce, chives, fennel, lemon mint, and tarragon. Make a light dressing so the greens tastes really come through: mix the olive oil, garlic, lemon juice, scallions, black sesame seeds, white sesame seeds, salt and freshly ground pepper to taste. Serve with lemon wedges and young nasturtium flowers.

Asian Slaw

Great burger topping or pita pocket stuffing.

2 lbs. napa cabbage, thinly sliced (discard leafy top)	2 large broccoli stems, thinly sliced	½ tsp. toasted sesame oil
2 large olive oil-packed roasted red bell peppers, thinly sliced	1 jicama, cut into thin matchsticks	4 tbsp. brown rice vinegar
		½ tsp. fructose
	2 tbsp. olive oil	1 tbsp. crystallized ginger, minced
		2 pinches sea salt

In a large bowl, toss peppers with cabbage. Mix in broccoli stems and jicama. Makes the dressing: blend the olive oil, toasted sesame oil, brown rice vinegar, fructose, crystallized ginger and sea salt. Pour over slaw and chill 1 hour to blend flavors. Makes enough for a topping for 8 tofu burgers or 6 pita pockets.

Nutrition per serving:	Vitamin C --------- 83 mg.	Fat ---------------- 4 g.	Magnesium ------- 43 mg.
Calories ----------- 117	Vitamin E --------- 6 IU	Cholesterol------- 0	Potassium --------- 399 mg.
Protein ----------- 3 g.	Carbohydrates ---- 18 g.	Calcium ---------- 57 mg.	Sodium----------- 140 mg.
Vitamin A -------- 234 IU	Fiber ------------- 6 g.	Iron -------------- 2 mg.	

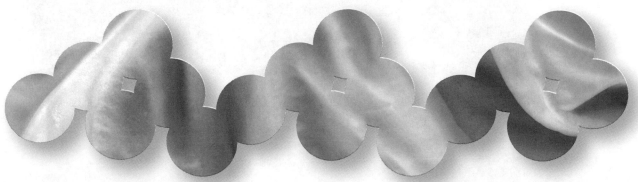

Entrées

Asian Brown Rice & Greens

4 cups cooked brown rice
½ cup chopped walnuts
2 tbsp. sesame seeds
2 cups baby bok choy
1 cup napa cabbage
1 cup baby spinach
1 onion, thinly sliced
1 carrot, diced

1 large head broccoli, diced
4 tbsp. grapeseed oil
1 tsp. crystallized ginger, minced
1 garlic clove, minced
2 cups bean sprouts (or sunflower sprouts)

2 tbsp. hoisin sauce
2 tbsp. soy sauce
2 tsp. toasted sesame oil
2 tsp. fructose
2 eggs
walnuts
sesame seeds

Have the cooked brown rice ready. Preheat a large wok. Toast the chopped walnuts and sesame seeds. Remove and set aside. Shred the bok choy, napa cabbage, and baby spinach. In the wok, heat the ginger and garlic in the grapeseed oil until fragrant. Add the carrots, onion and broccoli; sauté about 5 minutes. Add the greens and toss just until color changes, about 1 minute. Add the bean sprouts. Toss to coat. Add brown rice and mix all together. Turn off heat. Make a well in the center and add the eggs. Toss for 3 minutes until hot and set. Turn onto large serving platter. To make the sauce, mix the hoisin sauce, soy sauce, toasted sesame oil and fructose. Poor over rice and veggie mix. Top with walnuts and sesame seeds.

Sesame Ginger Chicken with Rice Noodles

1 cooked organic chicken breast, shredded
6 oz. package cellophane rice noodles, cooked
4 tbsp. olive oil
3 tbsp. honey
3 tbsp. soy sauce

2 tbsp. crystallized ginger, minced
4 tbsp. lime juice
1 tsp. toasted sesame oil
2 tbsp. sesame seeds
hot (or mild) pepper sauce
granulated garlic
2 tbsp. olive oil

2 cups baby bok choy, chopped
1 cup white daikon radish, shredded
2 – 3 pinches garlic-lemon seasoning
1 cup baby spinach leaves
1 carrot, shredded
1 red bell pepper, diced

Have the cooked, shredded chicken breast ready. Have the cellophane rice noodles, cooked briefly until soft and cooled, ready. Make the vinaigrette sauce: in a bowl, mix 4 tbsp. olive oil, the honey, soy sauce, crystallized ginger, lime juice, toasted sesame oil, sesame seeds, 2 dashes of hot (or mild) pepper sauce and 2 dashes granulated garlic. Heat 2 tbsp. olive oil in a wok until hot; add the bok choy and daikon radish; sauté with 2 – 3 pinches garlic-lemon seasoning for 2 minutes. In a serving bowl, mix the spinach leaves, carrot, bell pepper, and the chicken and cooked vegetables. Pour the vinaigrette sauce over the top and serve. Serves 6.

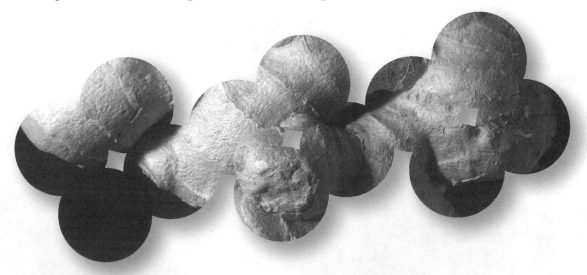

Veggies & Cheese in a Perfection Crust

⅓ cup plain low fat yogurt
⅓ cup water
1 tsp. baking soda
2 tsp. cream of tartar
½ tsp. sea salt
⅓ cup olive oil
4 tbsp. melted butter
¼ cup honey
1¾ cup unbleached flour
½ cup bran flakes

¼ cup oat flour
2 tbsp. toasted sesame seeds
6 cups mixed vegetables:
  bell peppers (any color),
    sliced
  cauliflower, chopped
  broccoli florets, chopped
  carrots, diced
  brown or white
    mushrooms, sliced

water chestnuts (jicama), sliced
11 oz. can cream of mushroom soup
½ cup white wine
3 tbsp. butter
2 tbsp. bottled barbecue sauce (or
  hickory sauce)
1 tbsp. soy sauce
low-fat cheddar, grated

Make the crust: Preheat oven to 450°F. In a bowl, whisk the yogurt, water, baking soda, cream of tartar, and sea salt. Mix in the olive oil, 4 tbsp. melted butter and honey. In a separate bowl, mix the unbleached flour, bran flakes, oat flour and toasted sesame seeds. Combine the 2 mixtures. Knead briefly on a floured surface, and roll or pat into a greased quiche pan. Prick bottom and bake for 5 minutes. Remove and cool for filling.

Preheat oven to 350°. Make the vegetable filling: In a large pot, bring 2 quarts of salted water to a boil. Add the mixed vegetables. Blanch until color changes, about 5 minutes. Drain well and place in the pie crust. Make the sauce: Mix the cream of mushroom soup with the white wine. Add 3 tbsp. butter, the barbecue sauce and soy sauce. Pour over veggies; cover with grated low fat cheddar. Bake until brown and bubbly. Makes 8 servings.

Nutrition per serving:			
Calories ----------- 387	Vitamin C --------- 44 mg.	Fat ----------------- 19 g.	Magnesium ------- 46 mg.
Protein ------------ 9 g.	Vitamin E --------- 3 IU	Cholesterol-------- 26 mg.	Potassium --------- 502 mg.
Vitamin A --------- 1010 IU	Carbohydrates ---- 43 g.	Calcium ----------- 126 mg.	Sodium------------ 514 mg.
	Fiber -------------- 4 g.	Iron --------------- 3 mg.	

Grilled Scallops Asian Style

Use long metal skewers for best results.

½ cup shredded,
  unsweetened coconut
2 papayas, peeled, seeded, cut
  into cubes
2 mangos, peeled, pitted, cut
  into cubes

1 lb. large sea scallops, rinsed
¾ cup orange juice
4 tbsp. lime juice
1½ tsp. Chinese 5-spice
  powder

1 tbsp. olive oil
1 small package (8 oz.) baby spinach
  leaves
granulated dulse (or crunchy soy
  bacon bits)

Preheat oven to 250°F. Toast coconut in oven until golden. Set aside. Preheat grill to medium heat. Thread papaya and mango cubes onto skewers for grilling. Thread sea scallops on separate skewers for grilling. Lay skewers on a lightly oiled hot barbecue grill. Cook until fruit is hot and scallops are opaque, ONLY 3 minutes per side. Watch closely… remove from heat; set aside.

Make dressing: In a large bowl, mix the toasted coconut with the orange juice, lime juice, Chinese 5-spice powder and olive oil. Add the baby spinach leaves; toss to coat.

Divide dressed greens on individual plates. Slide scallops and fruit from skewers to remaining dressing in the bowl. Stir to coat and spoon onto spinach. Sprinkle with granulated dulse or crunchy soy bacon bits. Makes 4 servings.

Healthy dessert options

Non-Dairy Papaya Ice Cream

Chill dishes for ice cream.

2½ cups vanilla RICE DREAM DESSERT

2 large papayas, peeled, seeded and mashed

In a blender, mix the RICE DREAM and mashed papayas until smooth. Pour the mixture into ice cube trays and freeze until solid. When frozen, place cubes in the food processor and process until creamy. Serve in chilled dishes. Makes 6 servings.

Orange Pudding

4 tbsp. grapeseed oil
6 tbsp. brown sugar
½ cup frozen apple-juice concentrate, thawed
½ cup egg substitute

1 cup whole wheat pastry flour
½ cup unbleached flour
1 tsp. ground allspice
1 tsp. non-aluminum baking powder

1 tsp. baking soda
2 tbsp. orange juice
2 tsp. orange zest
8 oz. grated carrots

Preheat oven to 350°F. In a bowl, combine the grapeseed oil and brown sugar. Add the apple juice concentrate and egg substitute and mix well (mix may look curdled).

In a separate bowl, combine the pastry flour and unbleached flour, allspice, baking powder and baking soda. Add to liquid ingredients and mix well. Add the orange juice, orange zest and grated carrots; mix gently. Pour batter into 9" round cake pan; bake 25 – 30 minutes, or until a tester inserted in center comes out clean. Makes 12 servings.

Wheat-Free Raisin Spice Cookies

¼ cup rice flour
¼ cup amaranth flour
1½ cups rolled oats
1 tbsp. crystallized ginger, minced
2 tsp. cinnamon

1½ tsp. nutmeg
½ tsp. allspice
1 tsp. baking pwdr
1 tsp. baking soda
½ cup apple sauce

½ cup frozen apple juice concentrate
1 tsp. vanilla
½ cup raisins
¼ cup dates, diced
2 eggs

Preheat oven to 400°F. In a bowl, mix the dry ingredients: rice flour, amaranth flour, rolled oats, ginger, cinnamon, nutmeg, allspice, baking powder and baking soda. In another bowl, combine wet ingredients: apple sauce, frozen apple juice concentrate, vanilla, raisins, dates and eggs. Mix all together. Drop by heaping tablespoons onto lecithin-sprayed baking sheets. Bake 12 – 15 minutes. Leave in the turned-off oven to cool and harden. Remove from baking sheets. Makes 24 – 30 cookies.

Nutrition per serving:
Calories ----------- 63
Protein ----------- 2 g.
Vitamin A --------- 8 IU

Vitamin C --------- 1 mg.
Vitamin E -----trace quantities
Carbohydrates ---- 12 g.
Fiber ------------- 1 g.

Fat ---------------- 1 g.
Cholesterol-------- 16 mg.
Calcium ----------- 26 mg.
Iron -------------- 1 mg.

Magnesium ------- 16 mg.
Potassium --------- 94 mg.
Sodium------------ 67 mg.

Overcoming Colon and Bowel Problems

Most diseases we endure today have their roots in poor drainage. Chronic constipation is the #1 gastrointestinal complaint in the U.S. Constipation affects as many as 4.4 million people and is responsible for 100,000 hospitalizations every year. The key to modern health is continually removing toxic wastes and pollutants from our bodies. It starts with back-up and fermentation in the colon, like a walking pressure cooker, and ends with the body actually *re-absorbing* unreleased waste material, which settles in weak cells unable to "clean house." Continuing accumulation of this poisonous build-up can result in disease.

Don't be fooled into believing new studies which failed to show a low fat, high fiber diet provided colon cancer protection. Experts now say they were flawed because they only measured short-term benefits while colon cancer can take decades to develop. Over the long term, a low fat, high fiber diet may be your best colon protector. Daily fresh vegetables and whole grains virtually guarantee a fully active elimination system, good digestion, low cholesterol and balanced blood sugar. Even a gentle, gradual change from a low fiber, low residue diet helps almost immediately, and it's better than a drastic program for relieving pain and inflammation in the colon. In fact, a slow, but complete switch to a high fiber diet over several months gives your body much better therapy than just adding a fiber supplement or a few fiber foods to your regular diet.

Do you have signs of colon and bowel problems?

Take this COLON PROTECTION TEST.

1. Bowel movements should be regular daily, and almost effortless.

2. The stool should be almost odorless (signalling increased bowel transit time with no fermentation).

3. There should be very little gas or flatulence.

4. The stool should float rather than sink.

Is the state of your colon putting you at risk for colon cancer?

People with chronic constipation or diarrhea are in a high risk category for colon cancer. Colon cancer is the third most common cancer for both men and women in the U.S. American colon cancer rates are much greater than the rest of the world! Over 146,000 Americans will be diagnosed this year. Over 56,000 people will die of colon cancer… even with all the advanced techniques of modern medicine.

What puts you at risk?

1. A lack of fiber. Colon cancer risk rises with age and overweight men are at the highest risk. An astonishing number of men eat a low fiber diet (even with all the media attention). Fiber is the transport system of the digestive tract, moving out food wastes out before they have a chance to form potentially cancer-causing chemicals.

2. A high fat diet. Fatty meats are the primary culprits. Harvard studies show that regular meat consumption increases colon cancer risk as much as 300%. Following a high meat diet like the Atkins Diet long term may be a recipe for colon disaster. One Harvard researcher noted that two years on the Atkins Diet "could initiate a cancer. It could show up as a polyp in seven years and as colon cancer in ten." Red meat animals are those more likely to have man-made hormone injections now linked colon cancer. Most red meat is barbecued today, a process that generates carcinogenic hydrocarbons on the meat surfaces.

3. Regular use of antacids, frequent rounds of antibiotics, over-use of laxatives. They may be doing you more harm than good. Antacids neutralize stomach HCl needed for food assimilation, and inhibit production of friendly digestive bacteria. Overusing laxatives for constipation irritates bowel membranes, and may almost bring normal systole-diastole activity to a halt. A vegetable fiber diet is both prevention and cure. Try an acidophilus supplement, like NUTRICOLOGY SYMBIOTICS WITH FOS, ¼ tsp. in water 3x daily, with 100 mg. B-complex.

You'll notice improvement in your waste elimination problems fairly quickly after diet improvement. There is no instant, easy route. It takes from 3 – 6 months to rebuild bowel and colon elasticity with good systole-diastole action. An herbal colon health formula can help in this effort for normalization.

The colon and bowel are the depository for all waste material after food nutrients are extracted. Unprocessed food decays and forms gases as well as 2nd, even 3rd generation toxins. Most naturopaths believe that this old, infected material in bowel pockets (diverticula), often re-absorbs into the body, becoming a breeding ground for putrefactive bacteria, viruses, parasites, yeasts and more.

90% of all disease is linked to constipation and colon toxicity from 3 areas:

1. Chemicals in our food and pollutants in the environment. A clean, strong system can metabolize and excrete many of these, but when we're constipated, they are stored as unusable substances. As more and different chemicals enter the body, they interact with those that are already there, forming mutant, second-generation chemicals far more harmful than the originals. Evidence in recent years shows that most bowel cancer is caused by environmental agents taken in through diet and air pollution.

2. Over-accumulated body wastes and metabolic by-products that are not excreted properly. Unreleased wastes can also become a breeding ground for parasite infestation. The human body is host to over 130 different types of parasites! An astounding figure.

3. Slow elimination time. Ideally, one should eliminate after each meal, but experts say the average American is 50,000 bowel movements <u>short</u> over a lifetime because our bowels are so sluggish. Bowel transit time should be about 12 hours. Slow elimination allows waste materials to ferment, become rancid, then recirculate in the body tissues as toxins, resulting in sluggish organ and gland functions, poor digestion, lowered immunity, and tissue degeneration.

Your body can tolerate a certain level of contamination. But when that level is passed, and immune defenses are low, toxic overload causes illness. The diet programs in this section include specifics for restoring both bowel and bladder areas, with watchwords to keep in mind so that problems don't return.

Healthy intestines are your body's second immune system.
These watchwords can keep it strong.

- Fiber foods, like prunes are the diet key—most experts recommend 40 – 45 grams daily: insoluble fiber isn't digested; it simply moves through your system, helping other foods move along with it.
- Follow a low fat, largely vegetarian diet, with plenty of intestinal brooms—fruits, whole grains, greens, veggies and cultured foods like yogurt.
- Avoid high fat, sugary, fried foods and dairy foods; they don't allow your body to get rid of waste easily.
- Drink 6 – 8 glasses of healthy liquids every day; avoid cow's milk.
- Have a regular daily time for elimination.

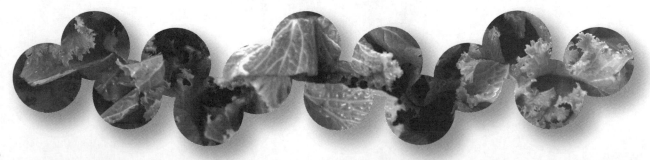

Diet to Rebuild Colon and Bowel Health
If you've had years of chronic constipation, start with a short 3-day colon cleansing juice diet.

The night before your restoration diet, make an easy fiber drink: mix equal parts of flax seed, pumpkin seed and oat bran in water. Let sit overnight. Take 2 tbsp. in the morning in juice. Or soak a mix of dried prunes, figs and raisins and blackstrap molasses. Take 2 tbsp. with yogurt or apple juice.

On rising: a glass of lemon juice and water, or a glass of aloe vera juice or Herbal Answers HERBAL ALOE FORCE juice with ¼ tsp. acidophilus added; or JARROW GENTLE FIBERS in apple or orange juice.

Breakfast: take 2 tbsp. of a dried fruit-molasses mix with yogurt or apple juice; add 2 tsp. nutritional yeast or LEWIS LABS FIBER YEAST to oatmeal or granola, top with apple juice; or have a bowl of fresh fruits with yogurt.

Mid-morning: take a fresh carrot juice or mixed vegetable juice, PURE PLANET CHLORELLA, FIT FOR YOU, INC. MIRACLE GREENS WITH FLAX, or CRYSTAL STAR® ENERGY GREEN RENEWAL™ drink; or green tea or CRYSTAL STAR® GREEN TEA CLEANSER™ to alkalize the system.

Lunch: have a fresh green salad with lemon/olive oil dressing, or yogurt cheese or kefir cheese; or steamed veggies and a baked potato with kefir cheese; or a fresh fruit salad with a yogurt or raw cottage cheese topping.

Mid-afternoon: have another fresh carrot juice, or GREEN KAMUT CORP. GREEN KAMUT; and/or green tea or slippery elm tea; and/or some raw crunchy veggies with a vegetable or kefir cheese dip, or soy spread.

Dinner: have a dinner salad with black bean or lentil soup; or a stir fry and miso soup with sea greens on top; or a baked vegetable casserole with yogurt cheese sauce; or spinach pasta with light lemon or yogurt sauce.

Before bed: have apple or papaya juice; or a glass of aloe vera juice.

Choose 2 or 3 supplements to help cleanse, then strengthen colon-bowel structure:
- **Cleanse old wastes:** CRYSTAL STAR® FIBER & HERBS COLON CLEANSE™ capsules 6 daily (1 – 3 months, complete cleanse); NATURE'S SECRET SUPERCLEANSE tabs; EARTH'S BOUNTY OXY-CLEANSE removes old hardened wastes. For a quick occasional cleanse: take 3000 to 5000 mg. vitamin C with bioflavonoids over a two hour period; or CRYSTAL STAR® LAXA-TEA™ to flush wastes gently over a 24-hour period; or ZAND CLEANSING LAXATIVE tabs.
- **Prevent constipation:** Omega-3 flax seed caps; magnesium 400 mg. daily; (Think twice about drugstore antibiotics, antacids or milk of magnesia; they kill friendly intestinal flora.) Probiotics prevent constipation, overcome antibiotic residues: JARROW CORP. JARRO-DOPHILUS + FOS; UAS DDS-PLUS WITH FOS; TRANSFORMATION PLANTA-DOPHILUS (for liver function); GARDEN OF LIFE PRIMAL DEFENSE.
- **Normalize digestive functions:** SOLARAY TETRA CLEANSE or NATURE'S WAY 5 SYSTEM CLEANSE; Fennel-ginger caps 4 daily; Garlic caps, 4 daily; Turmeric or goldenseal-myrrh extract drops in water enhance bile flow.
- **For a healthy, odor-free stool:** PLANETARY FORMULAS TRIPHALA; apple pectin tabs; Milk thistle seed, or dandelion extract enhances bile output and softens stool.
- **Natural laxatives:** Bee pollen 2 tsp. daily; senna leaf/pods (sparingly); una da gato caps 6 daily; cascara caps.
- **Enzyme therapy re-establishes pH balance:** CRYSTAL STAR® DR. ENZYME II: FAT & STARCH BUSTER™; Papaya enzymes digest milk proteins and sugars; Peppermint or ginger tea provides plant enzymes that balance digestion.

Bodywork and lifestyle improvements are critical to bowel regularity
- **Consider a catnip or dilute liquid chlorophyll enema** once a week to keep cleansing going. Note: Enemas may be given to children. Use small amounts according to size and age. Allow water to enter very slowly; let them to expel when they wish.
- **Consider a colonic irrigation to start your program.** A grapefruit seed extract colonic is very effective; a wheat grass retention enema is effective if there is colon toxicity. (Dilute to 15 – 20 drops per gallon of water.)
- **A brisk daily walk** can reduce your risk of developing colon cancer by 40 – 50%.
- **Get early morning sunlight on the body** every day possible for purifying vitamin A and vitamin D.
- **Apply warm ginger compresses** to lower spine and stomach to stimulate systol/diastol activity.
- **Be sure all food is well chewed.** Eat smaller meals more frequently rather than large meals.

Diet to Heal Irritable Bowel

Irritable Bowel Syndrome affects as many as *one in five* U.S. adults! A chronically inflamed, painful colon is often a result of food allergies (65%), usually a gluten reaction to wheat, cheese, corn, eggs, or other food sensitivity. Lactose intolerance symptoms mimic those of IBS and colitis. Fast foods (full of chemicals), fried foods (full of fat), refined foods (low in fiber) and sugars aggravate irritable bowel. Most victims are women between 20 and 40 with stressful jobs or lifestyles. Many also have bouts of candida yeast infection. New research shows that 78% of Irritable Bowel Syndrome patients have overgrowth of abnormal bacteria in the small intestine, aggravated by too many antibiotics which reduce immune response. Colon membranes become irritated, and the body forms pouchy pockets in reaction. In severe cases (ulcerative colitis), ulcerous lesions line the sides of the colon.

Natural therapies are effective and reduce the need for drugs. Many sufferers see dramatic results. Diet changes are a must. Healing herbs and supplements will not work without diet changes. If there is appendicitis-like sharp pain, seek medical help immediately.

Do you think you might have irritable bowel?

- Have you noticed unexplained weakness, lethargy and fatigue? Are you anemic?
- Do you have abdominal cramps, distention and pain within an hour after eating?
- Do you have recurrent constipation? alternating with bloody diarrhea? Is there mucous in your stool?
- Do you have rectal hemorrhoids, fistulas or anal fissures, or urgency to defecate?
- Have you lost weight lately without trying? Is your abdomen always distended even though you are thin?
- Are you a heavy smoker or caffeine user?
- Have you been under a great deal of emotional stress? Are you usually depressed and anxious?
- Have you recently taken one or more courses of antibiotics?

10-Day Diet to relieve irritable bowel...

During acute stage of irritable bowel pain:

Go on a mono diet for 2 days with apples and apple juice. (A 2-day vegetable juice-brown rice cleanse helps people sensitive to sorbital in apples.)

For the next 8 days:

Have 2 – 3 glasses of mixed vegetable juices throughout the day. Wheatgrass juice is a specific for ulcerative colitis. Have steamed brown and mixed vegetables for an early dinner each evening. Drink at least 6 – 8 glasses of pure bottled or mineral water throughout the day for best results.

On rising: take 2 fresh squeezed lemons, 1 tbsp. maple syrup in 8 oz. of water; or a glass of ALOE LIFE ALOE GOLD JUICE (add 1 – 2 tbsp. to 8 oz. of pure water); or apple juice.

Breakfast: have a fruit fiber mix of prunes, raisins and apples. Top with a little yogurt, vanilla kefir or apple juice; or have apple-alfalfa sprout juice for vitamin K; or a fiber drink like ALOE LIFE FIBERMATE.

Mid-morning: an IBS healing juice: 4 handfuls greens: 1 spinach, 1 parsley, 1 kale, and 1 arugula, 2 large tomatoes, ¼ head green cabbage, 4 carrots w/ tops, and 2 stalks celery w/ leaves, a 4 oz. tub fresh alfalfa sprouts and sprigs of fresh mint; or a green drink, like SUN WELLNESS CHLORELLA, or CRYSTAL STAR® ENERGY GREEN RENEWAL™.

Lunch: Have a simple green salad with a special Ginger-Flaxseed Dressing. For 2 cups: blend 1 cucumber chopped, 1 tbsp. flax seeds (or DESIGNING HEALTH OMEGA 3 BASIC POWDER—highly recommended), 1 tbsp. fresh grated ginger, 1 tsp. sesame oil, and 1½ cups water; have a veggie juice like Personal V-8 (page 18). Or take CRYSTAL STAR® CLEANSING & PURIFYING™ TEA with 2 CRYSTAL STAR® DR. ENZYME II: FAT & STARCH BUSTER™ caps.

Mid-afternoon: have a carrot juice; or green tea, or apple juice, or apple/alfalfa sprout juice. Or have a super-food green drink, like CRYSTAL STAR® ENERGY GREEN RENEWAL™ with 1 tsp. wheat germ added.

Dinner: have steamed brown rice and mixed steamed vegetables. Sprinkle with chopped dry sea greens (like dulse or kelp). Use 1 tbsp. flax or olive oil, and 1 tbsp. BRAGG'S LIQUID AMINOS. Or make a high fiber veggie broth: In 2½ cups water, cook 2 cups chopped fresh mixed vegetables, add 1 tsp. miso and 2 tbsp. chopped dried sea greens. Add REJUVENATIVE FOODS VEGI DELITE for friendly intestinal flora.

Before Bed: have a fiber drink like ALOE LIFE FIBERMATE at bedtime for 2 weeks; or another aloe juice drink; or papaya or apple juice; or RED STAR nutritional yeast broth for B vitamins; or a gentle cleansing booster like CRYSTAL STAR® BWL-TONE I.B.S.™ caps to soothe irritation while stimulating the body to eliminate wastes.

For long term healing:

Clean up your diet: Eat smaller, frequent meals. No large meals. Avoid coffee and caffeine foods. Eliminate nuts, seeds, dairy and citrus while healing. Cut back on saturated fat as much as possible. Eliminate refined sugars, sorbitol and wheat foods (the most irritating) of all kinds. Spicy foods are an irritant.

Eat a low fat diet with plenty of fiber, but low roughage. Cook foods lightly, never fry, few salts.

Eat cultured foods, like yogurt, kefir and REJUVENATIVE FOODS VEGI DELITE for friendly intestinal flora.

Eat fresh fruits, fruit fiber from prunes, apples and raisins, green salads with alfalfa sprouts for vitamin K, a light olive oil / lemon dressing, whole grain cereals like oatmeal or brown rice (not wheat), steamed veggies.

Choose 2 or 3 supplements to soothe and relieve irritable bowel pain:

- **Relieve pain and inflammation:** Take una da gato (cat's claw) extract, 3 capsules or 3 droppers daily (results in 5 days); peppermint oil is a specific for colitis and IBS, 2 capsules 3x daily, or 5 drops in tea. Try CRYSTAL STAR® GREEN TEA CLEANSER™ 2 cups daily with up to 5 drops peppermint oil added. Glutamine 500 mg. 4x daily; PLANETARY FORMULAS TRIPHALA INTERNAL CLEANSER caps or CRYSTAL STAR® BWL-TONE I.B.S.™ (results within 2 – 3 days).
- **For painful spasms:** CRYSTAL STAR® RELAX CAPS™, MUSCLE RELAXER™ caps or PMS CRAMP RELIEF™ extract; Wild Yam extract caps. Apply warm ginger compresses to spine and stomach.
- **Neutralize the allergen:** CRYSTAL STAR® BITTERS & LEMON CLEANSE™ drops, or Milk Thistle Seed drops in water each morning; GAIA TURMERIC CATECHU SUPREME; ALTA HEALTH CANGEST POWDER (for wheat allergies);
- **Soothe intestines:** Take chamomile tea 4 cups daily; slippery elm or pau d'arco tea as needed; NATURE'S ANSWER SEACENTIALS GOLD, an electrolyte replacement drink if there is diarrhea. High Omega-3 flax oil 3 caps daily.
- **Enzyme therapy restores the entire digestive system:** CRYSTAL STAR® DR. ENZYME WITH PROTEASE & BROMELAIN™ (between meals for colon lesions); Bromelain 1500 mg. daily; American Health papaya enzyme chewables; pancreatin 1400 mg. or ENZYMATIC THERAPY CHEWABLE DGL TABS before meals, PEPPERMINT PLUS (enteric-coated peppermint oil) between meals and GUGGUL-PLUS each morning. NATREN TRINITY POWDER in water to rebalance bowel flora.
- **Immune system support is crucial:** LANE LABS NATURE'S LINING TABS; NUTRICOLOGY PERM A VITE drink mix (with slippery elm, MSM, N-acetyl-d-glucosamine); or SOURCE NATURALS GLUCOSAMINE SULFATE 500 mg. for mucous membrane health. Royal Jelly with ginseng 2 tsp. daily. KAL COLOSTRUM to rebuild gut lining.

Bodywork and lifestyle improvements to relieve irritable bowel

- Do not take aspirin. Use an herbal analgesic, or non-aspirin pain killer.
- Avoid antacids. They often do more harm than good by neutralizing body HCl.
- Consciously practice relaxation techniques to reduce stress. Biofeedback and hypnotherapy work for IBS.
- Acupressure helps: Stroke abdomen up, across and down.
- For trapped gas: Try the Child Yoga pose.
- Effective gentle enema teas rid the colon of fermenting wastes and relieve pain: Peppermint, White oak bark, Slippery elm, Chamomile, Lobelia, Catnip (especially for kids).

Maintenance Recipes for a Colon/Bowel Healing Diet

Use these recipes on an ongoing basis once your initial healing diet is producing good results.

Breakfast

Hawaiian Morning Smoothie

1 small can papaya nectar	1 cup orange juice	2 pinches ginger powder
1 cup vanilla rice milk (or soy milk)	2 frozen bananas	1 tsp. spirulina powder

In a blender, mix the papaya nectar, vanilla rice milk, orange juice, frozen bananas, ginger powder, and spirulina powder. Makes 4 drinks.

Smooth Prunes

2 cups pitted prunes	1 tbsp. honey	nutmeg
1 pint plain or vanilla yogurt	½ tsp. vanilla	

Soak the pitted prunes in water in the fridge overnight. Discard the soaking water. In a blender, mix the prunes, yogurt, honey, and vanilla until smooth. Sprinkle with nutmeg. Makes 4 bowls.

A.M.-P.M. Fiber Drink

An excellent drink for daily regularity.

3 parts oat bran	½ part acidophilus powder	8 oz. of your favorite fruit juice
2 parts flax seed	¼ part fennel seed	1 banana
1 part psyllium husk powder		honey to taste

Combine fiber mix in the blender: oat bran, flax seed, psyllium husk powder, acidophilus powder, fennel seed. Store in an airtight container. To make 1 drink in the blender: add 1 heaping tablespoon fiber mix, about 8 oz. juice, 1 banana, honey to taste. Have one drink in the morning and one at bedtime.

Nutrition per serving:			
Calories ----------- 40	Vitamin C ---- trace quantities	Fat ---------------- 1 g.	Magnesium ------- 41 mg.
Protein ----------- 2 g.	Vitamin E ---- trace quantities	Cholesterol -------- 0	Potassium --------- 137 mg.
Vitamin A --------- 21 IU	Carbohydrates ---- 9 g.	Calcium ----------- 66 mg.	Sodium ----------- 5 mg.
	Fiber ------------- 4 g.	Iron -------------- 2 mg.	

Toasted Wheat Germ Muffins

High in fiber.

1 cup toasted wheat germ	2 tbsp. grapeseed oil	4 tsp. baking powder
½ cup plain yogurt	1 cup whole wheat pastry flour	½ tsp. sea salt
½ cup water		
1 egg		

Preheat oven to 375°F. Combine the toasted wheat germ, plain yogurt and water. Let stand 1 hour. Mix in an egg and 2 tbsp. grapeseed oil. Mix in the whole wheat pastry flour, baking powder, and sea salt. Fill lecithin-sprayed or paper-lined muffin tins ⅔ full. Bake 20 minutes or until a toothpick inserted in the center comes out clean. Makes 12 muffins.

Healing drinks

Fresh Lemon Mint Tea

A caffeine-free wake-up call.

1 handful fresh mint leaves, chopped

half a handful of fresh lemon mint leaves (or fresh lemon grass), chopped

⅓ cup fresh ginger, peeled and chopped

4 cups boiling water

6 tbsp. fresh lemon juice

6 tbsp. maple syrup (or honey)

Combine the mint, lemon mint, and ginger in a large teapot. Cover with 4 cups boiling water. Steep 20 minutes. Add the lemon juice and maple syrup. Makes 4 cups.

Green Tea Cleanser

Good hot or cold; full of antioxidants, Vitamin C.

4 tbsp. loose green tea (5 – 6 bancha green tea bags)

1 tbsp. burdock root pieces

3 slices crystallized ginger

1 tbsp. gotu kola

1 tbsp. hawthorn berries

1 tbsp. orange peel

1 tbsp. cinnamon-steeped honey (optional)

In a large teapot, steep 4 cups of hot water, green tea, burdock root pieces, crystallized ginger, gotu kola, hawthorn berries, and orange peel for 15 minutes. Strain out solids. Add the honey if desired. Makes 4 cups.

Constipation Cleanser

1 firm papaya

¼" slice ginger root, peeled

2 prunes

1 pear

In a juicer, juice all the ingredients. Makes 1 drink.

Soups, salads, appetizers

Spinach Dip For Raw Veggie Strips

1 bag fresh baby spinach, chopped

1 green onion, chopped

1 cup plain low fat yogurt

½ tsp. dill weed

In a blender, mix the baby spinach, green onion, plain low fat yogurt, and dill weed until fine chopped. Makes 1⅓ cups.

Velvety Vegetable Soup

2 yellow onions, sliced

2 ribs celery, sliced

2 tbsp. olive oil

4 cups organic low-fat chicken broth

2 russet potatoes, peeled & cubed

2 carrots, sliced

sea salt

pepper

fresh parsley, chopped

In a soup pot, sauté the yellow onions and celery in the olive oil for 5 minutes. Add the chicken broth, russet potatoes and carrots and cook on low heat until vegetables are soft. Pour soup into blender in batches and blend until smooth. Divide among soup bowls. Season with sea salt and pepper. Sprinkle with fresh parsley. Makes 4 servings.

Creamy "Cheese-y" Sauce for Steamed Veggies

½ cup lemon juice
4 tbsp. sesame seeds

1 carton kefir cheese (or rice cream cheese)
6 tbsp. honey

4 tbsp. Bragg's Liquid Aminos
½ tsp. lemon-pepper seasoning

In a blender, combine all ingredients until creamy. Makes 8 servings.

Nutrition per serving:			
Calories ----------- 104	Vitamin C --------- 4 mg.	Fat ----------------- 3 g.	Magnesium ------- 27 mg.
Protein ------------ 4 g.	Vitamin E ---- trace quantities	Cholesterol -------- 1 mg.	Potassium --------- 131 mg.
Vitamin A --------- 6 IU	Carbohydrates ---- 18 g.	Calcium ----------- 68 mg.	Sodium ------------ 431 mg.
	Fiber ------------- 1 g.	Iron -------------- 1 mg.	

Overnight Regularity Soup

Stores in the fridge easily for a week's worth of soup.

1 cup raisins
1 cup prunes
8 cups water

⅓ cup tapioca
juice of 1 lemon
honey

¼ cup apple juice

In a soup pot, bring the raisins, prunes, and water to a boil and add the tapioca. Cook over a low flame for 2 hours. Then, add the fresh lemon juice, honey and apple juice. Makes 5 servings.

Easy Lentil-Barley Stew

1 yellow onion, chopped
2 garlic cloves, minced
1 cup lentils, rinsed
1 cup barley

2½ quarts organic vegetable broth
2 cups celery, sliced
2 large carrots, sliced
½ tsp. dry sage

2 tsp. dried rosemary
5 – 6 tomatoes, chopped
sea salt
lemon-pepper seasoning

In a stew pot, sauté the yellow onion and garlic in 2 tbsp. grapeseed oil for 5 minutes. Add the lentils and barley, and stir for 5 more minutes. Add the organic vegetable broth, celery, carrots, sage and rosemary. Bring to a boil over high heat, stirring frequently. Reduce heat, cover and simmer, stirring occasionally, for 15 minutes.

Add the chopped tomatoes, cover and stir occasionally until lentils are tender to bite, about 15 minutes more. Season to taste with sea salt and lemon-pepper seasoning. Serves 4 – 6 people.

Lots o' Greens Salad

1 cup romaine lettuce, thinly sliced
1 cup napa cabbage, thinly sliced
½ cup cucumber, thinly sliced
½ cup green pepper, thinly sliced
½ cup carrots, thinly sliced

½ cup celery, thinly sliced
1 cup sunflower sprouts
1 cup trimmed snow peas
3 tbsp. soy sauce
3 tbsp. brown rice vinegar

2 tbsp. water or sake
¼ tsp. garlic clove, minced
¼ tsp. lemon peel, minced
¼ tsp. fresh ginger, minced

Make the salad. In a large mixing bowl, mix the romaine lettuce, cabbage, cucumber, green pepper, carrots, and celery. Add the sunflower sprouts and trimmed snow peas. To make the dressing, mix the soy sauce, vinegar, water, garlic, lemon peel, and fresh ginger. Pour over the greens and serve. Makes 6 servings.

Nutrition per serving:			
Calories ----------- 43	Vitamin C --------- 20 mg.	Fat ----------------- 1 g.	Magnesium ------- 21 mg.
Protein ------------ 4 g.	Vitamin E --------- 1 IU	Cholesterol -------- 0	Potassium --------- 228 mg.
Vitamin A --------- 1565 IU	Carbohydrates ---- 7 g.	Calcium ----------- 40 mg.	Sodium ------------ 424 mg.
	Fiber ------------- 2 g.	Iron -------------- 1 mg.	

Apple, Sprout & Carrot Salad

2 cups fresh alfalfa sprouts or
   sunflower sprouts
2 carrots, shredded
1 rib celery, diced

1 granny smith apple, cored
   and diced
2 tbsp. lime juice
¼ tsp. garlic-lemon seasoning

1 tbsp. toasted sesame oil
½ tbsp. soy sauce
1 tbsp. toasted sesame seeds

In a bowl, combine the alfalfa sprouts, carrots, celery, and apple. To make the dressing, mix the lime juice, garlic-lemon seasoning, sesame oil and soy sauce. Pour over the sprout mix and top with toasted sesame seeds. Makes 4 appetizer salads.

Entrées

Garlic-Rosemary Scented Salmon Steaks

2 tbsp. olive oil
2 garlic cloves, minced
4 large salmon steaks

3 tbsp. lemon juice
2 tbsp. fresh rosemary (½ tsp.
   dried rosemary)

lemon-pepper seasoning

In a skillet, sauté the garlic in the olive oil for 1 minute at medium-high heat. Add the salmon steaks and cook for 3 – 4 minutes on each side until browned. Pour the lemon juice over the fish and season with the fresh rosemary and lemon-pepper seasoning. Cover and simmer for 5 – 8 minutes, or until flesh flakes when tested with a fork. Makes 6 servings.

Sesame Chicken Salad with Pea Pods

8 oz. snow peas, trimmed
¼ cup green onions, thinly
   sliced
2 tbsp. sesame seeds
4 tbsp. olive oil
2 garlic cloves, minced

3 tbsp. lemon juice
1½ tbsp. soy sauce
1 tbsp. fresh ginger, minced
1½ tbsp. brown rice vinegar
3 cups cooked organic
   chicken breast, shredded

1 cup celery, diced
⅓ cup fresh cilantro leaves, chopped
1 bag mixed organic greens, any kind

Blanch the trimmed snow peas and green onions in boiling water for 1 minute only. Rinse under cold water to set color. Set aside. Dry toast the sesame seeds in a skillet until golden. Toss 2 tsp. of the seeds with the snow peas. Add the olive oil to remaining sesame seeds and sauté with the minced garlic, lemon juice, soy sauce, ginger and brown rice vinegar until fragrant. Add the shredded chicken, celery and cilantro. Chill and serve on greens. Makes 6 small salads.

Nutrition per serving:			
Calories ----------- 294	Vitamin C--------- 11 mg.	Fat ---------------- 12 g.	Magnesium ------- 65 mg.
Protein ----------- 35 g.	Vitamin E --------- 1 IU	Cholesterol-------- 80 mg.	Potassium --------- 497 mg.
Vitamin A --------- 19 IU	Carbohydrates ---- 13 g.	Calcium ----------- 47 mg.	Sodium------------ 168 mg.
	Fiber -------------- 3 g.	Iron -------------- 2 mg.	

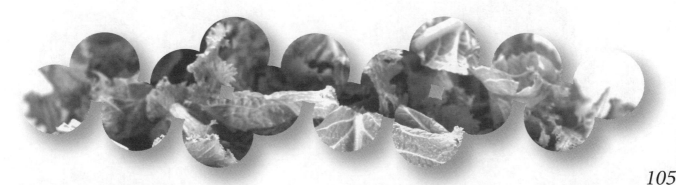

Quinoa Salad

Quinoa is higher in protein than any other grain.

1 cup quinoa	¼ cup celery, minced	1 tsp. grated lemon zest
2 cups water	¼ cup carrots, diced	¼ tsp. paprika
1 tsp. sea salt	4 tbsp. pine nuts	¼ tsp. ground cumin
½ cup raisins	¼ cup grapeseed oil	¼ tsp. ground coriander
2 tbsp. chives, chopped	1 tbsp. lemon juice	1 bag baby spinach leaves

Rinse the quinoa in a strainer to remove bitter edge. Set aside. Bring 2 cups of water to a boil with 1 tsp. sea salt. Add quinoa and cook over low heat until slightly chewy, about 10 minutes. Drain off any excess water. Put in a large mixing bowl and mix in the raisins, chives, celery, and carrots. Set aside. In a dry skillet, roast the pine nuts until golden; set aside. Make the dressing: in a small bowl, mix the grapeseed oil, lemon juice, grated lemon zest, paprika, ground cumin and ground coriander. Mix in the toasted pine nuts. Cover individual plates with baby spinach leaves and mound the quinoa salad on them. Pour dressing over and serve. Makes 4 salads.

Nutrition per serving:	Vitamin C --------- 15 mg.	Fat ----------------- 23 g.	Magnesium ------- 154 mg.
Calories ----------- 420	Vitamin E --------- 11 IU	Cholesterol -------- 0	Potassium --------- 754 mg.
Protein ----------- 11 g.	Carbohydrates ---- 48 g.	Calcium ----------- 77 mg.	Sodium ------------ 310 mg.
Vitamin A --------- 400 IU	Fiber -------------- 5 g.	Iron -------------- 7 mg.	

High Mineral Mu Shu Chicken

8 flour tortillas	1 tsp. fructose	6 large shiitake mushrooms, sliced
2 chicken breasts, skinned, deboned and cut into strips	1 shallot, minced	2 cups spinach, chopped
	½ tsp. ginger powder	2 eggs
	2 tbsp. sesame oil	hoisin sauce
½ cup sherry	1 tsp. toasted sesame oil	green onion, minced
2 tbsp. soy sauce	1 onion, sliced	toasted nori flakes
2 tbsp. sesame oil		

Wrap the flour tortillas in foil; warm in a 250°F oven for 15 minutes until soft.

Make the marinade: mix the sherry, soy sauce, sesame oil, fructose, shallot, and ginger. Marinate the chicken strips in this sauce for 1 hour.

In a skillet, sauté the sesame oil, toasted brown sesame oil, onion, and shiitake mushrooms. Pour off marinade from chicken pieces and add to the skillet. (Set chicken pieces aside.) Boil liquid down to ⅔ cup, about 2 minutes. Add chicken pieces and chopped spinach to mushroom mix. Add the eggs and stir until eggs are just set. Spoon some of the mixture over each tortilla. Top <u>each</u> with 1 tsp. hoisin sauce, 1 tbsp. minced green onion, 2 tsp. toasted nori flakes. Roll up and serve hot. Makes 8 servings.

Nutrition per serving:	Vitamin C --------- 5 mg.	Fat ----------------- 7 g.	Magnesium ------- 74 mg.
Calories ----------- 275	Vitamin E --------- 2 IU	Cholesterol -------- 60 mg.	Potassium --------- 501 mg.
Protein ----------- 14 g.	Carbohydrates ---- 34 g.	Calcium ----------- 156 mg.	Sodium ------------ 328 mg.
Vitamin A --------- 125 IU	Fiber -------------- 2 g.	Iron -------------- 4 mg.	

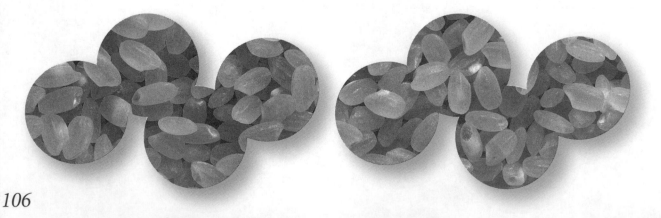

Tofu Shepherd's Pie

2 packages (24 oz.) firm tofu
6 large yellow Dutch potatoes
½ cup plain yogurt
½ cup cottage cheese
3 tbsp. butter
½ tsp. white pepper

½ tsp. sea salt
1 tbsp. soy sauce
1 large yellow onion, sliced
2 tbsp. olive oil
6 sliced mushrooms
½ tsp. dry basil

½ tsp. dry thyme
2 tsp. herbal seasoning salt
1 can condensed mushroom soup
white wine
1 cup frozen peas

Preheat oven to 375°F. Freeze the tofu. Thaw, squeeze out water; crumble in a large mixing bowl.

To make the mashed potato topping, bake the potatoes until soft and mash in a large bowl; then beat until fluffy with the yogurt, cottage cheese, butter, white pepper, sea salt and soy sauce. Set aside.

Make the filling: in a skillet, sauté the yellow onion and the crumbled tofu in the olive oil for 15 minutes. Add the sliced mushrooms, dry basil, dry thyme and herbal seasoning salt; sauté for 5 more minutes. Place in the bottom of an oiled round casserole dish or 9" x 13" baker. Dilute the condensed mushroom soup with white wine to make 2 cups. Spoon on top of the veggies. Scatter the frozen peas over the top. Spread on the mashed potato top. Bake for 35 minutes to heat and brown the potato crust. Makes 10 servings.

Healthy dessert options

Papaya Frosty

2 cups frozen papaya, cut in
  chunks
¼ cup lemon juice

1 cup water
½ cup brown rice syrup
12 ice cubes

1 tbsp. ginger syrup
4 cups water

In a blender, mix the frozen papaya chunks, lemon juice and 1 cup water. Add the brown rice syrup, ice cubes and ginger syrup; continue blending until very smooth. Pour into a large pitcher; add 4 cups water. Makes 6 servings.

Nutrition per serving:			
Calories ----------- 90	Vitamin C --------- 33 mg.	Fat ---------- trace quantities	Magnesium ------- 9 mg.
Protein ----------- 1 g.	Vitamin E --------- 1 IU	Cholesterol-------- 0	Potassium --------- 188 mg.
Vitamin A --------- 65 IU	Carbohydrates ---- 23 g.	Calcium ----------- 30 mg.	Sodium----------- 4 mg.
	Fiber ------------- 1 g.	Iron -------------- 2 mg.	

Bubbling Bananas in Lime Juice

4 bananas, thick sliced
1 tsp. grapeseed oil

3 tbsp. fructose
4 tbsp. lime juice

4 cups non-fat vanilla frozen yogurt

In a skillet, sauté the bananas in 1 tsp. grapeseed oil. Sprinkle with the fructose. Heat gently until fructose dissolves. Remove from heat; pour the lime juice over the bananas. Put on small dessert plates. Spoon the frozen yogurt on top of bananas. Makes 8 servings.

Nutrition per serving:			
Calories ----------- 173	Vitamin C --------- 8 mg.	Fat ---------------- 1 g.	Magnesium ------- 33 mg.
Protein ----------- 5 g.	Vitamin E ---- trace quantities	Cholesterol-------- 1 mg.	Potassium --------- 448 mg.
Vitamin A --------- 32 IU	Carbohydrates ---- 37 g.	Calcium ----------- 511 mg.	Sodium----------- 65 mg.
	Fiber ------------- 1 g.	Iron --------- trace quantities	

Heart Disease, Stroke and High Blood Pressure

Heart disease is still the biggest killer of Americans. A million of us die each year because of heart problems. Yet, most heart disease is 100% preventable with changes in diet and lifestyle. Almost unknown before the turn of the 20th century, today fully two-thirds of America suffers from some kind of cardiovascular disease—heart attack, coronary, hypertension, atherosclerosis, stroke, rheumatic heart and more. Natural therapies are proving to reduce mortality better than aggressive medical intervention or even the most advanced drug treatment. There has been a 28% reduction in U.S. heart disease deaths since 1987. Studies indicate this trend is largely the result of lifestyle changes to improve heart health… not high tech medical procedures or drug therapy.

Heart problems in women are different than those of men. They are hormone-dependent. (Heart attack signs are also different for men and women. See pages 111 and 113.) Beware of calcium channel blockers. They block many body functions and are implicated in aggravated cardiovascular problems. Research also shows that they raise the risk of suicide and breast cancer. Actively explore magnesium, Nature's calcium channel blocker, and CoQ-10 supplements with your physician (see High Blood Pressure, page 114 for more).

A word about heart surgery

Clearly, modern medicine has saved and extended lives. But is "heroic medicine" always the best choice when you aren't facing imminent death? Modern medicine was developed during war time when emergency treatment was the only way to deal with an emergency situation. So most medical procedures have a "battlefield mentality," prohibitively expensive, highly invasive, traumatic—often unnecessarily risky. Bypass surgery, the most popular surgical heart disease "solution," benefits less than 20% of heart patients. Patients experience no change in their life expectancy—compared to heart patients who had the same symptoms and did not get the surgery.

Know the facts before making the decision to have surgery or take heart drugs. Drugs and surgery can carry serious risks. Studies over the last 2 decades show that many patients do significantly worse after heart surgery than patients who use other treatments. Bypass surgery can cause depression and impaired memory that persists long-term. Most of us know someone for whom bypass surgery or a pacemaker became the beginning of the end of a normal lifestyle. My own father-in-law was one of those.

No matter how skilled or how advanced, surgery is never the whole answer. Your doctor knows this, too. All heart surgery MUST be followed by permanent changes in diet and lifestyle for ongoing heart health.

Why do Americans fall victim to heart disease when most heart disease is 100% preventable through simple diet and lifestyle changes?

Is our 20th century lifestyle so bad that we are literally killing ourselves? Perhaps.

First: There's still our sad American diet. While most Americans are trying to eat healthier, at best, we still only consume 3.6 servings of fruits and vegetables a day. Even worse, 25% of the "vegetables" we do eat are french fries—the most damaging for cardiovascular health! Low fiber is a big problem, despite all the media attention. The typical American eats less than one-third of the daily fiber recommended for cardiovascular health!

Second: There's our sedentary lifestyle. Lack of exercise makes us an open target for heart disease. Regular moderate exercise cuts risk for heart attack and stroke almost in half. Computers have changed our lives at every level. Federal statistics say up to 60 percent of us are not regularly active, 25 percent are not active at all!

Third: Americans are "stressed out," and our stress levels are rising. Most Americans feel overwhelmed on a regular basis. Financial or work-related stress in common. Chronic stress attacks your entire cardiovascular system. It causes coronary arteries to constrict, blood pressure to soar and cholesterol to build on artery walls. It's no wonder our hearts are about to explode!

Fourth: Smoking constricts arteries and can cause blood pressure to skyrocket, too. Researchers estimate that 150,000 heart disease deaths would be prevented each year if Americans just quit smoking! Heart attack risk is 5 times greater among smokers aged 35-39.

Is heart disease contagious? It may be.

The infectious bacteria *Chlamydia pneumoniae*, (a species of the bacteria that causes the STD, Chlamydia) may be a factor in heart disease, too. *C. pneumoniae* is a common cause of pneumonia, sinusitis and bronchitis. Here's where heart disease comes in. Blocked blood vessels are 20 times more likely to carry *C. pneumoniae* than unblocked vessels. One clinical trial finds that antibiotic therapy reduces the number of heart attacks in hospital heart patients. If you are recovering from coronary disease, a month long course of Echinacea-Goldenseal extract or CRYSTAL STAR ANTI-BIO™ caps may flush out infection trapped in blocked lymph glands and blood vessels.

Is gum disease tied to heart disease? Experts think so.

People with periodontal disease are 2.7 times more likely to have a heart attack than people with healthy gums! Gum disease allows toxic bacteria from excess plaque to enter the bloodstream, causing blood platelets to clump and accelerate atherosclerosis. The National Institutes of Health are now exploring the link between periodontal disease and heart attacks. If you already have gum disease or periodontitis, add CoQ10 to your daily healing program. It is a specific for teeth and gums, and your heart.

Rehabilitation Diet after a Heart Attack

The heart health diet below is for those who have survived a heart attack or major heart surgery. Coming back is tough. Sticking to a new lifestyle that changes not only your diet, but the way you handle every detail of your life is a challenge. Lifestyle changes are not easy, and they take time to accomplish. But they must take place for there to be permanent results. Use the diet on this page as a blueprint for a healthier heart. It focuses on food that have been proven successful against heart disease. It reduces dietary fats 30% or more, includes plenty of fish and seafood for Omega-3 oils, mineral-rich foods, particularly potassium and magnesium for cardiotonic action, is fiber-rich for a clean system, and subscribes to a little white wine before dinner for relaxation and digestion. Follow this diet for one to three months after an attack or surgery. Return to it any time as needed.

On rising: have grapefruit, apple or grape juice; or 2 lemons squeezed in water with maple syrup.

Breakfast: have fresh tropical fruits for extra potassium topped with a yogurt; mix 2 tbsp. each: lecithin granules, toasted wheat germ, nutritional yeast, sesame seeds, molasses and flax oil. Take 2 tsp. every morning on yogurt, or sprinkle on cereal, or whole grain toast. Add a little maple syrup, honey or apple juice to sweeten.

Mid-morning: have a potassium juice (page 16), or green drink like ALL ONE MULTIPLE VITAMINS & MINERALS GREEN PHYTOBASE, or CRYSTAL STAR® ENERGY GREEN RENEWAL™ drink with 1 tsp. BRAGG'S LIQUID AMINOS (green tabs OK, too. Take them with fresh carrot juice; or a mint tea).

Lunch: have baked onions, and a cup of miso soup with sea greens crumbled over the top; or a green salad with nuts, seeds, sprouts, and lemon/oil dressing; or baked tofu with brown rice and broccoli; or a black bean soup with a sandwich on whole grain bread; or a light seafood salad with spinach pasta for EFAs.

Mid-afternoon: have mint tea , or CRYSTAL STAR® STRESS ARREST™ tea with crackers and a veggie dip; or a circulation booster drink: Mix 1 cup tomato juice, 6 tbsp. wheat germ oil, 1 cup lemon juice, 1 tbsp. nutritional yeast.

Dinner: have a vegetarian casserole with brown rice, veggies, and a light sauce; or baked or grilled fish like salmon and tuna, or shellfish like oysters and scallops, with brown rice and steamed veggies; or a tofu - whole grain loaf with a green salad, or baked veggies with whole grain muffins or cornbread, and a little butter.

Before bed: fresh fruits, apple juice; or miso soup or a nutritional yeast broth.

Watchwords:

- Eat plenty of fish to balance blood viscosity for preventive effects.
- Add a brisk, daily walk.
- Do deep breathing exercises every morning.
- Boost peripheral circulation with dry skin brushing.
- Eat smaller meals with a little white wine to increase circulation. Eat magnesium-rich foods, like wheat germ, tofu, bran, broccoli and potatoes for heart regulation.
- Have a good daily laugh. A positive mental outlook can do wonders for your heart and your well-being.

Choose 2 or 3 supplements to enhance and accelerate your heart recovery program:

- **In an emergency:** 1 tsp. cayenne powder in water, or cayenne tincture drops in water may help bring a person out of a heart attack; or liquid carnitine as directed. Fifteen drops hawthorn extract every 15 minutes.
- **Tone the heart muscle:** NUTRICOLOGY COMPLETE HEART and CoQ-10 with Tocotrienols; LANE LABS PALM VITEE tocotrienols; ESTEEM CARDIOLIFE caps with CoQ10; Vitamin C with bioflavonoids, up to 5000 mg. daily for interstitial arterial integrity-elasticity, and to prevent TIAs (little strokes). EFAs from fish oil help tone arterial muscle); Health from the SUN TOTAL EFA also balance prostaglandins that regulate arterial muscle tone.
- **Improve blood flow:** METABOLIC RESPONSE MODIFIERS CARDIO-CHELATE w/ EDTA; WAKUNAGA KYOLIC SUPER FORMULA 106; or Gingko Biloba extract as vasodilators, 3x daily; CRYSTAL STAR® DR. ENZYME™ WITH PROTEASE & BROMELAIN or TRANSFORMATION PUREZYME to cleanse the bloodstream; NUTRICOLOGY BEST BLOOD OXYGENATION FORMULA.

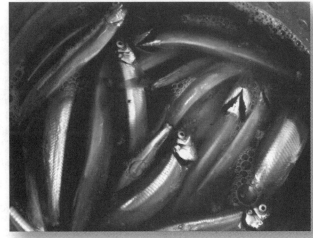

- **Antioxidants clear the cardiovascular system:** CRYSTAL STAR® HEART PROTECTOR formulas for men or women; Alpha lipoic acid 200 mg. or Grapeseed PCOs 300 mg. daily; N-acetylcysteine 100 mg. daily; or 2 tbsp. daily sea greens.
- **Cardiotonics for a strong, steady beat:** DOUGLAS LABS COQMELT daily or CoQ-10, 120 mg. daily; Carnitine 1000 mg.; Cayenne-Ginger caps; Siberian eleuthero caps 2000 mg. or tea daily; Wheat germ oil for tissue oxygen.
- **Reduce blood stickiness to prevent a heart attack:** Bromelain 1500 mg. to increase fibrinolysis; Chromium picolinate or SOLARAY CHROMIACIN for arterial plaque and insulin resistance; Omega-3 fish or flax oils 3x daily.

Important news for heart patients:

- **New research from Stephen Sinatra, M.D. shows** that the supplements, CoQ-10, L-Carnitine and D-Ribose, used in combination may help prevent and overcome heart disease. For detailed information, read *The Sinatra Solution* published by BASIC HEALTH. *For more recommended publications, visit www.healthyhealing.com*

Bodywork techniques relieve pain and improve circulation.

- **If you think you might be having a heart attack:**
- **IMPORTANT:** Get to an emergency medical center right away!
- Apply hot compresses and massage chest to ease acute angina.
- Chewing an aspirin immediately following symptoms of a heart attack, may be able to reduce mortality through its ability to reduce arterial blockage.
- **For prevention:**
- Take alternate hot and cold showers frequently to increase circulation.
- Smoking constricts arteries and can cause blood pressure to skyrocket. Researchers estimate that 150,000 heart disease deaths would be prevented each year if Americans just quit smoking. Is it time for you to quit?
- Take some mild regular daily exercise. Do deep breathing exercises every morning for body oxygen.

Heart problems for men and women are different

Until very recently, men and women's heart disease was considered largely the same. New research shows that men and women face very different challenges of heart disease. I've worked extensively to create natural healing programs that address the unique heart needs of men and women. Until the mid-'90s men's heart disease was virtually the only focus of conventional medicine study. (Consequently, male children now have a lower heart attack fatality rate than their fathers.) Yet, while about 500,000 men died each year from heart disease, even more, over 550,000, American women died. More frightening, studies reveal women receive less medical treatment despite having more symptoms.

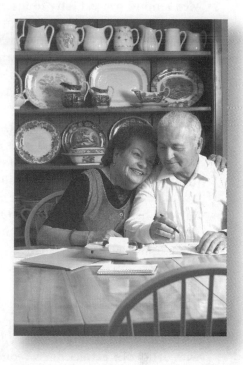

Heart disease is still the leading cause of women's death in America, accounting for half of *all* women's deaths and killing *5 times more often* than breast cancer. Heart disease for women, as for men, is linked to obesity, too little exercise and high cholesterol (even though tests show women have 60-70% less artery clogging plaque than men). It is also clearly hormone-related—a woman's highest risk is after menopause.

Many studies point to emotional health, stress, anger, and overwork as triggers of heart attacks for men. A Harvard study shows that men with the highest anger scores on personality tests are three times more likely to develop heart disease. Male pattern baldness and a protruding stomach also mean a higher risk of heart disease.

High blood pressure and atherosclerosis are the top cardiovascular problems that men face. High triglycerides (blood fats), related to a high fat diet and an overworked liver, can double a man's heart attack risk!

High blood pressure, often called "the silent killer," affects 1 in 3 of all American adults, especially African-American men. Coronary heart disease is 3 – 5 times more likely in people with high blood pressure! Atherosclerosis speeds up when blood pressure is high. Once atherosclerotic plaques form on your arteries, they restrict blood flow to organs and tissues leading to heart attacks, strokes, even gangrene.

Can donating blood regularly prevent a heart attack for a man? Yes, it can!

Men have twice as much iron in their bodies as women. Iron acts as a catalyst in cholesterol oxidation, linked to artery hardening and scarring. Recent studies show that men cut their risk for heart attack or stroke up to a third by reducing their excess iron when they regularly donate blood.

Does oral chelation reverse men's heart disease?

Intravenous chelation therapy with EDTA, though largely ignored by mainstream medicine, has been successful for arteriosclerosis for over 40 years. EDTA (*ethylenediamine tetra acetic acid*, a synthetic amino acid) binds to and flushes out arterial plaque and calcium deposits that cause artery hardening. Intravenous chelation is powerful but expensive. Oral chelation is cheaper and more convenient, a good option for men that improves blood flow and may even reverse some cardiovascular problems. Consider GOLDEN PRIDE ORAL CHELATION FORMULA #1 or METABOLIC RESPONSE MODIFIERS CARDIO-CHELATE.

New research shows heart attack symptoms are different for men and women!

Even with all the heart health information we have today, men and women still ignore heart attack symptoms… and, sadly, lose the first hours when treatment is so critical. See pg. 113 for women's heart attack signs.

Warning signs men should watch for:
• Pressure, or pain in the center of the chest lasting more than a few minutes
• Pain and numbness spreading to the face, neck or arms, usually on one side.
• Severe headache with light-headedness, sweating, nausea, skin paleness or shortness of breath.

A Man's Healthy Heart Program

- **Men tend to overeat fatty foods.** Hardening of the arteries is strongly tied to a diet high in butter, red meat, ice cream and eggs, the very foods many men overeat! Too much salt, a high stress lifestyle with little "downtime," and smoking are key factors. A low fat, high fiber diet is important for men's heart protection. It is essential for lowering high blood pressure. Reduce fatty dairy foods like ice cream and rich cheeses. Cut back on red meat, especially pork. A better choice? Eat seafood at least twice a week. An 11-year study covering over 22,000 male physicians found that eating seafood just once a week cuts men's risk of sudden cardiac death by 52%!

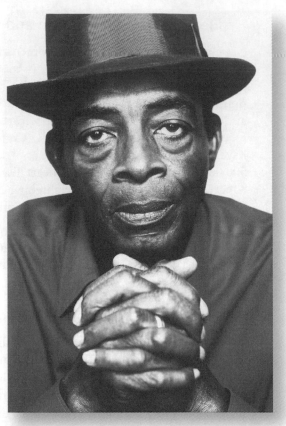

- **Use olive oil.** You can't fry in olive oil, but fried foods are so bad for your heart that this is a plus. Olive oil boosts healthy HDL cholesterol levels and removes blood fats. Try SPECTRUM NATURALS organic olive oil. Eat green foods—spinach, chard and sea greens, for magnesium therapy and EFAs, keys to heart regulation and health.

- **Men at risk for heart disease need more fiber!** Many studies show fiber reduces arterial plaque from atherosclerosis. An herbal fiber drink mix daily like JARROW GENTLE FIBERS along with artichoke extract helps reduce cholesterol, lower blood fats (triglycerides) and eliminate fatty build-up.

- **Add spices like garlic, onions, tumeric and cayenne peppers to your diet.** Garlic thins the blood, normalizes blood pressure, helps reduce serum cholesterol and arterial plaque build-up. Both onions and garlic stimulate healthy circulation. Cayenne peppers strengthen all cardiovascular activity, dilate arteries and reduce blood pressure. Tumeric, an anti-inflammatory spice, helps decrease cholesterol levels and prevents progression of atherosclerosis. Don't like spicy recipes? Consider a garlic product like WAKUNAGA'S KYOLIC FORMULA 106, with garlic, vitamin E, hawthorn and cayenne pepper. Boost circulation to thin "sticky blood" with FUTUREBIOTICS CIRCUPLEX.

- **Eat vitamin C rich foods like citrus fruits, broccoli or peppers.** Low blood levels of vitamin C are linked to atherosclerosis and increased heart attack risk. A new study shows that men with no pre-existing heart disease, but deficient in vitamin C have 3.5 times *MORE heart attacks* than men who are not deficient in vitamin C.

- **Herbal stress busters are a good choice for men.** They reduce anxiety linked to high blood pressure. Herbal formulas like CRYSTAL STAR® HEART PROTECTOR FOR MEN™ with gotu kola, passionflower and scullcap calm acute stress reactions. Siberian eleuthero is a primary adaptogen that builds body resistance to stress.

A Woman's Healthy Heart

Heart problems in women are hormone-dependent. A woman's highest risk for heart disease is during menopause. The risk rises noticeably every year for a woman in peri-menopause and goes on rising as she ages. Hundreds of thousands of hormone replacement therapy prescriptions are written every year by doctors trying to protect menopausal women from heart disease. Yet, the use of HRT to protect against heart disease is highly debatable. There is no conclusive evidence that estrogen protects against heart disease. The International Meeting on Atherosclerosis concludes that the heart protective benefits attributed to estrogen may result from population selection or changes towards healthier lifestyles during studies.

Research shows that synthetic HRT does NOT prevent heart attacks for women who already *have* heart disease. In fact, the latest studies show women who take HRT for over 5 years suffer *24% MORE heart attacks* than women who don't, and the risk is highest (a whopping 81% increase) during the first year on HRT. I believe there are better solutions for preventing heart disease naturally that don't carry these risks of HRT, with its links to uterine and breast cancer, blood clots and gallbladder disease.

Thinking about hormone replacement therapy to prevent heart disease?

- The most commonly prescribed hormone replacement drug, Premarin, actually suppresses folic acid, contributing to high homocysteine levels, a known risk factor for heart disease. New research shows synthetic progestins in combination with HRT drugs may cause dangerous coronary vasospasms linked to heart attack.
- Tests with some estrogen contraceptive pills actually increase a woman's risk of heart disease, heart attack, stroke and serious blood clotting problems.
- Some reports suggest that SERMs *(selective estrogen receptor modulators)* like Evista may protect against heart disease. But Evista should not be taken by women with congestive heart failure, common after menopause. Evista also increases risk of serious blood clots in the legs, lungs or eyes.

The biggest heart problems for women?

Statistics show that a woman is 50% MORE likely to die from a heart attack than a man! Women have heart attacks at older ages when they are in poorer health, with arteries less able to compensate for the partial death of heart muscle caused by a heart attack.

Heart attack symptoms may be different. Women should watch for shortness of breath, palpitations, fatigue; tooth, jaw and ear pain, even back pain, as well as chest pain.

Congestive Heart Failure, where the heart is unable to efficiently pump blood, affects over two million menopausal women today; and their risk for sudden cardiac arrest and death is up to 9 times higher than the general population! High iron stores after menopause may increase risk. New research shows NSAIDs *(Non-steroidal anti-inflammatory drugs)* may cause up to 20% of all heart failure cases. Alpha blocking blood pressure drugs may also be to blame. Symptoms to watch for: extreme fatigue and water retention (particularly bloated ankles). Consider CRYSTAL STAR® HEART PROTECTOR FOR WOMEN™ caps; or creatine 3000 – 5000 mg. daily.

Are you having a panic attack or a heart attack?

Women may confuse panic attacks with heart attacks during menopause because the symptoms seem so severe. Menopausal heart palpitations and nighttime anxiety attacks are extremely common. When I first began menopause, I remember waking up terrified that I was having a heart attack, but found out later that it was a panic attack. If symptoms persist, seek a qualified health practitioner.

Panic attack signs: these symptoms mean you may be having a panic attack. It should pass quickly.
- hyperventilating, shortness of breath, or bolting upright out of bed, especially in the wee morning hours.
- racing heartbeat, dizziness or feeling faint.
- feeling like you're "going crazy" or losing control, or being full of fear that has no basis in reality.

Herbs offer relief from nighttime panic attacks. I keep a herbal extract with herbs like hawthorn, arjuna, ashwagandha and passionflowers by my bed at night for immediate relief.

Heart attack signs: these symptoms may mean a heart attack. Seek medical attention immediately!
In addition to the symptom list for men (see page 111), women should watch for the following symptoms which can appear up to a month before the attack.
- Unexplained, unusual fatigue
- Poor sleep, usually accompanied by anxiety
- Unexplained shortness of breath, often without pain
- Unusual attacks of indigestion, often followed by or accompanied by, back pain, or teeth, jaw or ear pain

Note: A heart attack may be imminent for a woman if she has shortness of breath, often with palpitations, and breaks into a cold sweat, and if she has extreme weakness, usually accompanied by dizziness.

A Woman's Healthy Heart Program

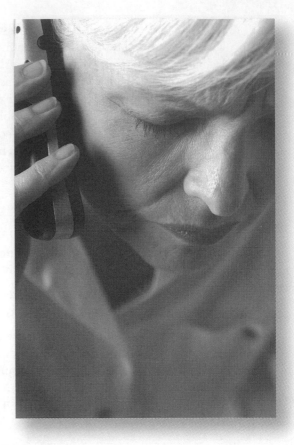

- **Sea veggies act as body tonics to restore female vitality after menopause.** They're loaded with fat-soluble vitamins like D and K that help make steroidal hormones like estrogen and DHEA which protect against heart disease. Sea veggies also dissolve fatty deposits in the cardiovascular system that precipitate heart disease.
- **Phytoestrogen foods like soy help maintain vascular function.** Soy foods not only lower cholesterol, but along with herbs, soy is a rich source of phytoestrogens for heart protection during menopause. My favorite phytoestrogen heart protector for post-menopausal women is a *dong quai/ damiana/ashwagandha* combination.
- **Have cold-water fish 3 times a week for heart-healthy omega-3 oils and EFAs.** Salmon is one of God's gifts, a rich source of omega-3 fatty acids and vitamin E. Wild salmon is a better source of EFAs than farmed salmon, and is much lower in hormone-disrupting PCBs (polychlorinated biphenyls).
- **Natural vitamin E,** like Lane Labs Palm Vitee with tocotrionols daily, cuts heart attack risk 77%!
- A daily herbal heart tonic helps protect against congestive heart failure, especially after menopause. Use a heart toning combination like Crystal Star® Heart Protector For Women™ with herbs like hawthorn, bilberry, motherwort, ashwagandha,
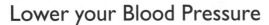
dong quai, gingko biloba, astragalus, red sage, and ginger root for 6 months as circulatory support; or try Heart Food Caps by Heart Foods or Complete Heart by Nutricology.
- **CoQ-10, up to 300 mg. daily,** or Douglas Labs CoQmelt strengthens the heart muscle and helps it work more effectively. (CoQ-10 is also a protector against breast cancer.)
- **EFAs (essential fatty acids) are important to women's heart health,** because they are critical for hormone balance… a big part of women's heart problems. EFAs help decrease blood platelet "stickiness." Evening primrose oil provides top quality EFAs. Spectrum Naturals high-lignan Organic Flax Oil is a good diet choice.
- **Eat brown rice regularly for heart smart B vitamins.** Brown rice as a valuable source of fiber, vitamins and minerals is superior to refined grains for heart health.

Lower your Blood Pressure

High blood pressure is a major health problem in America's fast-paced, high-stress world. High blood pressure affects 1 out of every 3 U.S. adults today, causes 60,000 deaths a year and directly relates to more than 250,000 deaths from stroke. It's the leading health problem for American women. New research shows that middle aged Americans actually have a 90% chance of developing high blood pressure. Less than half have their blood pressure under control, because over half don't know they have a problem! HBP is a silent condition that steals health and can steal life. It increases risk for heart attack, for congestive heart failure (especially in women) and kidney failure. It accelerates hardening of the arteries, damages blood vessels and speeds up aging of the brain.

What causes high blood pressure? Most cases are caused by arteriosclerosis and atherosclerosis (clogging arterial fats and increased fat storage), 90% of which are often the result of a calcium, magnesium or fiber deficiency - factors that can be controlled by diet and lifestyle improvement. Most sufferers are greatly overweight due to a high fat, high sugar diet; most have a high consumption of salt and red meat which raises critical copper levels. A high stress lifestyle is common, usually linked to smoking, excess alcohol and too much caffeine.

Key markers for high blood pressure: mucous and waste thickened blood, insulin resistance from poor sugar metabolism, thyroid metabolic imbalances, exhausted kidneys, auto-toxemia from chronic constipation.

Do you have high blood pressure?

In May 2003, the National Heart, Lung and Blood Institute revised their guidelines on normal blood pressure levels, putting 45 million Americans in new risk category called "pre-hypertensive."

Here are the new guidelines: Ideal blood pressure stays between 120 (systolic-the pressure exerted when the heart pumps) and 80 (diastolic-the pressure when the heart rests between beats) or slightly less. If the reading goes over 140/90, prehypertension is usually indicated. If the diastolic (or bottom) number goes over 104, severe hypertension is diagnosed. Your physician or a home blood pressure test kit can show your status.

Body signs and symptoms offer clues that your blood pressure may be high:

- frequent headaches and irritability? chronic constipation? (from calcium and fiber deficiency)
- dizziness? ringing in ears? heart arrhythmias? flushed complexion? red streaks in eyes? (auto-toxemia)
- fatigue? sleeplessness? depression? kidney malfunction? (insulin resistance, poor sugar metabolism)
- chronic respiratory problems? (from excess mucous and wastes)
- uncontrolled weight gain and fluid retention? (thyroid imbalance from increased fat storage, too much salt, red meat, and lack of exercise)

About magnesium… Nature's Calcium Channel Blocker

Actively explore magnesium, Nature's calcium channel blocker, and CoQ-10 supplements with your physician. I often receive questions about calcium channel blockers from people told by their doctors and pharmacists to take calcium channel blocker to break up calcified deposits in the arteries. In other words, calcium is the villain for heart health. Then, you hear from natural healers that calcium helps reduce blood pressure. It's the hero.

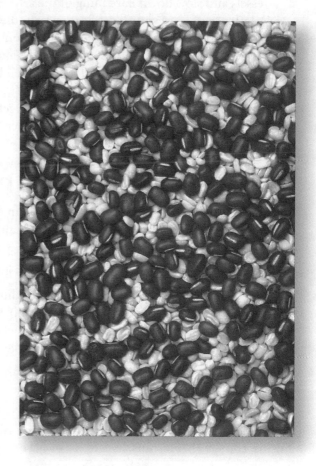

Here's how calcium channel blocking drugs work: They inhibit the entry of calcium into heart cells and smooth muscle cells of blood vessels. Without calcium, the cells cannot contract and the result is lowered blood pressure. But, calcium is an important mineral for heart health. Calcium regulates the proper contraction and relaxation of the heart, and inhibits heart spasms. Calcium also helps lower cholesterol.

Non-food calcium supplements (like calcium carbonate from oyster shells) aren't the best choice because they may cause too much calcium to overload the elimination system, potentially increasing risk for calcified deposits and stone formation. Calcium from herb and food sources is ideal because it comes with a protective ratio of magnesium to balance out the negative effects of calcium overload on the heart. Magnesium naturally blocks the entry of calcium into heart muscle cells, reducing vascular resistance and lowering blood pressure.

Magnesium is often called Nature's Calcium Channel Blocker. Foods like dark greens and sea greens, hot spices like cayenne, whole grains, nuts, seeds, and beans are all good, balanced sources of calcium and magnesium for heart health. Both minerals need to be present for optimum absorption, and food and herb sources provide this protective balance, naturally.

Guidelines to balance your blood pressure:

Clinical studies show that people with hypertension who make good life changes fare much better than those on anti-hypertensive prescription drugs. Vegetarians have far fewer blood pressure problems. Exercise is a key.

- **Cut the fat.** Harvard Medical research says a low-fat diet can lower blood pressure as much as drugs. Cut back on saturated fats (from meats and dairy) and trans fats (from snack foods and fried foods). *But don't cut out the good fats.* Foods high in essential fatty acids (EFAs) actually help reduce harmful blood clots in the arteries, and prevent cardiovascular damage with significant antioxidant and antibacterial activity. Include EFA rich foods like seafood (esp. salmon), sea greens (like nori and kelp), herbs like evening primrose or flax seed oil regularly.
- **Eliminate caffeine and nicotine for good.** Both are notorious for raising blood pressure.
- **Control your salt use.** The key to salt balance is drinking plenty of water. When your body perceives low water, it responds by retaining sodium to reduce further water loss, starting a vicious cycle of cravings for salty foods and liquids that ends in high blood pressure. (Constantly taking diuretics for high blood pressure can aggravate this cycle.) Tip: Natural sodium from celery actually helps flush table salt from your veins. If you're overloaded on salt, try a mixed veggie juice with high celery 2 – 3x daily.
- **Eliminate foods that provoke high blood pressure:** canned and frozen foods, cured, smoked and canned meats, peanut butter, soy sauce, bouillon cubes and condiments, fried chips and snacks, dry soups.
- **Eat vitamin C rich foods like peppers, kiwis, papayas, cauliflower and broccoli** to strengthen the blood vessels and slow down hardening of the arteries.
- **Get plenty of food source calcium in your diet.** Calcium deficiency often means high blood pressure.
- **Potassium is a good option.** Potassium controls heart rate, normalizes blood pressure fluctuations and flushes excess sodium in the body. Duke University studies reveal that hypertensive men who supplement with potassium regain health and reduce their blood pressure. Potassium is easily brought in through healing foods like sea vegetables (women), bananas (men), pomegranates, apricots, raisins, spinach, seafood and nuts. If your diet is strictly low-sodium, the sea vegetable nori (particularly nori that has been rinsed in fresh water before drying) has far less sodium than other sea vegetables.

Diet to Lower High Blood Pressure

A diet change is the best thing you can do to control high blood pressure. The rewards are high—a longer, healthier life—and control of your life. Avoid antacids that disrupt pH and invite your body to produce even more acid.

On rising: Have citrus juices or a potassium juice (pg. 16).

Breakfast: Make a mix of 2 tbsp. <u>each</u>: lecithin granules, toasted wheat germ, nutritional yeast, honey and sesame seeds. Sprinkle some on fresh fruit or mix with yogurt and add a tsp. New Chapter GINGER SYRUP; or have a poached or baked egg with bran muffins or whole grain toast, and kefir cheese or unsalted butter; or some whole grain cereal or pancakes with a little maple syrup.

Mid-morning: A green veggie drink, or natural V-8 juice or peppermint tea: or a cup of miso soup with sea greens snipped on top, or low-sodium ramen noodle soup; and some crunchy veggies with kefir cheese dip.

Lunch: Have one cup daily of fenugreek tea with 1 tsp. honey; then have a tofu and spinach salad with some sprouts and bran muffins; or a large fresh green salad with a lemon-flax oil dressing. Add plenty of sprouts, tofu, raisins, cottage cheese, nuts, and seeds; or have a light veggie omelet; or a seafood and vegetable pasta salad.

Mid-afternoon: Have a bottle of mineral water, or a cup of peppermint tea. Have a V-8 juice, or carrot juice; or a cup of miso soup with a hard boiled egg and whole grain crackers; or dried fruits; or an apple juice.

Dinner: Have apple or papaya juice before dinner. Then have a baked vegetable casserole with tofu and brown rice, and a small dinner salad; or a baked fish or seafood dish with rice and peas, or a baked potato; or a vegetable quiche (like broccoli, artichoke, or asparagus), and a light oriental soup; or some roast turkey and cornbread dressing with a small salad; or an Asian vegetable stir fry, with a light, clear soup and brown rice.

Before bed: Have a cup of miso soup, or nutritional yeast broth, apple juice, or some chamomile tea.

Choose 2 or 3 supplements to help normalize your blood pressure:

- **Regulate blood pressure:** Crystal Star® Heartsease H.B.P.™ caps, or Esteem Cardiolife Complex; Vitamin E therapy: Take 100IU daily for 1 week, then 400IU daily for 1 week, then 800IU capsules daily for 2 weeks. Add 1 selenium 200 mcg., and 1 Ester C with bioflavs each time. Hibiscus tea lowers blood pressure (1999 Journal of Ethnopharmacology). Optimal Health Pressure FX (88% effective in a Brazilian study).
- **Flavonoids tone arteries:** Hawthorn extract, especially for palpitation; Ginkgo Biloba extract or Cayenne-ginger caps for circulation; Grifron Reishi caps; Garlic caps 6 daily.
- **Naturally reduce edema:** Crystal Star® Tinkle™ caps (very effective); Dandelion extract drops in tea (fast acting). If taking diuretics, take vitamin C 1000 mg., potassium 99 mg., or Crystal Star® Ocean Minerals.
- **Reduce stress to control hypertension:** Nature's Secret Ultimate B daily with extra B$_6$ 100 mg., and niacin 100 mg. 3x daily. Crystal Star® Relax Caps™ with Calcium Magnesium Source™ caps; or CoQ$_{10}$ 60 mg. 3x daily.
- **Boost essential fatty acids:** Omega-3 fish or flax oils 3 daily; Evening Primrose Oil 3000 mg. daily.
- **Handle fats and dairy foods better:** Crystal Star® Dr. Enzyme 2: Fat & Starch Buster™; Bromelain 1000 mg. daily; Chromium picolinate 200 mcg. daily for insulin resistance; Planetary Triphala caps (very good results). Metabolic Response Modifiers Cardio Chelate with EDTA.

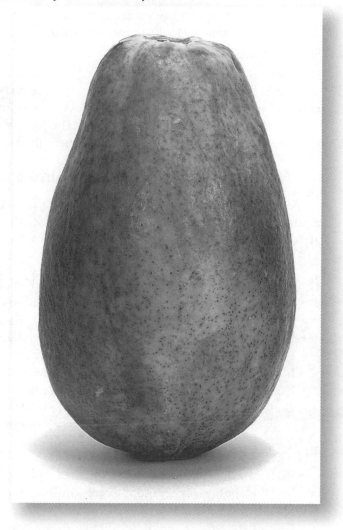

Bodywork techniques are a key to improving your circulation

- **Avoid tobacco in all forms** to dramatically lower blood pressure. Smoking constricts blood vessels, making your heart work harder. Smoking also aggravates high blood sugar levels.
- **Avoid Phenylalanine** (especially as found in Nutra-Sweet) and over-the-counter antihistamines that aggravate high blood pressure.
- **Eliminate caffeine and hard liquor.** They can cause adrenaline rushes that make blood pressure soar. (A little wine at night with dinner can actually lower stress and hypertension.)
- **Exercise is important.** Take a brisk 30 minute walk every day, with plenty of deep lung breathing.
- **Relaxation techniques are important.** Massage and meditation are two of the best for hypertension.
- **A dry skin brush all over the body** does wonders to stimulate better blood flow.
- **Reflexology point:** Pull middle finger on each hand 3x for 20 seconds each time, daily.

Diet to Lower Cholesterol

High cholesterol affects up to 60 million Americans, and it is a major factor for coronary heart disease. Cholesterol is a fat-related substance essential to every body function. Poor metabolism and over-indulgence in artery clogging foods leads to serious deposits in arterial linings, and to gallstones. There are two kinds of cholesterol. HDL (high density lipo-protein, or good) cholesterol, LDL/VLDL (low density and very low density lipoproteins, or bad) cholesterol. Both types are found only in your blood, not in food. People with cholesterol levels over 240 are 3 times as likely to die of cardiovascular disease. Research now links high cholesterol to increased risk of early Alzheimer's disease!

While statin drugs are widely touted for cholesterol reduction, research shows that taking them without making healthy lifestyle changes does not reduce rates of death, heart attacks or heart disease. Side effects of cholesterol-lowering drugs like Zocor, Mevacor and Pravachol include liver toxicity, kidney failure, impotence, stomach distress and vision impairment. The Journal of Clinical Pharmacology says these drugs also deplete CoQ_{10}, an essential co-enzyme that strengthens the heart and arteries, by up to 50%.

What level should your cholesterol be?

Cholesterol screening results can be complicated. Pay close attention to your results. High LDL cholesterol accumulated on arteries walls can eventually block the flow of blood to your heart or brain, resulting in a heart attack or stroke.

Is your cholesterol too high? Check these signs:
• Is your circulation poor? (from plaque formation on the artery walls)
• Do you get frequent leg cramps and pain?
• Do you lead a high stress lifestyle? Is your high blood pressure too high? (from a diet too low in fiber)
• Do you have bouts of difficult breathing? Are your hands and feet always cold?
• Is your skin and hair always dry? (from a diet without enough essential fatty acids)
• Do you get heart palpitations and dizziness alternating with periods of lethargy?
• Do you have multiple allergies and kidney trouble? (from a diet too high in saturated fats and sugars)

Here's what is tested in today's cholesterol screening.
• **LDL (low density lipoprotein),** the "bad" cholesterol, carries cholesterol through the bloodstream for cell-building, but leaves behind the excess on artery walls and in tissues.
- Ideal LDL levels are less than 130 mg./dL.
- Levels between 130 mg/dL to 159 mg./dL are borderline high.
- Levels 160 mg./dL and over are high.

Important: New research points out new LDL concerns. Almost half of all heart disease patients have pattern-B LDLs, smaller and denser than normal LDL'. Pattern-B LDLs enter into blood vessels 40% faster than normal LDLs, so fat is deposited on artery walls faster than it can be removed. Studies show people with more than 25% of pattern-B LDL cholesterol have three times the normal risk of heart diseases—even when their total LDL count is normal! New cholesterol screening shows pattern-B LDL cholesterol levels.

• **HDL (high density lipoprotein),** the "good" cholesterol, helps prevent narrowing of the artery walls by transporting excess LDL cholesterol to the liver for excretion as bile.
- Ideal HDL cholesterol levels are 60 mg./dL and above.
- Levels below 35 mg./dL are too low.

• **Triglycerides,** sugar-related blood fats that usually appear on your thighs and hips, increase the density of LDL cholesterol molecules. High triglycerides cause blood cells to stick together, impairing circulation and leading to heart attack. High triglycerides also elevate insulin levels, aggravating high cholesterol. Eliminating

sugar and reducing refined carbohydrates, like bread and pasta is critical to both high cholesterol and high triglycerides. For every ounce of triglycerides you eat you add 250 calories (the weight of a raisin).
- Ideal triglyceride levels are less than 200 mg./dL.
- 200 to 399 mg./dL is considered borderline.
- Levels above 250 increase your heart attack risk 50%.
- Levels 400 mg./dL and above are dangerous to health.

• **Total cholesterol:**
- Levels should be less than 200 mg./dL.
- Levels 200 to 239 mg./dL are borderline high.
- Levels over 240 mg./dL are high and put you at an increased risk for heart disease.
- Low cholesterol levels (below 180) affect 10% of Americans and can be dangerous, too. A new study by the University of Washington shows low cholesterol is a risk factor for hemorrhagic stroke!

Cholesterol Watchwords:

• **Cholesterol in eggs isn't the culprit.** Kansas State University research shows eating eggs in moderation has little impact on blood cholesterol levels. Eggs are still one of Nature's perfect foods, a whole food, with phosphatides to balance the cholesterol. The big contributor to high blood cholesterol levels is saturated fat and over-eating. Focus instead on plant foods like red yeast rice and Red Star nutritional yeast. Vegetarians who occasionally eat eggs and small amounts of low fat dairy are at the *lowest* risk for arterial or heart disease.
• **A low fat, high fiber diet is still the key to reducing cholesterol.** Reducing sugar is the key to lowering triglycerides and cholesterol. Fiber drinks like GREEN FOODS BERRY BARLEY ESSENCE, and herbal supplements like CRYSTAL STAR® SUGAR CONTROL HIGH™ capsules that balance blood sugar levels really help... usually with noticeable benefits in one to two months.
• **Focus on foods that lower bad cholesterol:** soy foods (with isoflavones), olive oil (recent research shows adults who consume 2 tbsp. of extra virgin olive oil a day for just one week have less LDL oxidation!), whole grains like oats, high fiber foods like fresh fruits and vegetables, beans, yogurt and cultured foods, and yams.
• **Substantially reduce or avoid cholesterol culprits** like animal fats, red meats, fried foods, fatty dairy foods like cheese and sour cream, salty, sugary snack foods (usually loaded with trans fats), and chemical laden foods.
• **Eat smaller meals, especially at night.** A little wine with dinner reduces stress and raises HDLs.
• **Take a morning cup of green tea** (or CRYSTAL STAR® GREEN TEA CLEANSER™), and a royal jelly/ginseng drink like PRINCE OF PEACE ROYAL JELLY - GINSENG VIALS for a month makes a noticeable difference in cholesterol levels.

Choose 2 or 3 supplements to help balance your cholesterol:

• **Balance LDL to HDL levels (the real secret):** Reishi extract drops; Red yeast rice; FUTUREBIOTICS CHOLESTA-LO; Policosanol, 5 – 30 mg. daily to inhibit LDL oxidation.
• **Support cardiovascular health:** Hawthorn extract 3x daily; GOLDEN PRIDE FORMULA ONE ORAL CHELATION with EDTA; or LANE LABS PALM VITEE tocotrienols.
• **Boost antioxidant intake:** CoQ_{10} 100 mg. daily; Grapeseed PCOs 100 mg. daily; or Bilberry extract 2x daily for PCOs; Microhydrin available at royalbodycare.com; American Health ESTER E 400 IU; Carnitine 1000 mg. daily.
• **Good fats balance out bad fats:** UDO'S PERFECTED OIL BLEND; Evening Primrose Oil 4000 mg. daily; Omega-3 rich FLAX OIL capsules daily.
• **Raise your HDL levels:** Panax ginseng and Suma root (both help protect the liver); SOLARAY ALFA JUICE caps; HERBS ETC. CHOLESTERO-TONIC.
• **Lower LDL, VLDL and triglyceride levels:** GRIFRON MAITAKE MUSHROOM caps; HEALTH FROM THE SUN BASIKOL WITH PHYTOSTEROLS (good results in Mayo clinic tests) or JAGULANA JIAOGULAN (good results in Chinese clinical tests); Cayenne-Ginger capsules 2 daily; KYOLIC AGED GARLIC EXTRACT, or Garlic-Fenugreek seed caps 6 daily (decreases bad cholesterol 10%); NUTRICOLOGY NAC (N-acetyl-cysteine) 1000 mg. daily, or SOLARAY GUGGUL-RED YEAST RICE caps (guggulipid lowers blood fats over all); Chromium 200 mcg. helps triglycerides.

- **Help the liver metabolize cholesterol:** Drink green tea or take Crystal Star® Green Tea Cleanser™; Milk Thistle Seed extract for 3 months; Dandelion root tea; Schiff Enzymall with ox bile daily. Solaray Lipotropic 1000. Esteem Cardiolife; Planetary Triphala caps.
- **Niacin therapy reduces harmful blood fats and benefits nerves.** (Not for use in cases of glucose intolerance, liver disease or peptic ulcer.) Flush-free niacin is OK. Dose: 1000 mg. daily; Nature's Way Niacin 100 mg. with glycine 500 mg. if sugar sensitive. Futurebiotics Cholesta-Lo with garlic and niacin.

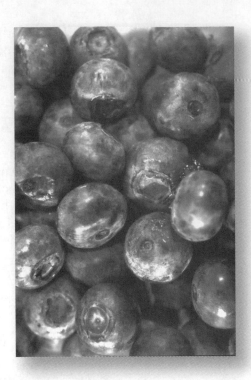

Bodywork techniques are a key to reducing your cholesterol

- **Reduce your body weight.** Many overweight people have abnormal metabolism. If you are 10 pounds overweight, your body produces an extra 100 mg. of cholesterol every day.
- **Exercise is preventive medicine for cholesterol.** Even if you cut your fat, you need to exercise to lower your LDLs. Take a brisk daily walk or other regular aerobic exercise to enhance circulation and boost HDL.
- **Eliminate tobacco use of all kinds.** Nicotine raises cholesterol levels.
- **Practice a favorite stress reduction technique at least once a day.** There is a correlation between high cholesterol and aggression. Men who are the most emotionally repressive have the highest cholesterol levels.

For more information on this topic, visit www.healthyhealing.com

Maintenance Recipes for a Healthy Heart Diet

Use these recipes on an ongoing basis once your initial healing diet is producing good results.

The diets and recipes that help prevent heart disease also improve congestive heart failure, heart palpitations, irregular blood pressure, cholesterol build-up, atherosclerosis, blood clots, hemorrhoids and varicose veins.

Breakfast

Apple Couscous for Breakfast

Light and satisfying

3 cups couscous, prepared according to package directions	½ cup chopped carrots	½ cup chopped apples
	1 tbsp. grapeseed oil	2 tbsp. raisins
	2 pinches herb salt	
3 tbsp. chopped almonds	2 pinches curry powder	

Sauté almonds and carrots for 3 minutes in the grapeseed oil. Combine with couscous and season with herb salt and curry powder. Top with apples and raisins. Makes about 4 cups.

Prune Walnut Muffins

1 cup whole wheat pastry flour	1½ tsp. cinnamon	2 eggs
½ cup toasted wheat germ	½ cup walnuts, diced	2 tbsp. frozen orange juice
½ cup Grapenuts	½ tsp. powdered ginger	concentrate
1 tbsp. baking powder	¼ tsp. nutmeg	3 tbsp. soft butter
¼ tsp. baking soda	½ cup plain yogurt	3 tbsp. honey
1 cup prunes, diced	½ cup water	

Preheat oven to 350°F. Mix the dry ingredients in a large bowl: flour, wheat germ, Grapenuts, baking powder and baking soda. Add fruits, nuts and spices: prunes, cinnamon, walnuts, powdered ginger and nutmeg. Mix wet ingredients in a large pan and heat until syrupy: yogurt, ½ cup water, eggs, orange juice, butter and honey. Add to dry ingredients in the bowl and combine until just gently moistened. Pour into grapeseed oil-sprayed muffin tins or paper-lined muffin cups and bake for 20 – 25 minutes or until a toothpick inserted in the center comes out clean. Makes 18 muffins.

Honeydew with Frosty Blueberries

½ cup honey	1 cup blueberries	crystallized ginger, minced
1½ tsp. vanilla	1 honeydew melon	

In a saucepan, heat the honey and vanilla. When honey starts to bubble, remove from heat, let cool slightly. Then gently stir in the blueberries until they are coated. Lift berries from honey with a slotted spoon and place on a tray in the freezer for 30 minutes (no more). Cut the honeydew in quarters. Place each quarter on a salad plate. Divide berries between melon pieces. Sprinkle with minced crystallized ginger. Makes 4 servings.

Healing drinks

Circulation Energy Tonic

Energize against aches and chills.

1 cup cranberry juice	4 tbsp. raisins	4 – 6 whole cloves
1 cinnamon stick	2 tbsp. honey	1 tsp. vanilla
1 cup orange juice	4 tbsp. almonds, chopped	4 – 6 cardamom pods

In a saucepan, combine all ingredients and heat gently for 15 minutes. Remove spices. Serve hot. Makes 4 drinks (2 day's supply).

Soy Protein Power Shake

2 cups honey-vanilla soy milk	3 tbsp. nutritional yeast flakes	2 tbsp. cocoa powder
2 frozen bananas	2 tbsp. bee pollen	1 tbsp. lecithin granules
4 tbsp. vanilla soy protein powder	2 tbsp. toasted wheat germ	1 tsp. cinnamon

Combine all ingredients in a blender and blend until smooth. Makes 2 shakes.

Soups, salads, appetizers

Vegetable Pickles

1 cup radishes, sliced
1 European hothouse
  cucumber, thinly-sliced

1 large carrot, thinly-sliced
½ tsp. sea salt

2 tbsp. umeboshi vinegar or
  seasoned brown rice vinegar
6 tbsp. sake

In a bowl, toss together radishes, cucumber, carrot and salt. Let sit at room temperature for 2 hours. Press vegetables gently in a colander to drain off liquid, then return to bowl. In a pan, bring vinegar and sake to a boil. Immediately remove from heat. Let cool; pour over veggies. Cover and chill for 24 hours. Serve in small lettuce cups that can be hand-held to eat. Makes 8 appetizers.

Low-Fat Hot Tuna Pâté

1 can water-packed white
  tuna, drained
1 tsp. lemon juice
1 tbsp. Dijon mustard

¼ tsp. lemon-pepper
  seasoning
1½ tbsp. sweet relish
1 tbsp. minced parsley

rye cocktail rounds

Preheat the oven to 325°F. In a mixing bowl, combine the tuna, lemon juice, mustard, lemon-pepper, relish and parsley. Spoon into lecithin-sprayed ramekins. Heat at 325° for 40 minutes or until browned. Serve right away with plenty of rye cocktail rounds. Makes 8 servings.

Nutrition per serving:			
Calories ----------- 103	Vitamin C--------- 11 mg.	Fat---------------- 1 g.	Magnesium ------- 6 mg.
Protein ------------ 9 g.	Vitamin E ----- trace amounts	Cholesterol-------- 0	Potassium --------- 60 mg.
Vitamin A --------- 6 IU	Carbohydrates ---- 16 g.	Calcium ----------- 159 mg.	Sodium------------ 375 mg.
	Fiber ------------- 2 g.	Iron -------------- 2 mg.	

California Falafel Salad

1 lb. extra firm tofu, cubed
8 oz. falafel mix or sesame
  burger mix
½ cup minced green onions

1 tbsp. olive oil
2 crumbled hard boiled eggs
1 cup thin-sliced celery
1 tbsp. sweet hot mustard

½ cup lemon mayonnaise
½ cup sweet pickle relish
shredded romaine lettuce

Boil tofu in 1 cup water for 5 minutes. Drain. Toss with falafel mix; set aside. Sauté green onions in olive oil for 2 minutes. Add ½ cup water and let simmer. Remove from heat. Add tofu and falafel mix. Toss to coat and set aside for a few minutes to absorb water. Add eggs, celery, mustard, lemon mayonnaise and relish. Stir just lightly to moisten. Chill for 1 hour and serve over shredded romaine lettuce. Makes enough for 6 salads.

Nutrition per serving:			
Calories ----------- 397	Vitamin C--------- 8 mg.	Fat---------------- 19 g.	Magnesium ------- 124 mg.
Protein ------------ 21 g.	Vitamin E --------- 1 IU	Cholesterol-------- 71 mg.	Potassium --------- 617 mg.
Vitamin A --------- 80 IU	Carbohydrates ---- 33 g.	Calcium ----------- 219 mg.	Sodium------------ 422 mg.
	Fiber ------------- 4 g.	Iron -------------- 11 mg.	

Turkey Almond Salad

The taste of a holiday turkey in a salad.

1 tbsp. shallots, minced
½ cup slivered almonds
½ cup whole wheat bread, cut in cubes
4 tsp. tamari

½ cup brown rice vinegar
⅓ cup grapeseed oil
1 tbsp. soy bacon bits
½ tsp. black pepper
2 cups cooked turkey, diced

1 cup celery, sliced
½ cup jicama, diced
spinach leaves, chopped

Preheat an oven to 350°F. On a cookie sheet, combine the shallots, almonds, bread cubes and toast in the oven until golden. To create the dressing, combine the tamari, rice vinegar, grapeseed oil, bacon bits and black pepper. Mix salad ingredients: turkey, celery and jicama. Toss with roasted mixture, and with dressing; serve over chopped spinach leaves. Makes 4 salads.

Salmon Wrapped Prawns

12 raw, peeled prawns
½ cup white wine

1 tsp. garlic-lemon seasoning
¼ tsp. hot pepper sauce

thin slices of smoked salmon
lemon wedges

Preheat broiler or grill. In a bowl, combine the prawns, white wine, garlic-lemon seasoning and hot pepper sauce. Allow to marinate in the refrigerator for at least 20 minutes.

Drain prawns; discard marinade. Cut thin smoked salmon into ½"-wide strips, 2" long. Wrap prawns and secure with toothpicks. Broil or grill about 6" from heat, until salmon is crispy on the edges. Watch closely. Serve with lemon wedges. Makes 12 appetizers.

Oats and Almonds Pilaf

1 cup sliced almonds
1 onion, diced
2 cloves garlic, minced

2 tsp. olive oil
1 cup oats
1¾ cup onion broth

6 tbsp. fresh parsley, chopped

Toast almonds in the oven for 10 minutes at 325°F. Stir and shake often.

Sauté the onion and garlic in the olive oil. Add oats and sauté until fragrant, about 5 minutes. Add onion broth; bring to a boil. Cover and simmer 15 – 20 minutes or until liquid is absorbed. Remove from heat. Fluff and mix in half of the parsley and half of the toasted nuts. Top with the rest of the parsley and almonds. Makes 3 servings.

Entrées

Fiber Veggie Toss

4 cups celery, sliced
1 cup snow peas, trimmed
2½ cups mushrooms, sliced
1 cup onions, thinly sliced
1 red bell pepper, slivered

1 tbsp. tamari
2 tbsp. arrowroot powder
1 tsp. sherry
1 tsp. fructose
½ tsp. hot chili oil

1 tbsp. grapeseed oil
1 tsp. toasted sesame oil
1¾ cups miso broth
crispy Chinese noodles

To prepare the sauce, combine the tamari, arrowroot powder, sherry, fructose and hot chili oil.

Heat a wok for a minute, then add the grapeseed oil and the sesame oil. Heat briefly and add the celery, bell pepper and onions. Sauté for 3 minutes. Add mushrooms, snow peas and miso broth. Add the sauce and bring to a boil. Simmer until thickened. Serve over crispy Chinese noodles. Serves 4 people as a main dish.

Highly Savory Eggplant

2 lbs. eggplant
2 tbsp. chopped dried onion
2 tbsp. ginger, minced
1 tbsp. garlic, minced
1 cup organic vegetable
  broth

¼ cup scallions, minced
2 tbsp. tamari
2 tbsp. balsamic vinegar
1 tbsp. sherry
½ tbsp. hoisin sauce
1 tsp. fructose

1 tbsp. arrowroot powder
½ tsp. toasted sesame oil

Preheat broiler. Peel and cut eggplant into strips. Salt, sprinkle with dried onion, and set in a colander to drain for 30 minutes. Rinse, then place strips on olive oil-sprayed baking sheets. Broil 3 – 4 inches from heat until browned. Turn strips over and brown other side, watching carefully. Insides should be soft.

Heat a large olive oil-sprayed wok. Add ginger, garlic and stir-fry for a few seconds, adding 4 – 6 drops toasted sesame oil to keep from sticking. Add broiled eggplant strips, broth, scallions, tamari, balsamic vinegar, sherry, hoisin sauce and fructose. Toss over high heat for 2 minutes. Stir in arrowroot powder dissolved in 2 tbsp. water and stir until thickened. Drizzle with ½ tsp. toasted sesame oil, toss briefly and transfer to warm serving dish. Makes 4 servings.

Nutrition per serving:			
Calories ----------- 136	Vitamin C --------- 7 mg.	Fat ----------------- 4 g.	Magnesium ------- 40 mg.
Protein ------------ 4 g.	Vitamin E --------- 1 IU	Cholesterol-------- 0	Potassium --------- 578 mg.
Vitamin A --------- 22 IU	Carbohydrates ---- 23 g.	Calcium ----------- 33 mg.	Sodium----------- 482 mg.
	Fiber -------------- 6 g.	Iron -------------- 1 mg.	

Tomato-Cheese Strata

1 tsp. olive oil
12 – 16 artichoke or spinach
  whole wheat lasagna
  noodles
5 eggs
1 cup plain yogurt

1 cup low-fat cottage cheese
½ cup red wine
½ tsp. lemon-garlic
  seasoning
½ tsp. pepper

1 cup low-fat mozzarella cheese
16-oz. jar julienne-cut, oil-packed
  sun-dried tomatoes
black olives, chopped
walnuts, chopped

Preheat oven to 350°F. Prepare an 8" x 11" baking pan by coating with a little olive oil.

Bring a large pot of salted water to boil. Add 1 tsp. olive oil so noodles won't stick, then add the lasagna noodles. Cook only 10 minutes (they'll cook more later). Drain and set aside.

Make the sauce while noodles cook. Mix the eggs, yogurt, cottage cheese, red wine, lemon-garlic seasoning and pepper.

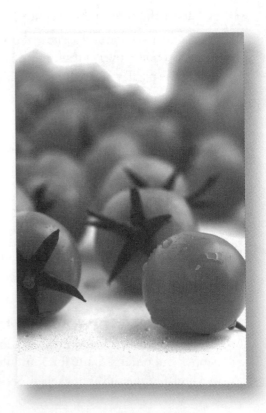

Assemble the strata. Line bottom of oiled baking pan with a layer of noodles. Sprinkle with mozzarella cheese. Scatter half of the sun-dried tomatoes over the cheese. Cover tomatoes with a scattering of chopped black olives. Cover olives with another layer of noodles, and repeat tomatoes. Pour sauce over and scatter chopped walnuts on top. Bake uncovered until edges are light brown and center is firm, about 45 minutes. Cool slightly to set; then cut in squares. Serves 8.

Rice Layers

3 cups brown basmati rice, cooked
1 tsp. tamari
1 tsp. dry basil
½ cup fresh parsley, minced

⅓ cup sliced almonds
3 large onions, diced
3 shallots, minced
2 tbsp. olive oil

1 red bell pepper, sliced in thin strips
low fat ricotta cheese
grated parmesan-reggiano cheese

Preheat oven to 350°F. Prepare an 8" x 8" square baking pan by coating with a little olive oil. Mix and toss the rice with the tamari, basil, parsley, and almonds. Sauté the onions and shallots in olive oil for 10 minutes. Add the bell pepper and sauté for 3 minutes. Assemble layers in the baking pan. Spoon a layer of rice over the bottom. Cover with a layer of ricotta. Cover with a layer of onions and peppers. Repeat layers. Cover top with parmesan-reggiano cheese. Bake 20 – 25 minutes then run under the broiler for 30 seconds to brown.

Try this: Just as good… broccoli-zucchini or mushroom and sliced turkey layers instead of onions and peppers. Makes enough for 6 people.

Lobster Salad with Ginger Dressing

8 oz. fresh pea pods
2 lobster tails (8 oz. each) or 16 oz. langostinos
baby greens

2 kiwi, peeled and thinly sliced
fresh strawberries, sliced
1 tsp. grated orange zest

¾ cup orange juice
2 tbsp. brown rice vinegar
2 tbsp. minced crystallized ginger

Trim and blanch pea pods in boiling water until color changes to bright green. Remove pods and rinse in ice water to set color. Return water to a boil, and add the lobster tails. Simmer covered until meat turns opaque in the center, about 7 minutes. Drain, clip fins and shell, and lift out meat. Slice meat into bite-size chunks and chill. Cover 4 salad plates with baby greens. Arrange kiwi slices in a ring over top. Fill the middle of the ring with the strawberries. Top with lobster and pea pods. Chill again while you make the dressing.

To make the Ginger Dressing, mix the orange zest, orange juice, rice vinegar and crystallized ginger. Pour over salad. Makes 4 servings.

Healthy dessert options

Fresh Ginger-Coconut Cookies

16 oz. shredded unsweetened coconut
¼ cup sesame seeds
3 tbsp. fresh ginger, peeled and grated (or crystallized ginger, minced)

½ cup red grape juice or cranberry juice
3 tbsp. crunchy peanut butter
1 pinch sea salt
½ cup date sugar

1 tbsp. unsweetened cocoa powder
2 tbsp. honey
2 tbsp. date sugar

Toast coconut and sesame seeds in the oven until golden. Save about ½ cup for rolling cookies in. Turn rest into a double boiler over simmering water and warm, adding the ginger, juice, peanut butter and sea salt. In another pan, melt ½ cup date sugar, cocoa powder and honey. Blend in coconut-juice mixture. Chill in the fridge. Roll 42 small balls. Mix 2 tbsp. date sugar with reserved coconut-sesame mix and roll cookies in the mix. Makes 42 ball cookies.

Nutrition per serving:			
Calories ----------- 96	Vitamin C ---- trace amounts	Fat ---------------- 8 g.	Magnesium ------- 17 mg.
Protein ----------- 1 g.	Vitamin E ---- trace amounts	Cholesterol -------- 0	Potassium --------- 87 mg.
Vitamin A --------- 1 IU	Carbohydrates ---- 7 g.	Calcium ---------- 14 mg.	Sodium----------- 18 mg.
	Fiber ------------- 2 g.	Iron -------------- 1 mg.	

Immune Defenses:
Dealing with Colds, Flu, Infections

Your immune response is critical. Your health throughout your life depends on it. Have you ever wondered why some people get sick more than others or why some seniors stay healthy in their later years while others are always sick? Even though you may have inherited a strong immune system, good nutrition, lifestyle and exercise play a significant role in maintaining robust immunity.

Every single person's immune system is unique, individual and personal in every way. Science has found it impossible to develop an "immunity drug." It would have to produce over 6 billion different drugs (the world's population today) to make one for everybody.

Integrate immune enhancing techniques into your life no matter how good you feel. Your immune system is challenged daily by at least 25,000 new chemicals that enter our environment every year - many of them from third world countries that don't have safeguards in place. These chemicals affect our air, our water, our food supply, and our basic hormone balance. We can't get away from them, their numbers are growing, and it means we live in an increasingly challenging world. A lot of us don't have very much to fight with. Today immune compromised fatigue diseases like candida albicans, chronic fatigue syndrome (CFS), fibromyalgia, Hashimoto's, lupus, sexually transmitted diseases, parasites, hepatitis and cancer are taking hold in almost epidemic proportions.

How can you stay well in a toxic environment?

It isn't easy. There is no "magic bullet," but there are tried and true "golden rules" that give you more control. Small but significant changes in your diet, and some simple natural therapies added to your daily life can add years to your health. Using natural therapies to build immunity is incredibly rewarding. You experience a feeling of empowerment, of control over the fate of your life, and a sense of well-being that comes from renewed health.

Your immune system is truly amazing

Immune defense is automatic and subconscious. It works on its own to set up a healing environment for your body. It is this quality of being part of us, yet not under our conscious control, that is the great power of immune response. It is as if God shows us his face in this incredibly complex part of us, where we can just glimpse the ultimate mind-body connection. Our immune system shows us that there is so much more to healing than the latest wonder drug. We can see that we are the ultimate healer of ourselves.

The immune system is the most complex and delicately balanced infrastructure of your body, your personal defense team that comes charging to the rescue at the first sign of an alien force—like a harmful virus, fungus, pathogenic bacteria or parasite. The immune system is always vigilant, constantly searching for proteins, called antigens, that don't belong in our bodies. It can deal with a wide range of them, even recognizing potential antigens, like drugs, pollens, insect venoms, malignant cells and chemicals in foods. It can identify and react to foreign tissue, such as transplanted organs or transfused blood, rejecting the tissue it perceives as harmful. In an allergic reaction, the immune system may even overreact, and respond to substances that really aren't harmful.

The workings of other body systems are well known, but the dynamics of the immune system are still largely a mystery. Part of the puzzle is its highly individual nature along with its incredibly complex character.

We know the main elements of the immune system itself: bone marrow, the thymus gland, the lymphatic system, the spleen, and a complex system of enzymatic proteins called the complement system. Mobilizing these elements can be a "big deal" for your body, requiring many of its resources. So nature in her wisdom gives you "first line of defense" shields to repulse infectious organisms—like your skin's protective acid mantle, and mucous membranes that line your respiratory, digestive and urogenital tracts. Disease happens when harmful microorganisms slip by these barriers and your immune response can't come to the rescue.

Here's how your immune system defends you. It's like a chain reaction.

1. **Lymphocyte defense cells**: Includes T-cells and B-cells, called "eater cells" or phagocytes. Lymphocytes form your body's overall defense system, attacking anything they perceive as foreign. But they don't identify microbes specifically, so some microorganisms, like pneumonia bacteria and viruses can slip past them. B-cells, though, can turn into plasma cells that produce specific antibodies, like immunoglobulins, that can neutralize specific invading antigens, including viruses. Lymphocytes and phagocytes also release chemicals called cytokines which send signals to integrate the immune system's efforts. Two well known cytokines are interferon, active against viral infections, and tumor necrosis factor (TNF), which destroys cells that grow abnormally, like cancer cells. When infected cells become inflamed, lymphocytes attack them in order to confine the pathogen. This defense backup is vital in resisting infections from mold-like bacteria, yeast, fungi, parasites and viruses.

2. **The thymus gland**: the major gland of your immune system, lays like a bib below your thyroid gland and above your heart. The thymus produces white blood cells responsible for "cell-mediated immunity." When diseases like tuberculosis slip inside past the defense lymphocytes, the immune system looks to cell-mediated immunity to prevent the spread of the infection. The thymus also converts regular white blood cells into immune-specialized T-cells, critical to our defense. How it does this is still a mystery to science. Even more interesting is the fact that when we reach the age of about seven, the thymus begins to shrink, possibly because it has completed this major work in the body. It may no longer be needed because once the T-cells leave the thymus, they become able to reproduce on their own—another one of nature's miracles!

3. **The lymphatic system**: like a secondary circulatory system, complements the bloodstream. Lymph nodes filter and remove infective organisms, with large cells called macrophages that engulf foreign particles like bacteria and cellular debris. The lymph doesn't have a pump, like the heart, to move fluids around, so lymph circulation depends upon your breathing and muscle movement—one of the reasons exercise is so important for any immune enhancing program. Exercise improves circulation in the lymphatic system so it can remove waste materials that block immune response. The spleen is the body's largest mass of lymphatic tissue. It destroys worn-out red blood cells and platelets, and serves as a reservoir for new ones. During a hemorrhage, the spleen comes to the rescue, by releasing stored blood and preventing shock.

4. **The complement system**: a complex series of 12 enzymatic proteins that circulate in the blood, reacts both to other immune substances and to antigens. The complement system promotes efficient T-cell function, by making lethal holes in harmful bacteria cells so they can be penetrated by the T-cells and B-cells, and by enhancing the immune inflammatory response.

5. **Fever, mucous, and the skin** also form part of the body's immune defenses. Mucous in the GI and respiratory tract kills both bacteria and viruses to keep the body protected against invasion. The skin contains sweat and sebaceous glands which produce substances capable of killing bacteria and fungus on contact.

A fever is actually one of Mother Nature's defenses. A slight fever is your body's normal mechanism for clearing up an infection or toxic overload quickly. You might get better faster when you're sick if you let Nature take its course for a little while. Fever helps to destroy bacteria and improves the flow of interferon to fight off viral infections. Your immune system raises body temperature to literally "burn out" harmful poisons, throwing them off through heat and then through sweating. The heat from a fever can also deactivate virus replication. (Modern orthodox medicine is rediscovering heating therapy for diseases as serious as AIDS.) Unless a fever is exceptionally high (over 103° for kids and 102° for adults) or long lasting (more than two full days), it may be a wise choice to let it run its natural course, even with children.

6. **Your liver**: your body's personal chemical plant for immune strength, the liver lays down the raw materials for your lymphatic system. It produces most of the lymph in the body, and the liver's special types of macrophages give the lymphatic system its power to filter harmful bacteria, especially harmful yeasts like candida albicans, and toxic compounds in the gastrointestinal tract.

What depresses your immune response?

- **Long term courses of drugs:**
  - antacids (allow infection by suppressing protective stomach acid, reducing nutrient assimilation)
  - antibiotics (destroy friendly bacteria vital to GI immunity)
  - anti-inflammatory drugs like acetaminophen, aspirin, ibuprofen (inhibit infection fighter white cells)
  - chemo and radiation drugs (weaken immune response, reduce nutrients, overload detox pathways)
- Long term pollutant exposure to smog, fluoride and chemicals (strains your body's detox mechanisms)
- Allergy-causing foods or chemicals. Allergies cause immunity to take a dive because immune defenses all channel to the allergen rather than to fight infection. (In turn, many allergies are the result of low immunity.)
- A diet high in refined, chemicalized foods. Low intake of protective, antioxidant, enzyme-rich fruits and vegetables. Fake fats like olestra are especially disrupting because they rob you of cancer-fighting carotenoids.
- A diet high in trans fats (deep fried foods, fast foods, and many snack foods), saturated fats and refined sugars. Trans fatty acids increase LDL (bad) cholesterol and decrease HDL (good) cholesterol, and are found at high levels in women with breast cancer. Saturated fats interfere with prostaglandin E1 which regulates immune T-cell activity. Sugary foods can suppress white blood cell immune activity for hours. Eating these foods regularly may mean your immune system takes a nose dive all day long!
- Excessive dieting (depresses interferon activity). Overeating also depresses immune response.
- Children born to parents who smoke, drink to excess or abuse drugs have more predisposition to illness.
- A lifestyle low on rest. Your body builds the most immune power during sleep. Poor sleep lowers the T-cell percentage in your blood. Killer cell activity is reduced by as much as 28% when sleep is cut by 4 hours!
- Not being breast-fed as a child. Breast milk is rich in antibodies, essential fatty acids and interferon that strengthen a child's developing immune system.
- Long lasting depression. Laughter lifts more than your spirits. It also boosts immune strength. Really! Laughter decreases cortisol, an immune suppressor, allowing the body's defense boosters to function better.
- Stress makes you unusually susceptible to low immune response. Listen to soft music. Your pulse rate will actually follow the mellow beat to de-stress your body. Enjoy a long bath, or get a massage therapy treatment. These relaxation techniques last a whole week in terms of reducing stress and enhancing immune response.
- Lonely, solitary people. Build a strong support system of family and friends into your life. Research from the Carnegie Mellon University shows that having friends actually lowers your risk of catching a cold by 30%!
- Couch potatoes. Exercise 2 – 3 times a week. Exercise improves immunity by increasing lymphatic flow and keeping oxygen high (disease doesn't readily attack in a high oxygen, high potassium environment). Tests on senior women show that those who exercise even moderately have marked improvement in immune response.

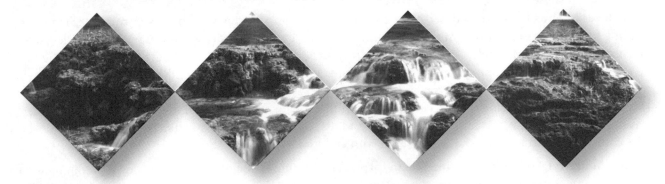

Is your immune response low?

It's difficult to measure immune health. Every person is different and immune response varies widely. Here's a quick personal quiz to monitor your immune status:
- Do you suffer from chronic infections, colds, respiratory problems or allergies? Are you always tired?
- Do you have chronic fatigue syndrome, Hashimoto's, lupus or fibromyalgia?

- Do you have irritable bowel syndrome (I.B.S.), leaky gut syndrome, chronic diarrhea or constipation?
- Do you have diabetes or liver disease? Have you ever been the recipient of an organ transplant?
- Have you had long-term antibiotics or steroid drug treatment? Do you have candida yeast infections?
- Do you have adult acne, rosacea or easy bruising (a sign of low collagen and protective vitamin C)?
- Have you recently undergone surgery, chemotherapy or radiation treatment?
- Do you have periodontal disease?
- Do you drink 2 or more drinks of hard alcohol 5 times a week or use recreational drugs regularly?
- Are you a smoker or are you exposed to second-hand smoke on a regular basis?
- Are you regularly exposed to smog, heavy pesticides, industrial heavy metals like cadmium or mercury?
- Do you eat meats—like pork or beef—that are injected with antibiotics and hormones?
- Do you have circulation problems or a history of claudication?
- Do you suffer from chronic stress, chronic insomnia, anxiety, panic attacks or depression?

Healing Diet to Restore Immune Strength

1. **Take a close look at the fruits and vegetables you're eating,** especially during the winter months when your body needs more substance from your diet. Warm weather fruits and vegetables like cucumbers, head lettuce, kiwis, melons, summer squash or tomatoes, are too light for winter (high risk season) health. Switch to vegetables and legumes- like carrots, potatoes, lentils, black beans and squash. Good winter fruits are cranberries, pears and apples. Apples are a hydrating energy food, full of enzymes to help you use the other foods you eat. Apples are rich in pectin, an amazing food fiber that binds to and helps eliminate gut toxins to keep your GI tract healthy. An apple a day may truly keep the doctor away. Cruciferous vegetables like broccoli, cabbage and cauliflower offer a megaload of nutrients for immune health, like vitamin C, beta carotene, calcium and fiber. They also have estrogen flushing activity against the environmental estrogens we get today from our meats and pesticides.

2. **Add more high fiber foods for high risk seasons.** Whole grains and sprouts are full of fiber. Sprouted seeds and grains are living foods, some of the healthiest foods you can eat. My favorite grain all year round is brown rice. In the winter, a combination of brown rice and root vegetables provides mineral building blocks and complex carbohydrates for strength. I make up a big pot of rice every 2 or 3 days with 1 teaspoon of miso for every cup of rice. Miso adds flavor and helps to set up an immune-enhancing environment in the body.

3. **Eat sea foods for essential fatty acids, vitamin E and omega-3 oils.** World Health Organization studies show that societies using fish and seafood as their primary source of fat and protein have much lower incidence of heart disease and cancer.

4. **Add to your healing enzyme supply during high risk seasons.** Food enzymes are basic to immune response for natural enzyme therapy. Foods like alfalfa sprouts, garlic, pineapple and papaya provide more of their enzymes to work with yours.

5. **Drink enough water.** Dehydration is at the root of a lot of disease, especially age-related conditions (like creaky joints, wrinkling skin, hemorrhoids, varicose veins and kidney stones). Consider bottled water or a high quality filtration system. City tap water may contain as many as 500 different disease-causing bacteria, viruses and parasites.

6. **Reduce fatty dairy foods to keep the body free flowing.** But include cultured dairy foods like yogurt, kefir, kefir cheese, cottage cheese and raw sauerkraut for friendly intestinal flora. Cultured foods help maintain the body's acid-alkaline balance, and strengthen the nerves and immune system. If you like wine, (a cultured food), have a little wine with dinner. More than an alcoholic drink, wine is a complex living food with absorbable B vitamins, and minerals like potassium, magnesium, organic sodium, iron, and calcium.

7. **Have a superfood drink twice a week.** Green superfoods like PURE PLANET CHLORELLA or SPIRULINA, GREEN FOODS GREEN MAGMA, CRYSTAL STAR® ENERGY GREEN RENEWAL™ supply a mini-transfusion to detoxify your blood.

7-Day Immune Stimulation Diet

Natural healing is not extravagant or heroic medicine; it is body normalization, rebuilding your body from the inside out. Your diet is the first place to start. Powerful immune-enhancing foods can be directed at "early warning" problems, like the ones you might have spotted in your quiz. Since immunity is the body system most sensitive to nutritional deficiency, good nourishment is the main key to keeping this system functioning at its peak. Incorporating some of these diet recommendations is well worth it. The inherited immunity and health of you, your children and your grandchildren is laid down by you and your choices.

On rising: Take 2 – 3 tbsp. cranberry concentrate in 8 oz. water or aloe vera juice; or an immune stimulating drink like CRYSTAL STAR® DR. VITALITY™ (green and white tea blend); or GARDEN OF LIFE GOATEIN drink mix.

Breakfast: Have a cup of green tea daily. Make an immune-stimulating mix of nutritional yeast flakes, lecithin granules, pumpkin seeds and flax seed. Sprinkle on your choice of whole grain granola with rice or soy milk, fresh fruit and yogurt, baked or poached eggs, or whole grain muffins or rice cakes with kefir cheese.

Mid-morning: a green superfood like CRYSTAL STAR® ENERGY GREEN RENEWAL™, GREEN KAMUT from GREEN KAMUT CORP. or GREEN FOODS GREEN MAGMA; or a fresh vegetable juice with 1 tbsp. green superfood like NUTRICOLOGY PRO-GREENS with EFAs or WAKUNAGA KYO-GREEN.

Lunch: have a leafy salad with lemon-flax oil dressing; or a whole grain sandwich with sprouts, nuts, seeds, veggies and yogurt or soy cheese; or a turkey or seafood salad or sandwich with yogurt dressing; or a cup of miso soup with brown rice and sea greens snipped in; or stir fry vegetables with onions, brown rice and tofu.

Mid-afternoon: have a carrot juice or a cup of immune stimulating herb tea like ginseng tea, and have some rice cakes with a soy spread or veggie dip.

Dinner: have baked or broiled seafood or fish with brown rice and veggies; or a high protein soup or sandwich on whole grain bread; or a light Italian spinach pasta meal; or an Oriental stir-fry with veggies and seafood, a clear broth soup with sea greens snipped on top; or a tofu and veggie casserole with brown rice and a low-fat yogurt, cheese and wine sauce.

Before bed: take a hot lemon and honey drink; or hot apple or cranberry juice; or green tea, or RED STAR nutritional yeast broth, or miso soup with sea greens.

Choose 2 or 3 supplements to stimulate the immune system:

- **Stimulate white blood cell activity with natural antibiotics:** ALLERGY RESEARCH GROUP LAKTOFERRIN WITH COLOSTRUM; Olive Leaf extract; NAC (N-acetyl-cysteine) 600 mg.
- **Immune modulators act as response tonics:** IMMUDYNE MACROFORCE, or NATURAL BALANCE MODUCARE caps for 2 months. Siberian eleuthero, Panax ginseng or Suma root; Propolis caps 4 daily during high risk seasons; NATURE'S WAY CELL MEND WITH IP-6; BIOSTRATH YEAST ELIXIR; ZAND HERBAL INSURE extract; FUTUREBIOTICS VITAL K.
- **Medicinal mushrooms enhance interferon production:** Reishi, shiitake and maitake mushrooms; PLANETARY FORMULAS REISHI SUPREME; GRIFRON MAITAKE D FRACTION; HERBS ETC. DEEP HEALTH WITH REISHI/SHIITAKE COMPLEX.
- **Enhance thymus gland activity:** NUTRICOLOGY ORGANIC THYMUS; NATURE'S PATH THY-LYTE; ENZYMATIC THERAPY THYMULUS; (Tap thymus with knuckles each morning to stimulate.)
- **Enzymes boost immune response:** CRYSTAL STAR® DR. ENZYME WITH PROTEASE & BROMELAIN™, 6 daily. BIOTEC CELL GUARD W/ SOD 6 daily for 6 weeks; TRANSFORMATION PUREZYME; Milk Thistle Seed extract.
- **Sea plants help remove toxins:** Sea greens of all kinds, 2 tbsp. daily, provide therapeutic iodine, potassium and sodium alginate to help purify your body; or take CRYSTAL STAR® OCEAN MINERALS™ caps, or IODINE, POTASSIUM, SILICA extract with sea plants; or BIOTEC PACIFIC SEA PLASMA tablets 6 daily; NATURE'S PATH TRACE-MIN-LYTE (sea greens).
- **Antioxidants build immune strength:** DIAMOND HERPANACINE HEALTHY HORIZONS with alpha lipoic acid; vitamin E with selenium; vitamin C or Ester C with bioflavonoids 3000 mg.; zinc 50 mg. daily; CoQ_{10} 200 mg. daily.
- **Probiotics restore GI immunity:** UAS DDS-PLUS; LANE LABS GI48; TRANSFORMATION PLANTADOPHILUS.

Bodywork and lifestyle improvements enhance immune response

- **Relaxation techniques are immune-enhancers.** A positive mental attitude makes a big difference in how the body fights disease. Creative visualization establishes belief and optimism. Massage therapy reduces stress.
- **Exercise keeps system oxygen high, circulation flowing.** Disease does not readily overrun a body where oxygen and organic minerals are high in the vital fluids. Reduce prescription drugs if possible, especially antibiotics and steroid drugs that depress immunity over the long term.
- **Stop and smell the roses.** Have one good laugh every day.
- **Limit or reduce antibiotics and steroids** that depress immunity.
- **Tobacco/nicotine in any form is an immune depressant.** The cadmium content causes zinc deficiency. It takes 3 – 6 months to rebuild immune response even after you quit.
- **Get a few minutes a day of early morning sunlight.** Avoid excessive sun. A sunburn depresses immunity.
- **Get quality rest,** immune power builds the most during sleep.

Healing Cold, Flu and Sinus Infections

Respiratory illnesses of all kinds are more than common in our society today. Americans catch about 66 million colds a year, costing the U.S. economy a whopping $40 billion a year! During high risk seasons, over one-third of the U.S. population has had a cold or flu within the last 2 weeks. Children in daycare are especially susceptible; they experience up to one dozen colds every year!

Your body is giving you a "cell phone call" when you get a cold. A cold is often your natural detox mechanism. Your body opens up and drains its elimination channels, by coughing, sneezing, diarrhea, etc. to relieve itself of wastes, toxins and bacteria that have built up to a point where your immune response can't overcome them.

Drugs and over-the-counter medicines only relieve the symptoms of infection. They do not cure it, and in my experience, often make the situation worse by depressing immunity, drying up needed mucous elimination, and keeping the virus or harmful bacteria inside the body. Most drug store remedies halt the body cleansing-balancing process, and generally make the cold last longer. Antibiotics are not effective against virally caused infections, and aspirin can enhance the reproduction of viral germs. Unfortunately, whatever temporary relief aspirin might afford, it may make it easier for viruses to multiply and spread.

A cold can be a friendly enemy—your wonderful immune system working to rebuild a stronger, cleaner system. The best way to get over a cold is to work with your body, not against it. Natural remedies are effective in speeding recovery and reducing discomfort for the vast majority of respiratory diseases.

Do you have a cold, or the flu?

Colds and flu are separate upper respiratory infections, triggered by over 200 hundred different rhino-viruses. Outdoor environment, drafts, wetness, temperature changes, etc. do not cause *either* a cold and flu. The flu is more serious, because it can spread to the lungs, and cause bronchitis or pneumonia. Nose, eyes and mouth are usually the sites of invasion from cold viruses. The most likely target for the flu virus is the respiratory tract. Viruses don't breathe, digest food or eliminate, but they replicate themselves with a vengeance. The following symptom chart can help identify your problem and allow you to deal with it better.

A cold profile looks like this:
- Slow onset. No prostration. Body aches, largely due to the release of interferon (an immune stimulator).
- Rarely accompanied by fever and headache.
- Sore throat, sinus congestion, listlessness, runny nose and sneezing.
- Mild fatigue and weakness as a result of body cleansing.
- Mild to moderate chest discomfort, usually with a hacking cough.
- Sore or burning throat common.

A flu profile looks like this:
- Swift and severe onset. Early and prominent prostration with flushed, hot, moist skin.
- Usually accompanied by high (102°-104°) fever, headache and sore eyes.
- Chills, depression and body aches.
- Extreme fatigue, sometimes lasting 2-3 weeks.
- Acute chest discomfort, with severe hacking cough.
- Sore throat occasionally.

For 92 million Americans (1 in 3), a chronic sinus infection is a daily energy drain. In some cases, a sinus infection can be serious, spreading to the eyes and threatening vision. When the thin, air-filled chambers of the sinuses become obstructed, mucous and infected pus collect in the sinus pockets causing pain and swelling. Chronic sinusitis, which may be a fungal infection, also results in nasal polyps and scar tissue. Suppressive over-the-counter sinus medications can both trigger a sinus infection by not allowing draining of infective material, and aggravate a sinus infection by driving it deeper into sinus cavities. Natural healing methods revolve around relieving the cause of the clogging and inflammation.

Do you have chronic colds? An ounce of prevention is worth a pound of cure.
- A daily walk works wonders! It revs up immune response, brings in oxygen, keeps your mood positive.
- Take vitamin C 1000 mg. every hour during the day in powder form with juice… take zinc lozenges as needed.
- Smoking or alcohol suppress immunity. Refined foods, sugar, and dairy foods increase thick mucous.
- Nutrient absorption is less efficient during a cold. A vegetarian diet is much easier on your digestion.
- Drink 8 glasses daily of fruit and vegetable juices, herb teas and water to flush toxins out of the system.
- Take a hot bath or sauna to release toxins though the skin. Increase room humidity.
- Go to bed early, and get plenty of sleep. Most regeneration of cells occurs between midnight and 4 a.m.
- Use Xlear nasal wash every day to help keep bacteria from multiplying.

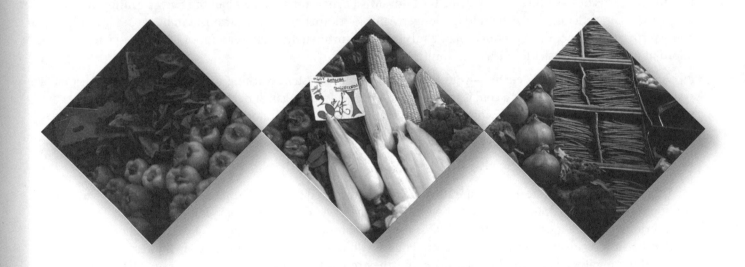

Do you have a sore throat due to a cold, or a more serious strep throat?
- Strep throat onset is rapid; onset of a sore throat that comes before a cold is slow.
- Strep throat is very sore; the throat is not so sore if it's part of a cold.
- Strep throat is accompanied by an ache-y fever; a sore throat that's part of a cold has only mild achiness.
- Strep throat is accompanied by swollen lymph nodes; with a cold, lymph nodes aren't sore.
- Antibiotics work for strep throat; they don't usually work for a cold.
- Strep throat is hoarse, with inflamed vocal chords; sore throat due to a cold has a raspy, breathy voice.
- Strep throat is linked to pneumonia or ear infection; sinusitis accompanies a sore throat with a cold.

Cleansing Diet for Colds, Sore Throat, Sinus Infections

Avoid white flour, sugar and dairy foods. They increase production of thick mucous. When the acute stage has passed, eat light meals, including plenty of fresh and steamed vegetables, fresh fruits and juices, and cultured foods for friendly intestinal flora. Light meals with rich plant nutrients are the easiest to assimilate.

Start with a 24-hour mucous elimination diet. You'll get better results if you allow your body to rid itself first of toxins and mucous accumulations. Green drinks and vegetable broths promote mucous elimination.

Before you begin: make up garlic syrup: soak a chopped garlic bulb in 1 pint honey and water overnight; take a tsp. every hour during your 24-hour cleanse. Take grapefruit or cranberry juice throughout the day, or CRYSTAL STAR® CLEANSING & PURIFYING™ TEA to combat infection.

On rising: take a glass of lemon juice, honey and water with a pinch cayenne pepper each morning to thin mucous secretions.

Breakfast: take a potassium juice (page 16), or aloe vera juice. Take CRYSTAL STAR® D-CONGEST™ spray for nasal congestion; and take 3 garlic capsules and ½ tsp. vitamin C or Ester C powder in water.

Mid-morning: have a fresh carrot juice; or dilute pineapple juice, or a pineapple/papaya juice, or cranberry/apple juice; and/or a cup of comfrey/fenugreek tea, green tea or CRYSTAL STAR® DR. VITALITY TEA.

Lunch: have a hot vegetable, miso or onion broth, or CRYSTAL STAR® RESTORE YOUR STRENGTH™. Take CRYSTAL STAR® D-CONGEST™ spray for nasal congestion; and take 3 garlic capsules and ½ tsp. vitamin C or Ester C powder in water.

Mid-afternoon: take another green drink like BARLEANS GREENS, or CRYSTAL STAR® RESTORE YOUR STRENGTH™. Zinc lozenges under the tongue, or CRYSTAL STAR® ZINC SOURCE™ throat rescue drops in water as a nasal rinse for sinusitis or on back of the tongue to kill throat bacteria. Or use NEW CHAPTER GINGER WONDER syrup as a gargle.

Dinner: have a potassium drink, or miso soup with sea greens; or a glass of carrot juice; and take 3 garlic capsules and ½ tsp. vitamin C or Ester C powder in water.

Before bed: take a hot lemon and honey drink; or hot apple or cranberry juice; green tea or CRYSTAL STAR® DR. VITALITY™ TEA; or miso soup each night.

Healing Diet for Colds and Sinus Infection

After your congestion cleanse, follow this diet for 3 – 5 days. It's loaded with vitamin C, and can produce symptomatic relief from many respiratory problems in under 48 hours. Have plenty of leafy greens. Eat plenty of plain yogurt. Drink 8 glasses of healthy liquids, fruit and vegetable juices, broths, herb teas (especially green tea and peppermint tea), and water to relieve congestion and other symptoms. (1 – 2 tsp. BRAGG'S LIQUID AMINOS may be added to any broth or juice.) All respiratory infections benefit from a non-clogging diet.

Eat light meals—fresh and steamed vegetables, fresh fruits and juices, and cultured foods like REJUVENATIVE FOODS VEGI-DELITE for friendly intestinal flora. Boost immunity with glutathione foods: avocado, asparagus, watermelon, oranges, peaches, and green superfoods like chlorella and barley grass. Add plenty of garlic, onions and mustard. Avoid dairy foods, starches and refined foods—the breeding ground for congestion.

On rising: take a cranberry, apple or aloe vera juice; or lemon juice in hot water with 1 tsp. honey.

Breakfast: take green tea, or a cup of CRYSTAL STAR® GREEN TEA CLEANSER™, or CRYSTAL STAR® RESTORE YOUR STRENGTH™ drink, PURE PLANET CHLORELLA or GREEN FOODS GREEN MAGMA to regenerate immune response; and take garlic/ginger tea with ½ tsp. ascorbate vitamin C or Ester C powder.

Mid-morning: Balance intestinal structure with GARDEN OF LIFE GOATEIN protein drink; or have a fresh carrot juice; or a glass of cranberry/apple juice; or a cup of miso soup with sea greens snipped on top; or CC POLLEN DYNAMIC TRIO drink, or CRYSTAL STAR® ENERGY GREEN RENEWAL™ drink.

Lunch: a green salad with lemon/oil dressing gives your bowels a good sweeping; and/or a hot vegetable, miso or onion broth, or REJUVENATIVE FOODS VEGI DELITE cultured veggies; or steamed veggies with brown rice; take garlic/ginger tea with ½ tsp. ascorbate vitamin C or Ester C powder.

Mid-afternoon: have a cleansing alfalfa/mint tea, or another green drink like WAKUNAGA KYO-GREEN.

Dinner: have miso soup with sea greens; or tofu/veggie casserole with sea greens; or a veggie stir fry with brown rice, sea greens, miso soup. Take garlic/ginger tea with ½ tsp. ascorbate vitamin C or Ester C powder.

Before bed: take a hot water, lemon and honey drink; or hot apple or cranberry juice; or miso broth.

Choose 2 or 3 supplements to stimulate the immune system while offering symptom relief:

- **During initial stage:** MERIX HEALTH C & F CAPS WITH VIRACEA (highly recommended); CRYSTAL STAR® ANTI-BIO™ caps, 6 daily; Vitamin C crystals, ¼ tsp. every half hour to flush toxins; Colloidal Silver drops every 3 hours.
- **During acute phase:** PLANETARY FULL SPECTRUM OLIVE LEAF EXTRACT; HERBS ETC. ECHINACEA TRIPLE SOURCE; CRYSTAL STAR® ZINC SOURCE™ throat spray or BEEHIVE BOTANICAL PROPOLIS THROAT SPRAY every 2 hours. Echinacea extract to flush lymph glands; ENZYMATIC THERAPY ESBERITOX chewables; elderberry-mint-yarrow tea; CRYSTAL STAR® DR. ENZYME WITH PROTEASE & BROMELAIN™ as an anti-inflammatory, immune booster.
- **A great "cold" cocktail!:** To aloe vera juice: add ¼ tsp. vitamin C crystals, 2 tsp. NATURE'S WAY SAMBUCOL ELDERBERRY SYRUP, ½ tsp. turmeric powder, 1 capsule echinacea, ½ tsp. propolis extract.
- **Congestion cleansers:** Cayenne-ginger caps; Echinacea-goldenseal caps; Dandelion rt. tea; CRYSTAL STAR® D-CONGEST™ spray; ZAND DECONGEST extract.
- **For strep throat:** CRYSTAL STAR® ANTI-BIO™ extract every hour; NUTRIBIOTIC GRAPEFRUIT SEED extract in water; Zinc lozenges kill throat bacteria; or CRYSTAL STAR® ZINC SOURCE™ drops directly on throat; take vitamin C 5000 mg. daily, and Lysine 1000 mg.; ZAND HERBAL LOZENGES; PLANETARY OLD INDIAN COUGH SYRUP.
- **For a bad sore throat, try one of these gargles:** 1. lemon juice and brandy; 2. black tea; 3. liquid chlorophyll in water with pinch cayenne; 4. lemon juice and sea salt in water; 5. cider vinegar and honey in water.
- **For sinusitis:** XLEAR NASAL WASH (highly effective); BOIRON SINUSITIS TABS; EUROPHARMA SNEEZE-EZE (outstanding, immediate results); NUTRIBIOTIC NASAL SPRAY & EAR DROPS.
- **Essential oils:** 1. Eucalyptus opens sinus passages. 2. Wintergreen relieves nasal congestion. 3. Mint or chamomile relieve headaches. 4. Tea tree oil and oregano oil combat infection and thin mucous.
- **Chest rub:** 15 drops essential oils like oregano, tea tree, or eucalyptus in 1 oz. of jojoba oil; rub on the chest.
- **Inhalant:** add 6 drops of essential oils to a quart hot water—inhale the steam.

Bodywork can help you feel much better.

- **Regular exercise encourages immune response.** Even just a short walk every day, puts cleansing oxygen into the lungs, restoring vitamin D in the body, and fresh air into the brain.
- **Take a hot 20 minute bath or sauna at the onset** of a cold, flu or any respiratory problem to stimulate the body's defenses and increase elimination of toxins through the skin. Apply hot ginger compresses to chest.
- **Stimulate easier breathing by massaging** and gently scratching the lung meridian from the top of the shoulder to the end of the thumb to clear chest mucous. Massage therapy opens up blocked body meridians.
- **A catnip enema** can cleanse infection from strep throat.
- **Sinusitis:** Nasal salt irrigation clears breathing: add ½ tsp. sea salt to 1 cup warm water. Fill a dropper with liquid, tilt your head and fill each nostril; then blow your nose. Apply Tiger Balm or Chinese White Flower oil to sinus area.

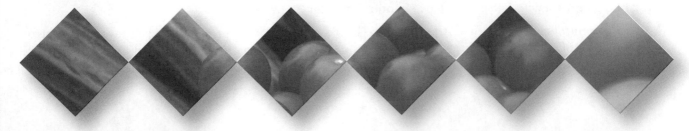

Healing Flu, Bronchitis and Pneumonia

Like a cold, the flu is an upper respiratory infection by a rhinovirus. Unlike a cold, flu infections are more severe, longer-lasting and highly contagious. Some people become incapacitated for weeks at a time. 36,000 people die every year from influenza-related diseases. For complete recovery, flu treatment works best in stages.

The ACUTE, infective stage (aches, chills, prostration, fever, sore throat, etc.), usually lasts for 2 – 4 days.

The RECUPERATION, healing stage, (replenishes natural resistance), usually lasts for 1 – 2 weeks.

The IMMUNE RECOVERY stage usually lasts 2 – 3 weeks, especially in high risk seasons. Recovery from flu is often slow with a good deal of weakness. Beware. Colds and flu are different. It's important to know what ails you before you can treat it. See pages 131-132 for the differences.

About the Flu Vaccine… is it necessary? does it work?

Two consecutive years of flu vaccine shortages have Americans in a panic. One of the saddest cases in 2004 was of an elderly woman who died after collapsing and hitting her head while standing in line for over 4 hours waiting for her shot. Is the panic really justified?

With a death toll of 36,000 annually in the U.S., the flu can be deadly, especially for the elderly, pregnant women, people with HIV/AIDS, and children whose immune systems aren't fully developed. Still, it is not generally the flu that kills people. It's pneumonia or another bacterial infection that takes hold when immune response takes a dive from the flu.

The Centers for Disease Control and Prevention reported in 2004 that the vaccine had no or low effectiveness against influenza or influenza-like diseases. Some experts in the medical community feel flu shots are actually worthless. Consider this quote: "There is no evidence that any influenza vaccine thus far developed is effective in preventing or mitigating any attack of influenza… they are worthless." Dr. J. Anthony Morris, research virologist and former Chief Vaccine Control Officer of the FDA. Today's medical experts do not suggest a flu vaccine for healthy, young people.

Although rare, the flu vaccine can produce side effects and adverse reactions:
• Guillain Barre syndrome
• Mild body aches and slight fever
• Dangerous for those allergic to eggs

Having a strong immune system is the best protection against the flu. Many herbs help greatly in that process. The herbs elder, andrographis, garlic; the homeopathic remedy, oscillococcinum; and the trace mineral, selenium, are all proven flu remedies to choose from. Further, washing hands regularly with soap and water and avoiding people who are sick can go a long way to helping you stay "flu-free." For all of my detailed recommendations to help overcome flu, bronchitis and pneumonia, please see pg. 136.

What about Bronchitis?

Chronic bronchitis is an inflammatory infection of the bronchi. Experts see it as a direct result of prolonged exposure to irritants like cigarette smoke and environmental chemicals. The typical victim is forty or older, with low immunity from stress, fatigue or smoking. Viral bronchitis affecting women is very hard to treat, lasts from 3 weeks to 5 months, and does not go away on its own. Chronic bronchitis can be incapacitating and lead to serious lung disease. Acute bronchitis is generally self-limiting, like a bad chest cold, with eventual complete healing.

Pneumonia and pleurisy are inflammatory lung diseases. Bacterial pneumonia is caused by staph, strep or *pneumo-bacilli*; it responds to antibiotics, both medical and herbal. Viral pneumonia is an acute systemic disease caused by virulent viruses; it does not respond to antibiotics. Herbal antivirals have shown some success. Pleurisy, an inflammation of the pleura membrane surrounding the lungs, often accompanies pneumonia. Pneumonias drastically weaken the immune system. It can take 3 months to recover strength and up to 2 years to be able to resist a cold without falling victim to another bout of pneumonia.

Do you have Flu, Bronchitis, or Pneumonia?

Here are some ways to tell. Also, see page 132 for flu symptoms.

Acute Bronchitis: deep chest cold; slight fever; headache, nausea, lung and body aches; hacking, mucous-producing cough.

Chronic Bronchitis: bronchial tissue inflamed; mucous thick and profuse; difficult breathing from clogged airways; repeated attacks of acute bronchitis; chest congestion; mucous-y cough and wheezing for 3 months; fatigue, weakness and weight loss.

Pneumonia: inflamed lungs and chest pain; aggravated flu and cold symptoms, worsening after 5 days; swollen lymph glands; difficult breathing; heavy coughing and expectoration; back and body aches; chills and high fever; sore throat; inability to "get over it"; fluid in lymph and lungs; great fatigue which remains for six to eight weeks even after recovery.

Flu, bronchitis and pneumonia can be serious diseases. Do not risk your health if you have major difficulty breathing. Short term heroic medicine may be necessary. Newer broad spectrum drugs can sometimes give your body a "breather" from the infection trauma and are less harmful to normal body functions than most primary antibiotics. Ask your physician.

Healing Diet for Flu, Bronchitis and Pneumonia

Diet Watchwords

1. Get rid of the infected, thick mucous with the cleansing diet below for 1 – 3 days. Then follow a vegetarian, light "green" diet, high in vegetable proteins, low in meat, dairy foods and animal fats, for 3 weeks to allow lungs to heal easily. Avoid sugars, dairy foods, starchy and fatty foods during healing to reduce congestion (these foods allow a place for the virus to live).

2. Take cleansing broths, hot tonics, high vitamin C juices, vegetable juices and green drinks. Avoid alcohol.

3. Take flax seed tea each night during acute stages to cleanse the colon (where infected mucous builds up).

4. During the recuperation stage: Have a salad every day, cultured foods: Rejuvenative Foods Vegi Delite Sauerkraut, yogurt and kefir, for friendly flora replacement, and steamed vegetables with brown rice for strength.

5. Avoid alcohol and tobacco—they are immune suppressors. Avoid caffeine foods—they inhibit iron and zinc absorption.

6. As an emergency measure for sinusitis, take fresh grated horseradish root in a spoon with lemon juice. Hang over a sink immediately to expel large quantities of mucous.

7. If you just can't seem to "get over it:" make up 1 gallon of Crystal Star® Cleansing & Purifying™ Tea; take 5 to 6 cups daily with 15 Fiber & Herbs Colon Cleanse™ capsules daily until the virus is removed (about 1 week).

The night before you begin…

Take a gentle herbal laxative. Make a onion-honey syrup: Put 5 – 6 chopped onions and ½ cup honey in a pot and cook over very low heat for two hours. Strain and take 1 tbsp. every two hours for the next 3 days.

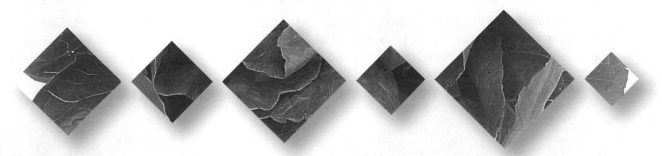

The next day...

On rising: Take a hot lemon-maple syrup-water drink each morning, or a cup of green tea, or aloe vera juice to rebalance body chemistry; or a potassium juice (pg. 16), or CRYSTAL STAR® RESTORE YOUR STRENGTH™ drink.

Breakfast: have grapefruit juice with 1 tsp. green superfood, like ESTEEM GREEN HARVEST or WAKUNAGA KYO-GREEN; or pineapple juice, a natural expectorant—add 1 tbsp. of a green superfood like SUN WELLNESS CHLORELLA.

Mid-morning: take a carrot juice or mixed fresh vegetable juice such as Personal Best V-8 (page 18).

Lunch: have a green drink like GREEN FOODS GREEN MAGMA or CRYSTAL STAR® ENERGY GREEN RENEWAL™.

Mid-afternoon: CRYSTAL STAR® D-CONGEST™ spray or mullein tea with NEW CHAPTER GINGER WONDER SYRUP.

Dinner: have a Potassium broth (page 16), or NATURE'S PATH TRACE-MIN-LYTE for electrolytes. Or make an electrolyte broth, rich in zinc, vitamin A, C, potassium and magnesium: In 2½ cups water, cook 1½ cups mixed vegetables (carrots, broccoli, dark leafy greens, celery and parsley), with 1 tbsp. miso. Strain and take broth.

Before Bed: have cranberry or celery juice, or a cup of miso soup with 1 tsp. RED STAR nutritional yeast.

Choose 2 or 3 supplements to help you overcome flu and bronchitis faster:

- **Acute flu stage:** CRYSTAL STAR® VIREX™ caps to raise body temperature to reduce virus replication (with CRYSTAL STAR® DR. ENZYME WITH PROTEASE & BROMELAIN™ for best results); Boiron Oscillococcinum (take at first sign for best results); Vitamin C crystals: ¼ tsp. every half hour to bowel tolerance to flush out infection. Andrographis drops; LIFE RISING YIN CHIAO; NUTRIBIOTIC GRAPEFRUIT SEED extract drops; or Olive leaf extract capsules 2 – 6 daily.
- **Flu infection fighters:** CRYSTAL STAR® ANTI-BIO™ caps (anti-viral support) every 2 hours until improvement; NATURE'S PATH SILVER-LYTE ionized silver; EAST PARK FLU BAN OLIVE LEAF caps or OREGANO oil capsules, 3x daily; HEALTH FROM THE SUN FLUGUARD (antiretroviral boxwood); MERIX HEALTH PRODUCTS C &F CAPS (fast acting); BONESET TEA (or homeopathic *Eupatorium Perfoliatum*) or NATURE'S WAY SAMBUCOL elderberry syrup, inhibits flu virus.
- **Relieve bronchitis inflammation and infection:** Oregano oil as directed. CRYSTAL STAR® ANTI-BIO™ caps 6x daily; Reishi mushroom extract, or PLANETARY REISHI MUSHROOM SUPREME, for T-cell defense. EIDON SELENIUM DROPS (to prevent virus mutation) or CRYSTAL STAR® IODINE, POTASSIUM, SILICA™ extract for bio-available silica; Zinc lozenges deactivate throat virus activity or CRYSTAL STAR® ZINC SOURCE™ throat rescue spray.
- **Speed up recovery time:** Glutamine 1000 mg. 3x daily; astragalus or reishi mushroom extract 4x daily; Garlic-ginger tea 2 cups daily or WAKUNAGA AGED GARLIC EXTRACT; Cayenne/bayberry caps normalize glands; LANE LABS ADVACAL reduces achiness (a sign the body is drawing on bone calcium); Chamomile tea (relieves pain).
- **Restore immune response:** NUTRICOLOGY NAC a powerful immune booster, 1000 mg. daily, or NUTRICOLOGY LACTOFERRIN WITH COLOSTRUM; Panax ginseng or astragalus to boost lymphocytes and interferon; C'EST SI BON CHLORENERGY; OPCs from white pine or grapeseed, 100 mg. 3x daily; CoQ-10, 200 mg. daily.
- **Expectorants relieve irritating mucous:** CRYSTAL STAR® D-CONGEST™ spray; YOGI BREATHE DEEP tea; ESTEEM BREATHE EASY caps; Lobelia extract drops in water; NAC (N-acetyl-cysteine), or NUTRICOLOGY NAC 2 daily.

Bodywork can help you feel much better

- **Take a sauna:** follow with a brisk rubdown, chest-back percussion with a cupped hand to loosen mucous.
- **Apply your choice below to feel better faster:**
  - alternating hot and cold witch hazel compresses to the chest. Use eucalyptus oil in a vaporizer.
  - a hot cayenne/ginger poultice: Mix powders: ½ tsp. cayenne, 1 tbsp. lobelia, 3 tbsp. slippery elm, 2 tbsp. ginger and enough water to make a paste. Leave on chest 1 hour.
  - a mustard plaster to chest to stimulate lungs and draw out poisons: Mix 1 tbsp. mustard powder, 1 egg, 3 tbsp. flour and water to make a paste. Leave on until skin turns pink.
  - tea tree oil on the chest, or apply EARTH'S BOUNTY O₂ OXY-SPRAY on the chest.
- **Do deep breathing exercises daily,** morning and before bed to clear lungs especially during recovery. Breathe in, pushing abdomen out, then from chest to completely fill upper and lower lungs.
- **Get plenty of rest.** Get a complete massage therapy treatment to cleanse remaining pockets of toxins.

Maintenance Recipes for a Immune-Building Diet

Use these recipes on an ongoing basis once your initial healing diet is producing good results.

Breakfast

Honey Apple Pancakes

1¼ cups whole wheat pastry
   flour
1 tsp. baking powder
¼ tsp. apple pie spice

¼ tsp. sea salt
¼ tsp. baking soda
1 egg
¾ cup apple juice

2 tbsp. honey
1 tbsp. grapeseed oil

Preheat a griddle to hot. In a bowl, mix the whole wheat pastry flour, baking powder, apple pie spice, sea salt and baking soda. In another bowl, mix the egg, apple juice, honey, and grapeseed oil.

Stir mixtures together until slightly lumpy. Ladle onto hot oiled griddle, turn when bubbles appear and cook for 1 more minute. Makes 8 servings.

High Protein Fruit Breakfast Mix

For enzymes and skin tone.

Fruit Mix #1

½ cup fresh papaya, chopped
½ cup fresh strawberries,
   chopped

¼ cup almonds, toasted and
   sliced
¼ cup toasted sesame seeds
¼ cup prunes, chopped

¼ cup dried papaya (or dried
   pineapple), chopped
¼ cup vanilla yogurt

Fruit Mix #2

½ cup fresh grapes, sliced
½ cup fresh pineapple, sliced
¼ cup walnuts, toasted and
   chopped

¼ cup toasted sunflower
   seeds
¼ cup dried prunes, chopped

¼ cup raisins
¼ cup vanilla yogurt

Topping

2 tbsp. toasted wheat germ
2 tbsp. crystallized ginger,
   chopped

2 tsp. honey
2 tsp. lecithin granules

2 tsp. lemon juice
2 tsp. nutritional yeast flakes

Pick whichever fruit mixture appeals to you, and combine all ingredients in a bowl. Mix well. To make the topping, combine all of the topping ingredients in a small bowl and mix well. Pour the topping over either fruit mix. Makes two or three servings.

Nutrition per serving:			
Calories ----------- 466	Vitamin E --------- 9 IU	Cholesterol-------- 1 g.	Potassium --------- 744 mg.
Protein ----------- 14 g.	Carbohydrates ---- 63 g.	Calcium ---------- 178 mg.	Sodium----------- 41 mg.
Vitamin C--------- 52 mg.	Fiber ------------- 9 g.	Iron ------------- 4 mg.	
	Fat---------------- 21 g.	Magnesium ------- 156 mg.	

Healing drinks

Cold and Flu Tonic to Clear Head Congestion

4 cloves garlic, minced (or 2 tsp. garlic-lemon-sesame seasoning)
¼ tsp. cumin
¼ tsp. black pepper

½ tsp. hot mustard powder
1 tbsp. olive oil
1 cup water
1 tsp. turmeric
½ tsp. sesame salt

½ tsp. ground coriander (1 tbsp. fresh cilantro)
1 cup cooked split peas (or 1 cup frozen peas)

In a dry pan, toast the minced garlic, cumin, black pepper, and hot mustard powder until aromatic. Add the olive oil and stir well. Toast a little to blend. Add the water, turmeric, sesame salt, ground coriander, and cooked split peas. Simmer gently 5 minutes; then mix all ingredients in a blender. Makes 2 drinks.

Nutrition per serving:	Vitamin E --------- 1 IU	Cholesterol-------- 0	Potassium --------- 379 mg.
Calories ----------- 170	Carbohydrates ---- 23 g.	Calcium ----------- 34 mg.	Sodium----------- 540 mg.
Protein ----------- 9 g.	Fiber ------------- 4 g.	Iron -------------- 2 mg.	
Vitamin C--------- 3 mg.	Fat---------------- 4 g.	Magnesium ------- 38 mg.	

Morning Immuni-Tea

1 cup water
3 slices fresh ginger, peeled

2 tbsp. dried sage leaves (or 1 handful fresh sage leaves)

15 drops echinacea root extract
15 drops milk thistle seed extract

In a large teapot, simmer 1 cup water, the fresh ginger root and sage for 20 minutes. Strain. Add the echinacea extract and milk thistle seed extract. Makes 1 cup.

Virus Fighter Broth

¼ daikon radish, chopped with leaves

¼ burdock root, chopped
1 carrot, chopped

3 dried shiitake mushrooms, sliced

In a soup pot, cover the daikon radish, burdock root, and carrot with water. Soak the sliced shiitake mushrooms. Save soaking water and add to soup pot with sliced mushrooms. Simmer one hour. Add 1 dropper of echinacea or usnea extract. Makes 2 bowls.

Onion-Miso Antibiotic Broth

1 onion, chopped
½ tsp. sesame oil

1 stalk celery with leaves, diced
1 qt. vegetable broth

4 tbsp. miso
2 green onions, diced

Sauté the chopped onion in sesame oil for 5 minutes. Add the celery with leaves and sauté for another 2 minutes. Add the vegetable broth, cover, and simmer for 10 minutes. Add the miso and green onions. Remove from heat. Makes 6 small bowls of broth.

Nutrition per serving:	Vitamin E ---- trace quantities	Cholesterol-------- 0	Potassium --------- 84 mg.
Calories ----------- 49	Carbohydrates ---- 7 g.	Calcium ----------- 20 mg.	Sodium----------- 239 mg.
Protein ----------- 3 g.	Fiber ------------- 1 g.	Iron -------------- 1 mg.	
Vitamin C--------- 3 mg.	Fat ----------- trace quantities	Magnesium ------- 9 mg.	

Cold Defense Cleanser

Make this broth the minute you feel a cold coming on. It may prevent it.

1½ cups water	½ tsp. cayenne	1 tbsp. lemon juice
1 tbsp. honey	1 tsp. ground ginger	1 dropperful echinacea extract
1 tsp. garlic powder	3 tbsp. brandy	

In a soup pot, simmer the water, honey, garlic powder, cayenne, ground ginger, brandy, and lemon juice. Add 1 dropperful echinacea extract just before taking. Makes 2 drinks. (Best in small sips).

Soups, salads, appetizers

Fresh Goulash Salad

1 cup tomatoes, diced	4 tbsp. green onion, diced	a pinch of cayenne pepper
1 cup zucchini, grated	a few pinches of thyme, basil,	4 tbsp. sunflower seeds
1 cup corn kernels	oregano and marjoram	juice of ½ lemon
4 tbsp. bell pepper, chopped	1 tomato, chopped	

In a large mixing bowl, mix the diced tomatoes, grated zucchini, corn kernels, chopped bell pepper, green onion, and the herbs. Make a fresh goulash sauce: In a blender, mix the chopped tomato, cayenne pepper, sunflower seeds, and lemon juice. Pour over the salad. Makes 4 salads.

Wild Spring Herb and Flower Salad

½ head romaine lettuce, chopped	⅓ cup young nasturtium leaves	¼ cup orange mint leaves
½ head frisee, chopped	½ cup arugula leaves	¼ cup lemon balm leaves
½ head red leaf lettuce, chopped	¼ cup sweet violets	2 tsp. baby dill, chopped
	⅓ cup sweet violet leaves	2 tbsp. sea greens (toasted)
	¼ cup fresh dandelion leaves	2 tbsp. olive oil
		2 tbsp. balsamic vinegar

In a large mixing bowl, mix the romaine lettuce, frisee, red leaf lettuce, nasturtium leaves, arugula leaves, sweet violets, sweet violet leaves, fresh dandelion leaves, orange mint leaves, lemon balm leaves, baby dill and toasted sea greens. Pour the olive oil and balsamic vinegar over the salad. Makes 6 salads.

Four Mushroom Immune Booster

1 tbsp. sesame oil	3 oz. maitake mushrooms	3 spears Belgian endive, finely sliced
2 garlic cloves, minced	3 oz. portobello mushroom	½ head red leaf lettuce, chopped
2 tsp. pickled ginger, minced	2 tbsp. balsamic vinegar	1 head radicchio, chopped
3 oz. oyster mushrooms	¼ cup soy sauce	
3 oz. shiitake mushrooms	¼ cup seasoned stock	

In a skillet, sauté the minced garlic and pickled ginger in 1 tbsp. sesame oil. Add the oyster mushrooms, shiitake mushrooms, maitake mushrooms and portobellos, and balsamic vinegar. Sauté for another 4 minutes. Add the soy sauce, seasoned stock; and simmer for another 2 minutes. In a bowl, mix the Belgian endive, red leaf lettuce, and radicchio. Divide mix between salad plates; pile on mushroom mix. Sprinkle with dulse flakes. Makes 6 servings.

Creamy Rice Salad

1½ cups salted water	½ cup lemon-lime yogurt	½ tsp. sesame salt
6 oz. white basmati rice or golden rose rice	½ cup green onions, thinly sliced	1 cup cocktail tomatoes, halved
1 cup frozen green peas	¼ cup parsley, chopped	1 cup hothouse cucumber, diced
½ cup low-fat mayonnaise	¼ tsp. lemon-pepper seasoning	½ cup celery, diced
		Bibb lettuce leaves

In a large soup pot, bring the salted water to a boil. Add the rice and return to boil. Cover and cook over low heat until water is absorbed and rice is tender, about 40 minutes. Remove from heat, add the frozen green peas, fluff with a fork; set aside. Make the dressing. In a bowl, mix the low-fat mayonnaise, lemon-lime yogurt, green onions, parsley, lemon-pepper seasoning, and sesame salt. Let sit to allow flavors to bloom. Stir the halved tomatoes, diced hothouse cucumber, and diced celery into dressing. Add dressing and veggies to rice blend; toss to mix. Serve in large bowls lined with Bibb lettuce leaves. Makes 6 servings.

Nutrition per serving:	Vitamin C --------- 20 mg.	Fat ----------------- 1 g.	Magnesium ------- 22 mg.
Calories ----------- 169	Vitamin E --------- 1 IU	Cholesterol-------- 1 mg.	Potassium --------- 314 mg.
Protein ----------- 6 g.	Carbohydrates ---- 35 g.	Calcium ----------- 65 mg.	Sodium------------ 268 mg.
Vitamin A --------- 88 IU	Fiber -------------- 3 g.	Iron -------------- 1 mg.	

Traditional Healing Chicken Soup

4 lbs. uncooked organic chicken	4 leeks, quartered	¾ tsp. pepper
5 carrots, quartered	4 celery ribs, cut in 2" lengths	2 qts. organic chicken stock
3 parsnips, quartered	2 whole bay leaves	4 cups water
	1 tsp. sea salt	

Rinse the organic chicken pieces and put in a large soup pot with the carrots, parsnips, leeks, celery ribs, bay leaves, sea salt, pepper, organic chicken stock, and water. Bring to a boil slowly. Reduce heat and simmer, uncovered, skimming off fat and foam until chicken is tender—about 1 hour. Strain; transfer chicken and veggies with a slotted spoon to a platter. Cover. Return broth to soup pot and boil until liquid is reduced to 6 cups, about 30 minutes. Season again. Remove bones from chicken, tear into bite size pieces. Divide chicken and vegetables between soup bowls. Pour broth over and serve. Makes 6 – 8 servings.

High Mineral Grilled Red Onions

2 tsp. dry mint	1 tsp. sea salt	4 large red onions, sliced in thin rings
2 tsp. dry oregano	4 tbsp. balsamic vinegar	
1 tsp. honey	3 tbsp. olive oil	olive oil

In a large shallow dish, mix the mint, oregano, honey, sea salt, balsamic vinegar and olive oil. Add the red onion rings; let marinate, covered and refrigerated overnight, turning once. Heat a BBQ grill until it's quite hot. Remove onions; discard marinade. Brush with olive oil; grill in a BBQ basket, turning once, for about 8 minutes or until tender. Season to taste; serve hot. Makes 6 servings.

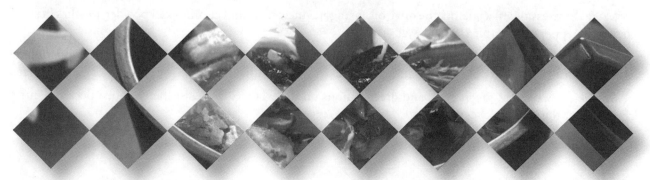

Pear and Chevre Salad with Toasted Walnuts

½ cup walnut pieces	½ tsp. garlic-lemon seasoning	1 bunch watercress
1 tsp. grapeseed oil	2 pinches white pepper	8 oz. mild goat cheese (chevre), or
½ cup walnut oil	2 heads Boston or Bibb lettuce	feta cheese
1 tbsp. red wine vinegar	1 bunch arugula	3 ripe pears, peeled, thin sliced

In a skillet, pan roast the walnut pieces in 1 tsp. grapeseed oil until fragrant. In a small bowl, make the dressing: mix the walnut oil, red wine vinegar, garlic-lemon seasoning and pinches of white pepper. Stir in walnuts.

In a large bowl, tear heads of Boston or Bibb lettuce, arugula and watercress and toss together. Divide onto salad plates. Crumble the goat cheese or feta over greens. Place pear slices around the cheese. Pour dressing over. Makes 8 salads.

Entrées

Quick Homemade Vegetable Stew

4 tbsp. soy bacon bits	8 oz. package frozen baby	1 head green cabbage, shredded
3 garlic cloves, minced	lima beans	1 tbsp. tamari
2 tsp. olive oil	16 oz. package French cut	½ tsp. black pepper
1 lb. potatoes, cut into cubes	green beans	1 tsp. sea salt
2 carrots, sliced		a small handful fresh parsley,
4 cups salted water		chopped

In a skillet, sauté the soy bacon bits and minced garlic in 2 tsp. olive oil until aromatic. Add the cubed potatoes and carrots; saute, stirring frequently, for 5 minutes. Set aside.

In a large soup pot, bring the salted water to a boil. Add the frozen baby lima beans, and French cut green beans. When water returns to a boil, add the sautéed veggies, and simmer for 15 minutes. Add the shredded green cabbage and simmer for 10 more minutes. Season with the tamari, black pepper, and sea salt. Sprinkle with chopped parsley. Makes 6 servings.

Layered Chicken Salad

⅓ cup olive oil	1 small bunch spinach,	½ cup grated low-fat soy cheddar or
¼ cup tarragon vinegar	washed and torn	swiss cheese
½ tsp. ground cumin	2 large beefsteak tomatoes,	⅓ cup fresh parsley, chopped
1 tsp. chili powder	thinly sliced	½ cup green peas, steamed
a few pinches of sesame salt,	1½ cups cooked organic	3 green onions, minced
black pepper and nutmeg	chicken breast, diced	⅓ cup chopped pecans, toasted
1 head Romaine lettuce, shaved		

Make the dressing: In a jar, mix the olive oil, tarragon vinegar, ground cumin, chili powder, pinches of sesame salt, black pepper and nutmeg. Shake well.

Cover bottom of a large clear salad bowl with shaved Romaine. Cover lettuce with the spinach and tomatoes. Cover tomatoes with the cooked chicken. Cover chicken with the grated low-fat soy cheddar or Swiss cheese.

Sprinkle the parsley, green peas, and green onions on the salad. Cover with the chopped pecans. Pour the dressing over the salad. Makes 6 servings.

Vegetable Jambalaya

12 oz. fresh firm tofu, frozen	1 red bell pepper, diced	½ tsp. dry sage
2 cups Italian plum tomatoes, chopped	1½ cups organic vegetable broth	½ tsp. marjoram
1 cup dry red wine	1 cup uncooked brown basmati rice	1½ tsp. lemon-pepper seasoning
2 tbsp. olive oil	12 oz. package baked tempeh, cut in bite-size pieces	½ cup arugula leaves, chopped
3 cloves garlic, minced		hot pepper sauce
1 yellow onion, diced	½ tsp. dry thyme	
1 rib celery, diced		

Thaw tofu and crumble in a bowl. Set aside. Marinate 2 cups chopped Italian plum tomatoes in 1 cup dry red wine for 1 hour. Set aside.

In a soup pot, sauté the garlic, yellow onion, celery, and red bell pepper in 2 tbsp. olive oil for 10 minutes. Add the organic vegetable broth and bring to a boil. Add the rice, tempeh pieces, crumbled tofu, marinated tomatoes and wine marinade. Add enough water to cover ingredients. Return to a boil, reduce heat and simmer 50 minutes, stirring occasionally, until rice absorbs the liquid. Season with the thyme, sage, marjoram, and lemon-pepper seasoning. Fluff with a fork. Top with the arugula leaves and dashes of hot pepper sauce. Makes 6 servings.

Healthy dessert options

Blueberry Cobbler

3 cups blueberries	¼ tsp. cinnamon	2 tsp. brown sugar
¼ cup currants	¼ tsp. vanilla extract	3 tbsp. whole wheat pastry flour
1 tbsp. brown sugar	1 cup rolled oats	1½ tbsp. soft butter

Preheat oven to 325°F. In a medium bowl, combine the blueberries, currants, brown sugar, cinnamon and vanilla extract. Mix gently. Transfer to an 8" square baking pan. In a bowl, combine the rolled oats, brown sugar, whole wheat pastry flour and butter. Mix with fingers until mixture is crumbly. Spoon onto blueberry mixture. Bake 45 minutes until brown. Cool before serving. Makes 4 – 6 servings.

Pineapple-Cranberry Bars

1½ cups fresh cranberries	2 eggs	½ tsp. nutmeg
1½ cups orange juice	2½ cups whole wheat pastry flour	1 cup chopped walnuts
4 tbsp. butter	2 tsp. baking powder	¾ cup shredded coconut
2 tbsp. maple syrup	1 tsp. baking soda	¾ cup crushed pineapple, drained
1 tsp. grated orange zest	½ tsp. cinnamon	

Preheat oven to 350°F. Have ready a grapeseed oil-sprayed 9" x 13" baking pan. In a skillet, sauté the cranberries and orange juice until cranberries pop. Beat in a bowl the butter, maple syrup, grated orange zest, eggs and the cranberry-orange juice mix. In another bowl, stir together: the whole wheat pastry flour, baking powder, baking soda, cinnamon and nutmeg. Mix both together and stir in the chopped walnuts. Spoon into baking pan. Top with a mixture of the shredded coconut and drained pineapple. Bake for 20 – 25 minutes or until a toothpick comes out clean. Cool and cut. Makes 24 bars.

Osteoporosis: Building Bone with a Mineral-Rich Diet

Few things age a person as quickly as osteoporosis (porous bone), a disease that robs bones of their density and strength, making them thinner, more prone to break. Eventually, bone mass decreases below the level required to support the body. Over 28 million Americans suffer from osteoporosis today, and experts from the National Osteoporosis Foundation predict 40 million Americans will suffer from osteoporosis by the year 2015.

Long considered a woman's problem, because of its female hormone involvement, osteoporosis affects from 35 to 50% of women in the first 5 years after menopause. For women, osteoporosis risk is greater than the combined risks of breast, uterine and ovarian cancers. In fact, half of all women over 50 will suffer an osteoporosis-related fracture in her lifetime. Most of these are vibrant women at the height of their careers with no outward signs of poor health. Most have no idea their bones are becoming weaker and more brittle until they actually break. Bone loss is greatest in the high weight-bearing bones—hips, spine and ribs.

Osteoporosis also affects men, just at a later age, with less ferocity. Some bone loss occurs in both sexes around 45 years of age. But a greater testosterone supply and more bone tissue offer men some protection from osteoporosis. Yet today's men, in ever-increasing numbers are suffering from the disease. In America, by age 75, one-third of all men are affected by osteoporosis. One in eight men will suffer an osteoporosis-related fracture.

The Fosamax Problem

Over 800,000 women in the U.S. today take Fosamax *(Alendronate sodium)*, the first non-hormonal drug approved to treat osteoporosis. Fosamax belongs to a class of drugs called "bisphosphonates" which inhibit the action of osteoclasts, the cells in the skeleton that break down bone. When Fosamax was FDA approved in April of 1997, the public was ecstatic. Preliminary reports found Fosamax could reduce height loss and risk of fractures without any serious side effects.

However, as Fosamax made its way into the American public at large, its downfalls became glaringly clear. Esophageal injury caused by this drug is a real threat with at least 250 reports linking Fosamax. Of these, 51 cases were considered serious. I have heard from these women myself. Ulcers in the esophagus, severe chest pain, blurry vision, difficulty swallowing, headaches, and gastrointestinal distress are other side effects of Fosamax therapy. The latest research shows that if left untreated, eye inflammation resulting from Fosamax use could lead to blindness!

Taking Fosamax with NSAIDs (non steroidal anti-inflammatory drugs) or aspirin is a really bad idea as risk for gastrointestinal problems can skyrocket from both drugs! Leading health experts now believe Fosamax actually *blocks* bone resorption, the process which removes weakening bones to allow space for new healthy bone growth, a definite concern for people with osteoporosis trying to build strong bones. Over time, women using this drug may actually see an increase in fractures due to bone weakening. In addition, Fosamax stays in the body 10 – 15 years after taking it, so residual effects from the drug may continue to surface for years!

Are you at risk for osteoporosis?

Check the following risk factors:
- Post-menopausal with family history of osteoporosis (high risk for women who have not had children).
- Women and men over 75 years; women over 45 with a history of calcium and vitamin D deficiency.
- A consistently high consumption of tobacco, coffee and animal protein.
- Long courses of steroid drugs. Research shows that over a long period of time these drugs tend to leach potassium from the system, weakening the bones.

- Long use of synthetic thyroid. The drug Synthroid increases risk for both osteoporosis and high cholesterol, and may also aggravate weight problems.
- Women who had their ovaries removed before menopause, who had an early menopause (before 45 years old), or those with a history of irregular periods. Hormone and calcium deficiencies are common in women with irregular menstrual cycles, those who exercise excessively or who have eating disorders.

A bone mineral density (BMD) test is best. If you think you're at risk, ask your physician or local pharmacy about bone mineral density screening. **Other early warning signs to watch for:**
- Bone loss is greatest in the spine, hips and ribs, so osteoporosis begins to show up as chronic back and leg pain. Bone pain may also occur in the spine, affecting the cranial nerves.
- Look for loss of bone in the jaw and tooth sockets. Bone may draw away from the teeth, causing them to loosen, or fall out. Look for unusually frequent dental problems, too.
- Vision defects or facial tics may also occur due to bone marrow obliteration.

Note: Use pH paper (sold in most laboratory supply stores or college book stores) to test your urine. A habitual reading below pH 7 usually means calcium and bone loss. Above pH 7 indicates a low risk. You can also get a bone mineral density (BMD) measurement test through your doctor or local pharmacy. The new DEXA (Duel Energy X-ray Absorptiometry) bone density tests enable doctors to measure bone strength without being confused by muscle, fat or skin. By doing this, the DEXA method is able to more accurately measure bone strength in the spine and hips, where the majority of disabling fractures occur.

Why is the rate of hip fractures in the United States so high? Our bone-stealing diet and lack of exercise are the heart of the problem. Highly processed, additive-laden foods set the stage for bone loss.

Is your diet "bad to the bone," putting you at risk for osteoporosis?

- **Is your diet low in minerals?** You're endangering your bones and your digestion. Minerals are critical for a strong skeleton, and they're the bonding agents between you and your food. Low minerals means low thyroid function and poor collagen protein development, also part of osteoporosis. Over 50% of American women suffer from calcium deficiency alone.
- **Is your diet low in fresh foods**? Then your body is low in essential enzymes. Osteoporosis is at least in part, a result of enzyme deficiency. I find this is especially true for older men who try to correct digestive problems with handfuls of antacids.
- **Is your diet excessively high in protein?** There is a clear relationship between high protein consumption and osteoporosis. Popular high protein diets today severely restrict whole grains and carbs, so your bones may be dangerously low in calcium. The American Dietetic Association says "when protein consumption is doubled, calcium loss increases 50%!" Animal protein is an even bigger danger for osteoporosis. The kidneys pull calcium from the bones trying to rid the body of the excess nitrogen found in animal protein. Studies of vegetarians and non-vegetarians from age 60 – 90, reveal that the mineral content in meat eaters' bones decreased 35% over time, while mineral content of a vegetarian's bones decreased only 18%.
- **Is your diet is high in red meats, sodas, caffeine foods and alcohol?** Your body's pH is critical to healthy bone. Just as the body works to maintain a normal temperature of 98.6°, so your metabolism works to maintain normal blood pH at around 7.3. The blood tries to balance body pH by withdrawing calcium from your bones, so these foods create over-acid blood which puts you at risk for bone loss. As much as 60 mg. of alkaline minerals like calcium can be leeched from the skeleton every day to help neutralize overly acidic blood pH. Over time, this mineral loss can translate into major bone loss from demineralization.

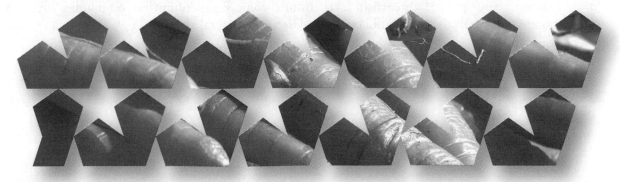

About 80% of your diet should be alkaline; about 20% acid-forming foods.

- Alkaline foods: All vegetables, most fruits, sea greens, sprouted seeds and beans, seeds (except sesame), almonds, grains like millet, quinoa, amaranth and buckwheat, olive oil, herbs and herb teas.
- Acid-forming foods: Animal foods (meat, fish, poultry, dairy), wheat, oats, white rice, breads, acid fruits like cranberries and strawberries, sunflower, safflower and grapeseed oils, the herb stevia (a sugar replacement).
- Acid-forming foods to avoid: Sugar, sweeteners like saccharin and Nutrasweet, candy, soft drinks, all processed and chemicalized foods, white flour products, nuts (except almonds) and nut butters, alcoholic beverages, and commercial vinegar containing foods. USDA research finds that men who consume five cans of cola a day for three months absorb less calcium, increasing risk for bone deterioration and breaks! Soda consumption has doubled since the 1970s, a major reason while osteoporosis incidence is only growing in our society. High levels of phosphorous in meat and highly processed foods also deprive the body of calcium.

Important news about bone loss risk factors...

If your diet is high in milk and dairy products you may be MORE at risk for osteoporosis! Most of us have been told from childhood to drink milk for strong bones. Advertising tells us that dairy foods are the best source of dietary calcium for bone protection. The ads don't tell you that it's been a hotly debated myth in the natural foods industry for years. The truth about drinking milk for strong bones? A twelve year, Harvard Health study of over 78,000 women reveals that high intake of milk and dairy products does not reduce bone breaks. In fact, proteins in milk can cause calcium loss through the urine. Beyond calcium loss, for up to 25% of all Americans, lactose intolerance means little calcium and minerals in dairy foods is even digested. Further, most commercial milk today is loaded with fat, hormone-disrupting chemicals and antibiotics, no good for health.

Your weight loss diet may be weakening your bones. A recent study shows that for each 10% drop in weight, there is a two-fold increase in the risk of hip fractures in older women. When blood calcium levels become low from a severe weight loss diet, your bones release their calcium to keep the rest of the body running smoothly. Even taking calcium supplements may not be enough to maintain bone mass during dieting. Women who crash diet regularly show up with estrogen deficiency, also involved in bone loss. Doubly discouraging is the fact that many studies show most women gain all of their weight back after strict dieting. After many years of developing natural weight loss programs, I find dieters get better results when they add minerals via green drinks and vegetable juices. Women who drink high mineral juices don't gain the lost weight back, either as quickly or as much. Since a majority of American women say they're on a weight control diet most of the time, a low fat diet, while adding high mineral drinks from food or herb sources to avoid bone loss is a better weight loss choice.

Beyond diet, your lifestyle influences osteoporosis.

- Lack of exercise stunts healthy bone growth. Too little sunlight means less vitamin D is available for bone building.
- Smoking interferes with your body's calcium and estrogen production. Women smokers have 10% lower bone density and are more vulnerable to fractures than non smokers.
- Depression may cause bone loss. People with a history of severe depression have 15% less bone density in their lower spines than non-depressed people.
- Overusing steroids, antibiotics or tobacco, and too much alcohol severely reduces mineral absorption.
- Stress may raise your risk. High cortisol levels from chronic stress inhibit bone building, suppress the production of androgens that help build bones, and decrease mineral absorption.

- Ovary removal puts you at greater risk for osteoporosis.
- Fluoridated water is a risk factor. New studies link hip fractures to fluoridated water. Fluoridated water literally leeches calcium from the bones. The Journal of American Medical Association says hip fracture rates are much higher in people living in fluoridated communities. New studies prove that fluoride's cumulative effect on bone is devastating. Increased hip fractures have been reported in at least nine studies from five countries even at relatively "low" water fluoride levels. The World Health Organization says "individuals consuming between 2 – 8 mg. of fluoride/day (2 – 8 liters of fluoridated water), can develop the pre-clinical symptoms of skeletal fluorosis," (arthritis-like symptoms). Drinking the recommended 6 – 8 glasses a day of water may put you at risk. Fluoride comes from other sources than your water. Fruits and vegetables (from fluoridated irrigation water), juices, soft drinks, beverages, and dental products all increase your fluoride intake.

Can you beat osteoporosis without drugs? How do hormones fit into the picture?

Clearly estrogen is involved in bone-building and bone loss. Estrogen has been the mainstay of orthodox medicine therapy for decades. Yet while some tests find estrogen does inhibit bone cell death, other tests find that as many as 15% of women on estrogen therapy continue to lose bone! Most experts agree that declining estrogen levels after menopause do not by themselves cause osteoporosis. I believe hormone balance (not merely replacement) is the key. We know progesterone is a key to laying down and strengthening bone, and may even help reverse osteoporosis in some women. Thyroid function and collagen development are critical as well. Low androgen hormone levels of DHEA and testosterone play a role in men's osteoporosis.

Ipriflavone, synthesized from isoflavones (plant estrogens), is a new leader in natural osteoporosis treatment. Studies find ipriflavone inhibits bone cell death and may even increase new bone growth. Three different long term studies from Italy show that 200 mg. of ipriflavone 3 times daily is effective against bone loss.

Can progesterone creams derived from wild yam roots really stave off osteoporosis? Progesterone actually enhances bone formation, something estrogen cannot do. In a recent study on women with osteoporosis, a bone scan showed up to *5% new bone density* in an eighteen month period after the women used a natural wild yam progesterone cream, along with a good nutritional program. A four-year study shows that plant-derived progesterone creams increased bone density anywhere up to 40% for women from 45 to 60 years of age. Results were even better when a germanium supplement was added orally. I respect the work of California physician John Lee M.D., who found some women with severe osteoporosis experience an amazing 30% increase in bone density after using progesterone cream in combination with lifestyle therapy. In the most severe cases, a small amount of bioidentical estradiol, in combination with progesterone cream, produced the best results.

A man's testosterone supply protects against osteoporosis. Can extra testosterone help women arrest osteoporosis? Testosterone drugs are not a good option for women. Male characteristics such as voice deepening, facial and chest hair growth surface quickly.

What about calcium? It's a cornerstone treatment for osteoporosis. Calcium is the most abundant mineral in the body, and 98 percent of all calcium is stored in our bones. But calcium isn't the only mineral involved in bone. Two-thirds of the magnesium in the body is also contained in the bones. Osteoporosis is the result of much more than a calcium deficiency and preventing osteoporosis is more than adding more calcium to your diet.

Do you have a calcium deficiency?

Calcium deficiencies show up pre-menstrually as back pain, cramping, or tooth pain. (A calcium supplement before your period helps these symptoms disappear if this is your problem.) Note: women who think they are helping themselves by taking calcium-containing antacids may be doing just the opposite. Antacids are linked to easy fractures because they block stomach acids, which some specialists say, causes reduced bone growth and poor nutrient absorption.

Boost all your minerals instead! Other minerals, like silica and magnesium are just as important to bone health. Bone strength is best enhanced when calcium is used with other nutrients, such as B vitamins, magnesium, silica, manganese and boron, especially for older women who do not retain calcium very well by itself.

You need a constant supply of mineral-rich foods and nutrients to replenish the organic matrix of bone. Organically grown foods, sea plants and herbs are becoming the best way to get them. Foods and herbs are used by the body's own enzyme action, as a whole, (not a partial substance), and this is a key to their effectiveness. Vegetarians traditionally have denser, better-formed bones, because the most usable minerals come from leafy greens, sprouts, whole grains, soy foods, eggs, and vegetable complex carbohydrates.

Want to know your mineral status?

EIDON'S MINERAL BALANCING program analyzes your mineral levels through hair analysis tests, and designs you a personalized mineral supplement program to get your body back in balance. Call 800-700-1169 to learn more.

A Healing Plan for (almost) Unbreakable Bones

Successful intervention against osteoporosis isn't a pill… it's a program.

Osteoporosis is far more complex than was thought even just 5 years ago. Bone and cartilage are living tissue, an ever-changing infrastructure. Osteoporosis involves both mineral and non-mineral elements, so your bones need a full range of support nutrients. Although it is a life-threatening disease, osteoporosis is a lifestyle disease… that means we can do something about it. Bone loss can be arrested; remaining bone can be preserved; new bone mass can even be rebuilt with a vigorous osteoporosis intervention program. Once you know what contributes to bone weakening, and what contributes to bone building, you have the power to keep your bones strong. The most successful treatment involves not only normalizing hormone levels, but also improving lifestyle and dietary habits that we know accelerate bone loss. It's not just a case of adding estrogen, progesterone or even testosterone.

Osteoporosis Intervention Diet

Don't let osteoporosis steal your health! Nutritional therapy offers a broad base of both treatment and protection. Natural therapies can literally transform people crippled by osteoporosis. Start with diet improvements.

1. **Eat vitamin C-bioflav rich foods:** kiwis, oranges, grapefruit and potatoes enhance collagen production. Bioflavonoids boost collagen/connective tissue: Vitamin C or Ester C with bioflavs. up to 5000 mg. daily.

2. **Eat calcium, magnesium and potassium-rich foods:** broccoli, seafoods, eggs, yogurt, kefir, carrots, dried fruit, sprouts, miso, green and black beans, leafy greens, tofu, bananas, apricots and molasses. Mineral-rich veggies and herbs like oatstraw, burdock, dandelion and borage seed come without heavy protein, and offer high levels of vitamin K, which helps calcium attach to bone tissue. Try Bone Strength Snack Balls: Mix 1 cup sesame tahini, ½ cup honey, 2 tbsp. powdered ginseng, 3 tbsp. powdered dong quai, 3 tbsp. bee pollen, 1 tbsp. spirulina or barley grass, ½ cup ginseng/royal jelly/honey blend, ½ cup chopped walnuts, ½ cup raisins. Roll into a paste. Make balls. Roll in toasted amaranth, grapenuts, and 3 tbsp. dry dulse flakes. Chill.

3. **Skip the salt and add sea greens like nori, wakame, dulse or kombu to your diet.** 2 tbsp. daily, chopped on salad, soup, rice, even pizza, offer bone building minerals and vitamins, like D, E and K to boost adrenal production of steroidal hormones like estrogen, progesterone and DHEA—prime supports for bone health. Try a supplement like CRYSTAL STAR® OCEAN MINERALS™ caps or NATURE'S PATH TRACE-MIN-LYTE (sea plants and electrolytes).

4. **Add more deep green veggies.** They provide all essential minerals for rebuilding bone. Use green superfoods. Green foods have a pH close to 7 which buffers uric acid and lactic acids, and helps the body change from catabolic (breaking down) to anabolic (building up) bone mass. Try CRYSTAL STAR® ENERGY GREEN RENEWAL™, NUTRICOLOGY PRO GREENS WITH EFAs, FIT FOR YOU, INTL. MIRACLE GREENS, or JUST BARLEY.

5.   **Reduce protein from red meat and dairy foods.** They disrupt pH balance and lead to mineral loss. Get protein from fish, legumes, vegetables and sea greens instead. Drink juices like carrot and orange instead for extra calcium. One 8 oz. glass of fresh carrot juice has 400 mg. bioavailable calcium.

6.   **Avoid:** sugar, salty snack foods, hard alcohol, caffeine (except green or white tea or Crystal Star® Dr. Vitality™, which has bone building properties), tobacco, and nightshade plants that interfere with calcium absorption.

7.   **Boost collagen,** the protein that forms building blocks for bone and cartilage: A daily cup of fresh pineapple juice deters osteoporosis by providing manganese, which the body uses to make collagen. Sea veggies are good sources of manganese. Or try Lane Labs Toki™ Collagen Replacement Drink (noticeable results for bones).

Choose 2 or 3 osteoporosis protection supplements to really make a difference:

- **Balance your hormones** (don't just add estrogen): Ipriflavone 600 mg. daily, or Metabolic Response Modifiers Osteo-Max 200 mg. ipriflavone with 200 mg. MCHC; Crystal Star® Pro-est Balance™ roll-on, or Pure Essence Fem Creme. Take with Nutricology Germanium 150 mg. daily for best results (good activity). Crystal Star® Male Performance™ caps, 4 daily, for men.
- **Boost your minerals (not just calcium):** Lane Labs Advacal Ultra (clinically proven to increase bone density in the spine); Calcium citrate 1500 mg./magnesium 1000 mg. with boron 3 mg. (too much boron alone actually causes bone loss); Flora Vegesil for 6 months, or Ethical Nutrients Bone Builder with Silica (silica is the main mineral for bone regeneration via collagen-calcium production). Crystal Star® Calcium Magnesium Source™ and Iodine, Potassium, Silica Source™ extract. Trace Mineral Research Concentrace; or horsetail or nettles tea.
- **Boost mineral absorption:** Vitamin D 1000IU; marine carotene 100,000IU, or Phycotene Microclusters available at royalbodycare.com; zinc 30 mg.; boron 3 mg.; vitamin K 100 mcg.; Alacer Emergen-C or Nature's Path Trace-lyte for electrolytes and pH balance.
- **Boost bone health with EFAs:** Crystal Star® Evening Primrose Pearls, 6 daily; Spectrum Naturals 1300 mg. EPO; Barlean's Omega Twin flax-borage; Nature's Secret Ultimate Oil.
- **Add enzymes to boost nutrient absorption:** for men, Herbal Products Dvlpt. Power Plus Enzymes or Nature's Secret Rezyme; for women, Crystal Star® Dr. Enzyme™ with Protease & Bromelain; Transformation Digestzyme.
- Floradix Calcium, Magnesium, Vitamin D & Zinc herbal syrup. Note: Low stomach acid diminishes calcium absorption. Herbal "bitters" encourage the body to produce more stomach acid.

Bodywork is critical for bone density growth.

- **Smoking leaches bone nutrients:** Smoking a pack a day results in a 10% loss in bone density. Smoking also appears to interfere with estrogen production.
- **Get early morning sunlight** on the body every day possible for vitamin D to enhance bone.
- **Avoid:** fluorescent lighting, electric blankets, aluminum cookware all tend to leach calcium from the body.
- **Exercise is as important as a good diet for bones:** Exercise is a nutrient in itself. Duration of exercise is more important than intensity. Note: if you already have low bone density, start on a weight bearing exercise program after improvements from diet changes are seen in your bone scans in order to avoid injury. The best exercises are often water workouts. The water limits overdoing it, and is very forgiving to fragile bones. Numerous studies make it clear that physical exercise (at least one hour of moderate exercise 3 times a week) can prevent bone loss and actually increase bone mass. A lack of exercise doubles the rate of urinary and fecal calcium excretion, resulting in a significant negative calcium balance.
- **Pump a little iron for your bones:** People who do regular weight bearing exercises have denser bones than those who don't. Your bones can rebuild themselves, but only when they're used. A sedentary lifestyle increases osteoporosis risk. Power walking is good for bones, so are aerobic workouts, like Tae Bo, or weight bearing exercise 3 – 4 times a week (especially for men and women under 35 whose bone mass is still growing).

Building Strong Bones

Your bones are alive! Bone is living tissue that interweaves a mineral, inorganic matrix, and a non-mineral, organic matrix framework. A solid mineral base is of prime importance to bone health. Healthy bones are critical to your body's mineral needs because they act as your body's mineral reservoirs when it doesn't get enough minerals from your food.

Minerals and trace minerals are the building blocks of your cells, the basic elements your body needs for proper metabolism. Minerals are the bonding agents between the body and food. Without them, the body cannot absorb or utilize nutrients. Minerals regulate pH balance, transport body oxygen, and control electrolytic movement between cells, nerves and tissue. They play a key role in heart health, sugar and blood pressure regulation, and cancer prevention. Even small mineral deficiencies imbalance your body by mobilizing needed elements *out* of the various body 'reservoirs' to compensate. Immediate effects of this process are irritability, nervousness, or depression. A mineral-poor diet can mean osteoporosis, premature aging, hair loss, brittle nails, dry, cracked skin, forgetfulness, food allergies, back pain, PMS, poor motor coordination, joint deformity, difficult pregnancy, taste and smell loss, slow learning, poor attention span, and the inability to heal quickly. This is only a partial list. Minerals are important!

Our bodies don't make minerals. They must be taken in through food, drink or mineral baths. Unfortunately, today's fruits and vegetables lack good mineral quality. Years of pesticides, non-organic fertilizers, and chemical sprays have leached them out of the soil. High stress lifestyles and habits inhibit mineral absorption. Eating too much meat protein and too many preserved and over-refined foods, a lack of vitamin D from sunlight, and too little exercise, are involved in our lack of minerals. Excessive steroid and antibiotic use, tobacco, and too much alcohol, all contribute to mineral depletion and weakening of bone structure.

We begin to think about our bones as we age, but nearly 87% of teenage girls and 64% of teenage boys aren't getting enough calcium, let alone other bone-building nutrients. Extending those nutrient deficiency numbers means over half of America's future women, and one in eight men will develop osteoporosis fractures.

Mineral needs clearly increase as the body ages, requiring more digestive and enzyme help. Calcium is not even the main mineral for bone regeneration; silicon is. Pay extra attention to your bone health. New French research shows a significant correlation with increased hip fractures and fluoride in drinking water. Most of America's tap water (64%) is already fluoridated, with pending legislation on the books for the rest of our cities. If you have prematurely gray hair, it may be a sign you have decreased mineral bone mass.

Do you have weak bones?

Ask your local pharmacy about bone mineral density screening, and ask yourself the following questions.
• Do your bones break easily? And heal slowly?
• Do you have lots of dental plaque? Do you have gum disease? Do your teeth shift? Are they loose?
• Do you have prematurely gray hair (before 40)? Or unusually thin skin?
• Do your nails break easily and often?
• Are your muscles weak? Are your joints and tendons sore? Do you have chronic lower back pain?

Critical nutrients for strong bones:

• **Calcium:** green leafy vegetables, sea greens and seafoods are rich sources of calcium.
• **Silica:** strengthens bone connective tissue by crosslinking collagen strands. Silica is in mother's milk, leafy greens, brown rice, bell pepper. Herb sources: horsetail, boneset, oatstraw, dandelion, alfalfa, sea vegetables.
• **Magnesium:** involved in bone biochemical reactions. Chlorophyll-rich plants are rich in magnesium.
• **Vitamins:** B-6, B-12, folic acid and K help activate osteocalcin, the major noncollagen protein in bone. Leafy greens are excellent sources of vitamin K. Vitamin D from sunlight stimulates the absorption of calcium.
• **Enzymes:** transport nutrients, remove wastes, increase calcium absorption and other bone nutrients.

Strong Bones High Mineral Diet

Get serious early about taking care of your bones. Deposit structure building nutrients in your bone banks so you don't end up with low bone strength. Teenagers build the majority of their skeleton bones during adolescence. Most women stop building bone mass between 21 – 35 years of age. Bone mass for these women can decrease by about 1% a year. At menopause, bone loss can rise up to 5% each year. There is no accelerated phase of bone loss for men, yet they still have age-related bone loss.

On rising: a green protein drink - GREEN KAMUT GREEN KAMUT or JUST BARLEY in apple or orange juice.

Breakfast: mix 2 tbsp. each: toasted wheat germ, sesame seeds, RED STAR YEAST and lecithin granules. Sprinkle 2 tsp. on your breakfast foods—yogurt with fresh fruits, poached or baked eggs on whole grain toast, or whole grain cereal or pancakes with apple juice, soy milk, honey or yogurt.

Mid-morning: a potassium juice (page 16), CRYSTAL STAR® RESTORE YOUR STRENGTH™ drink; or carrot juice and miso soup with sea greens snipped on top; and crunchy veggie sticks with kefir cheese dip.

Lunch: have a veggie omelet and a carrot/raisin salad or a three bean salad; or a green salad with spinach, peppers, sprouts and lemon-oil dressing; or a veggie sandwich with avocado, soy cheese on whole grain bread.

Mid-afternoon: have a hard boiled egg with a yogurt dip and an herb tea like rose hips, nettles, dandelion, or a green drink like NUTRICOLOGY PRO GREENS; or have low-fat cheese with whole grain crackers, and bottled water.

Dinner: have a mushroom, asparagus, or broccoli quiche; or baked salmon with brown rice and peas; or a light Italian veggie pasta meal with tomatoes and onions; or a stir-fry with veggies and brown rice, and miso soup. Have a glass of wine for extra boron *before* dinner—liquids with meals inhibit mineral absorption.

Choose 2 or 3 supplements to boost your bone strength:

- **Build bones with more bone nutrients:** Herbs are a good bone-builders. Add silica: CRYSTAL STAR® IODINE, POTASSIUM & SILICA™; EIDON SILICA; BODY ESSENTIALS SILICA GEL, collagen formation. Add calcium: LANE LABS ADVACAL ULTRA (good clinical results); CRYSTAL STAR® CALCIUM MAGNESIUM SOURCE™ caps or extract; FLORA CALCIUM.
- **Improve assimilation of bone nutrients:** Magnesium, 400 mg. daily (esp. if celiac disease); Vitamin D 400IU daily; B-complex 100 mg. with extra B-6 100 mg., 400 mcg. Manganese, 5 mg.; Betaine HCl 650 mg.; ENZYMEDICA DIGEST or CRYSTAL STAR® DR. ENZYME™ WITH PROTEASE & BROMELAIN (provides amino acids that help calcium uptake).
- **Healthy glands mean good bones:** Estrogen-progesterone balancing herbs: CRYSTAL STAR® FEM SUPPORT™ CFS drops or PRO-EST BALANCE™ roll-on; MOON MAID PRO-MENO WILD YAM CREAM or royal jelly-ginseng capsules; DHEA 25 mg. daily; PURE ESSENCE LABS FEM CREME; INDIUM-EASE up to 694% higher gland mineral uptake.
- **For suspected bone cancer:** yarrow tea, or NATURAL ENERGY PLUS CAISSE'S TEA, or FLORA FLOR-ESSENCE tea.
- **Help your body remodel your bones:** LANE LABS ADVACAL ULTRA (highly recommended); JARROW HYDROXYAPATITE caps; Vitamin A & D 25,000IU/1000IU daily; NATURAL BALANCE IPRIFLAVONE (menopausal women); Vitamin E 400IU; CoQ$_{10}$ 60 mg. 2x daily; Bilberry extract (bioflavonoids); EIDON'S MINERAL BALANCING PROGRAM (recommended).
- **Effective bone knitters and healers:** HOMEOPATHIC ARNICA MONTANA, or apply B & T ARNIFLORA gel for swelling; REAL LIFE RESEARCH TOTAL B LIQUID; Nettles caps or Horsetail extract; Tape on a comfrey poultice for 3 days; change daily. Glucosamine-Chondroitin capsules 1000 mg. daily; or shark cartilage 1400 mg. daily.

Bodywork is critical for bone health

The British journal LANCET states: Some medicines put bone health at risk if you take them for a long period of time: L-thyroxine, a thyroid stimulant; steroid drugs like hydrocortisone, cortisone, prednisone; phenytoin and phenobarbital (anti-seizure drugs); heparin, a blood thinner; furosemide, a diuretic; and NO-DOZ, a stimulant. Some drugs can hamper your body's ability to maintain and repair bone: Ibuprofen, NSAIDS like NAPROXEN, FENCLOFENAC, INDOMETHACIN, SULINDAC, KETO-PROFEN, DICLOFENAC, ASPIRIN, PIROXICAM, FLURBIPROFEN, ASOPRO-PAZONE.

Exercise and Bodywork:

- Aerobic exercise and light weight training are primary bones builders and strengtheners.
- Get some sunlight on the body for natural vitamin D. Swim or walk in the ocean when possible.
- Don't smoke. It increases bone brittleness and inhibits bone growth.
- Avoid aluminum cookware, deodorants and fluorescent lighting that leach calcium from the body.

For more information on this topic, visit www.healthyhealing.com

Maintenance Recipes for a Bone-Building Diet

Use these recipes on an ongoing basis once your initial healing diet is producing good results.

Breakfast

Carrot & Raisin Oatmeal

2 carrots	½ cup raisins	½ tsp. cinnamon
½ tsp. sea salt	⅔ cup oat bran	
4 cups water	1⅓ cups rolled oats	

In a food processor, shred the carrots. Mix them with the sea salt and add to 4 cups water. Bring to a rapid boil. Reduce heat to a simmer and cook 4 minutes. Add the raisins, cook for 3 minutes. Stir in the oat bran, rolled oats, and cinnamon. Cook stirring until thick, about 5 minutes. Serve at once. Makes 4 serving.

Nutrition per serving:	Vitamin C --------- 5 mg.	Fat ----------------- 2 g.	Magnesium ------- 58 mg.
Calories ----------- 220	Vitamin E --------- 1 IU	Cholesterol-------- 0	Potassium --------- 455 mg.
Protein ------------ 8 g.	Carbohydrates ---- 47 g.	Calcium ----------- 47 mg.	Sodium------------ 238 mg.
Vitamin A --------- 1015 IU	Fiber -------------- 7 g.	Iron -------------- 3 mg.	

Brown Rice Pilaf with Baked Eggs

1 tbsp. butter	¾ tsp. poultry seasoning	½ cup grated parmesan-reggiano
⅔ cup shallots, minced	½ cup shredded Swiss cheese	cheese
1⅓ cups brown basmati rice	4 eggs	sea salt and cracked pepper to taste
2 cups organic low-fat chicken broth	plum tomato, slices	

Preheat oven to 400°F. Use a 10 – 12" oven-safe frying pan to make the pilaf. Sauté the butter and shallots until golden, about 3 minutes. Add the basmati rice and stir until grains are lightly toasted, 2 minutes. Add the chicken broth and poultry seasoning; stir, and bring to a boil. Cover, reduce heat and simmer until grains are tender to bite, about 12 minutes. Add the shredded Swiss cheese. Using the back of a spoon, make 4 deep wells in rice. Slide 1 egg into each well. Lay the plum tomato slices around eggs. Move to the oven and bake until egg whites are opaque and yolks have desired texture, about 8 minutes. Sprinkle the pilaf and baked eggs with grated parmesan-reggiano cheese. Use a wide spatula to scoop out pilaf and eggs, 1 at a time, and put on plates. Season with sea salt and cracked pepper to taste. Makes 4 servings.

Healing drinks

High Protein & EFAs Coconut Milk Drink

2 cups chopped fresh
   pineapple

15 oz. can unsweetened
   coconut milk

1 banana
½ cup orange juice

Combine all ingredients in a blender and serve over ice. Makes 3 drinks.

Daily Carrot Juice Cleanse

4 carrots
½ cucumber

2 ribs celery w/ leaves

1 tbsp. dry dulse, chopped

Combine all ingredients in a juicer. Makes 2 large drinks.

Sweet, Low-Fat Protein Drink

Rich in vitamin C, potassium, antioxidants.

1 cup vanilla soymilk or rice
   dream
2 bananas

3 ripe kiwi fruit
1 cup pineapple-coconut
   juice

1 cup seedless grapes
2 tbsp. honey

Combine all ingredients in a blender. Makes 2 large drinks.

Soups, salads, appetizers

Sea Green-Stuffed Mushrooms

Cook gently so mushrooms stay juicy.

24 button mushroom caps
½ cup dried arame sea
   greens, crumbled

6 dried shiitake mushrooms
1 tsp. toasted sesame oil
1 small onion, diced

2 tbsp. lemon juice
2 tbsp. teriyaki sauce
1 tbsp. crystallized ginger, minced

Preheat oven to 350°F. Wipe the button mushrooms, mince stems, leaving the caps whole. Set aside. Soak the arame and shiitake mushrooms in water—just enough to cover them—for 15 minutes. Drain and rinse well. Discard shiitake woody mushroom stems. Cover shiitakes and arame again with water. In a saucepan, bring to a boil; then simmer 15 minutes. Drain. Squeeze out liquid and mince both vegetables. In a skillet, heat the sesame oil and sauté the diced onion and minced mushroom stems for 5 minutes. Add the arame and shiitakes, lemon juice, teriyaki sauce, crystallized ginger; simmer for 5 minutes. Stuff button mushroom caps with the mixture; cover, bake for 20 minutes. Serves 8 people as an appetizer.

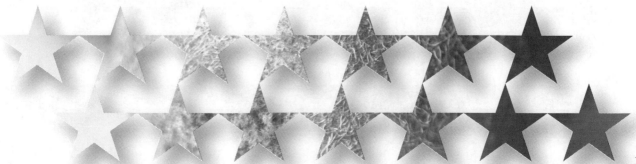

Mineral-Enzyme Summer Salad

2 tbsp. lime juice
½ tsp. of sea salt
4 tomatoes, diced
3 avocados, diced
3 green onions, thin-sliced

¼ tsp. garlic-lemon
   seasoning
lemon-pepper seasoning to
   taste
1 tbsp. olive oil

¼ tsp. ground cumin
1 tbsp. lime juice
1 (6 oz.) package baby spinach leaves
1 cucumber, peeled and diced
2 tbsp. fresh cilantro, chopped

In a non-metallic bowl, mix the lime juice and sea salt. Fold in the tomatoes, avocados, green onions and garlic-lemon seasoning. Season with lemon-pepper and set aside. In a bowl, whisk the olive oil, ground cumin, and lime juice. Toss with the baby spinach leaves and cucumber. Divide among plates. Spoon on the avocado mixture and sprinkle with the chopped fresh cilantro. Makes 4 servings.

High Mineral Spinach Salad

1½ cups whole wheat bread
   cubes
1 tbsp. soy bacon bits
2 tbsp. balsamic vinaigrette
2 tbsp. parmesan cheese

1 (6 oz.) bag baby spinach
   leaves
1 cup green cabbage,
   shredded
1 cup red cabbage, shredded

1 cup tofu cubes
1 cup water-packed artichoke hearts,
   sliced
½ cup balsamic vinaigrette

Preheat oven to 400°F. In a baking dish, mix the bread cubes, soy bacon bits, balsamic vinaigrette and parmesan cheese. Bake for 10 minutes until light brown. Set aside. Wash the spinach leaves and toss in a salad bowl with the green cabbage, red cabbage, tofu cubes, sliced artichoke hearts. Pour on ½ cup balsamic vinaigrette; marinate 30 minutes. Toss with the toasted crouton blend and serve. Makes 6 servings.

Baby Artichoke Quiches

2 (11 oz.) jars water-packed
   artichoke hearts, drained
   and chopped
2 cups low fat cottage cheese
2 eggs

¼ cup low fat plain yogurt
¼ cup water
1 cup grated parmesan
   cheese

½ cup fresh parsley leaves
1 tsp. garlic-lemon seasoning
paprika

Pan-spray 12 muffin cups. Preheat oven to 375°F. In a blender, mix the cottage cheese, eggs, yogurt, water, parmesan, parsley and garlic-lemon seasoning. Line muffin cups with the chopped artichokes. Divide the cheese mixture between cups. Sprinkle with paprika. Bake for 30 minutes until puffy and brown. Serve warm. Makes 12 servings.

Nutrition per serving:	Vitamin C --------- 8 mg.	Fat ---------------- 2 g.	Magnesium ------- 30 mg.
Calories ----------- 107	Vitamin E --------- 1 IU	Cholesterol-------- 44 mg.	Potassium --------- 217 mg.
Protein ----------- 12 g.	Carbohydrates ---- 7 g.	Calcium ----------- 176 mg.	Sodium------------ 235 mg.
Vitamin A--------- 58 IU	Fiber ------------- 3 g.	Iron -------------- 1 mg.	

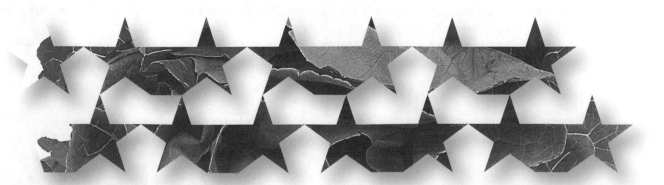

Dairy-Free Creamy Broccoli Soup

Intense flavor.

¼ cup grapeseed oil
2 pinches ground coriander
6 cups broccoli stems and
  florets, diced

2 ribs celery, diced
1 yellow bell pepper, diced
herbal seasoning salt
white pepper

organic vegetable broth or chicken
  broth
chopped fresh parsley, cilantro or
  mint (choose one)

In a soup pot, heat the grapeseed oil and ground coriander. Add the diced broccoli, celery and yellow bell pepper. Season with an herbal seasoning salt, and white pepper. Cook 30 minutes. Make the soup: In a blender, purée broccoli mix in batches with 1 cup organic vegetable broth or low fat chicken broth. Strain soup through a sieve into a large bowl and discard any fibrous material that sticks to the sieve. When all broccoli mix is pureed, pour soup back into the pot and reheat, thinning with more broth if needed. Ladle into bowls and top with chopped fresh parsley, cilantro or mint. Each topping gives a different taste to the soup. Serves 6.

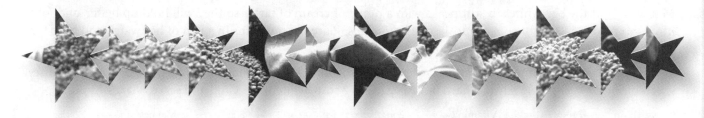

Sesame Mushroom Soup

Rich, non-dairy and high in protein.

2 tbsp. grapeseed oil
1 large onion, diced
1 tsp. ginger, grated
½ tsp. dry basil (or 1 tbsp.
  fresh basil, chopped)
a pinch cayenne pepper
2 cups mushrooms, sliced

3 stalks celery, thin sliced
½ tsp. sesame salt
¼ tsp. black pepper
4 cups tomatoes, chopped
½ cup organic vegetable
  broth

½ cup white wine
3 tbsp. sesame tahini
2 tbsp. peanut butter
1 cake very firm tofu, cubed
fresh cilantro, chopped

In a large soup pot, sauté the onion, ginger, basil and cayenne pepper in 2 tbsp. grapeseed oil until fragrant. Add the sliced mushrooms, celery, sesame salt, and black pepper, and sauté for another 7 – 10 minutes. Add the chopped tomatoes, organic vegetable broth, white wine, sesame tahini, peanut butter; and simmer for 15 – 20 minutes. Add the cubed tofu and heat through. Serve hot with chopped fresh cilantro. Serves 6.

Sweet Carrot Cream

2 tbsp. grapeseed oil
½ tsp. lemon-garlic seasoning
1 cup vegetable broth
1½ lbs. carrots, sliced
2 ribs celery sliced

3 cups leeks, sliced (mostly
  white parts)
1 cup plain yogurt
5 cups vegetable broth
⅓ cup fresh parsley, chopped
¼ tsp. nutmeg

¼ tsp. white pepper
1 tsp. brown sugar
½ cup carrots, minced
¼ cup plain yogurt
½ tsp. sea salt
1 tbsp. fresh mint, chopped

In a large soup pot, bring the grapeseed oil, lemon-garlic seasoning and 1 cup vegetable broth to a simmer. Add the sliced carrots, celery, and leeks and simmer 5 minutes. In a blender, purée this mixture with 1 cup plain yogurt until smooth. Return to soup pot. Add 5 more cups vegetable broth, the fresh parsley, nutmeg and white pepper. Heat gently. In a saucepan, sauté brown sugar for 3 minutes until caramelized. Add the minced carrots, ¼ cup plain yogurt, sea salt, and a bit more white pepper. Cook for 10 minutes until carrots are tender-crisp. Mix into hot soup. Serve in soup bowls. Sprinkle with fresh mint. Serves 6 people.

Crab Puffs

1 lb. crab meat	2 pinches white pepper	½ cup plain yogurt
2 tbsp. butter	2 eggs	¼ cup light mayonnaise
2 tbsp. unbleached flour	¼ tsp. paprika	2 tbsp. green onions, chopped
½ cup plain yogurt	1 cup kefir cheese or low fat	2 tbsp. sweet pickle relish
4 tbsp. water	cream cheese	1 hard boiled egg, crumbled
4 tbsp. white wine	1 pinch cream of tartar	2 tbsp. white wine
½ tsp. sea salt		

Preheat oven to 350°F. Drain the crab meat and set aside. In a skillet, melt the butter and stir in the flour and simmer until bubbly. Mix in ½ cup plain yogurt, the water and 4 tbsp. white wine, the sea salt and 2 pinches white pepper. Stir until a smooth sauce forms. Remove from heat.

In a bowl, separate 2 eggs. Beat the egg yolks until frothy. Add a little of the heated sauce to the yolks to warm them, then add them back to the sauce in the skillet and stir in well. Add the paprika, kefir cheese and the crab. Mix well. Beat the egg whites to stiff peaks with a pinch of cream of tartar so they will hold up better, and fold into crab mixture. Pour or spoon into 12 oiled ramekins. Place the ramekins in a pan of hot water, and bake for 40 – 45 minutes or until puffs are high and firm.

To make an easy Homemade Tartar Sauce: in a bowl, mix ½ cup plain low fat yogurt, the light mayonnaise, green onions, sweet pickle relish, a hard boiled egg, and 2 tbsp. white wine. Chill and serve. Makes 12 puffs.

Nutrition per serving:	Vitamin C --------- 2 mg.	Fat ----------------- 5 g.	Magnesium ------- 23 mg.
Calories ----------- 146	Vitamin E --------- 1 IU	Cholesterol-------- 104 mg.	Potassium --------- 254 mg.
Protein ------------ 13 g.	Carbohydrates ---- 5 g.	Calcium ----------- 109 mg.	Sodium------------ 267 mg.
Vitamin A --------- 93 IU	Fiber ------------- 1 g.	Iron -------------- 1 mg.	

Entrées

Tofu Tamale Casserole

3 tbsp. olive oil	6 – 8 tomatoes, chopped	¼ cup red wine
2 garlic cloves, minced	1 (4 oz.) can green chilies,	2 tbsp. chili powder
1 onion, diced	chopped	½ tsp. cumin powder
1 lb. firm tofu, crumbled	1 cup corn kernels	½ tsp. pepper
1 red bell pepper, diced	½ cup vegetable broth	low-fat jack cheese, grated
1 cup cooked brown rice	1 cup yellow cornmeal	2 tbsp. green olives, minced

Preheat oven to 350°F. In a large wok, sauté the garlic, diced onion, tofu, and red bell pepper in 3 tbsp. olive oil until brown. Remove from heat; stir in the brown rice, chopped tomatoes, green chilies, corn kernels, vegetable broth, yellow cornmeal, red wine, chili powder, cumin powder and pepper. Pour mixture in casserole dish. Bake for 45 minutes. Remove from oven; sprinkle with grated low fat jack cheese and 2 tbsp. minced green olives to cover top. Bake for 15 more minutes until bubbly. Makes 6 – 8 servings.

Nutrition per serving:	Vitamin C --------- 45 mg.	Fat ----------------- 11 g.	Magnesium ------- 110 mg.
Calories ----------- 287	Vitamin E --------- 2 IU	Cholesterol-------- 5 mg.	Potassium --------- 586 mg.
Protein ------------ 16 g.	Carbohydrates ---- 33 g.	Calcium ----------- 222 mg.	Sodium------------ 240 mg.
Vitamin A --------- 229 IU	Fiber ------------- 5 g.	Iron -------------- 8 mg.	

Tofu Pasta Sauce

A meaty-textured sauce.

8 oz. firm tofu or tempeh, cubed
½ cup unbleached flour
sea salt
pepper
2 tbsp. olive oil

2 garlic cloves, minced
2 yellow onions, diced
1 orange bell pepper, diced
1 red bell pepper, diced
4 oz. cremini mushrooms, thin-sliced

1 tsp. dry basil
1 (28 oz.) can roma tomatoes with juice
1 tbsp. honey
½ tsp. tarragon
½ tsp. oregano

In a bag, shake the tofu with the flour, sea salt and pepper. In a skillet, brown this mixture in the olive oil. Remove and set aside. Keep skillet hot; sauté the garlic and yellow onions until fragrant. Add the orange bell pepper, red bell pepper, cremini mushrooms and basil; sauté for 5 minutes. Add tofu back to skillet. Then add the roma tomatoes with juice, honey, tarragon and oregano. Bring to a boil. Reduce heat. Cover and simmer 10 minutes; uncover and simmer 10 minutes. Serve hot over spaghetti or rotelli. Makes 8 servings.

Vegetable Herb Stew

1 red potato, cut into ¼"-thick pieces
4 cups organic vegetable broth
1 onion, chopped
1 clove garlic, minced
3 tbsp. olive oil

1 carrot, diced
1 rib celery, diced
8 oz. mushrooms, sliced
½ tsp. thyme
½ tsp. dill weed
½ tsp. dry basil
½ tsp. herbal seasoning

½ tsp. pepper
1 cake tofu, cut in cubes
¾ cup white wine
2 tbsp. sherry
1 tbsp. soy sauce
1 cup frozen peas

In a large soup pot, cook the red potato pieces in the vegetable broth until tender. In a saucepan, sauté the onion and garlic in 3 tbsp. olive oil 5 minutes. Add the carrots, celery, mushrooms, thyme, dill, basil, herbal seasoning and pepper, and sauté for 5 minutes. Add this mixture to the potato stock; simmer 20 minutes. To the soup pot, add the tofu, white wine, sherry and soy sauce, and stir. Remove from heat; add the frozen peas and let sit for 5 minutes while peas warm. Makes 6 – 8 servings.

Potato-Green Bean Salad with Dulse Flakes

Dulse tastes a lot like bacon, great with beans and potatoes.

1 lb. red potatoes, thin-sliced
8 oz. frozen French-cut green beans, cooked

2 tbsp. olive oil
2 tbsp. sesame seeds
½ cup scallions, thin-sliced

1 tbsp. lemon juice
1 tbsp. dulse flakes
¼ tsp. black pepper

Steam the red potatoes for 10 minutes until just tender; add the green beans. Cover, remove from heat and set aside. In a skillet, heat the olive oil and sauté the sesame seeds until golden. Add the scallions, lemon juice, dulse flakes, and black pepper; sauté until fragrant. Toss with potatoes and beans. Serve hot. Makes 4 servings.

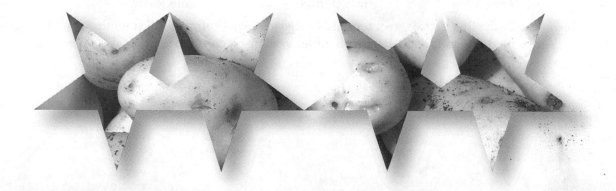

Sesame-Seared Salmon with Radicchio

4 thick salmon fillets, skinned	1 tbsp. olive oil	2 tbsp. lemon juice
bottled teriyaki sauce	3 small heads radicchio, shredded	1 tsp. garlic-lemon seasoning
⅓ cup sesame seeds	3 tbsp. olive oil	1 tsp. ginger, minced
		½ tsp. cracked black pepper

Preheat oven to 450°F. Coat the salmon fillets with bottled teriyaki sauce. In a dry skillet, toast the sesame seeds until golden. Press salmon fillets onto seeds to coat both sides. Heat 1 tbsp. olive oil in the skillet. Sear salmon fillets about 2 minutes each side. Place fillets in a baking pan and bake for about 6 – 8 minutes. Heat 3 tbsp. olive oil and the lemon juice in the skillet and sauté the shredded radicchio for 3 minutes. Add the garlic-lemon seasoning, ginger and black pepper. Turn radicchio onto plates and top with a crusted salmon fillet. Makes 4 servings.

Healthy dessert options

Sugar-Free Orange Scones

2 cups unbleached flour	2 tbsp. maple syrup	2 tbsp. frozen orange juice concentrate, thawed
2 tsp. baking powder	½ cup frozen orange juice concentrate, thawed	½ tsp. almond extract
½ tsp. baking soda	½ cup vanilla soymilk	2 tbsp. orange honey
¼ tsp. sea salt	grated zest of 1 orange	sliced almonds
¼ cup grapeseed oil		
⅓ cup orange honey		

Preheat oven to 350°F. In a bowl, mix the unbleached flour, baking powder, baking soda and sea salt. Stir in ¼ cup grapeseed oil. Add the orange honey, maple syrup, ½ cup orange juice concentrate, the vanilla soymilk and the orange zest. Mix lightly; allow to sit for 10 minutes. Pat dough into rectangles about ½" thick. Place on a grapeseed oil-sprayed baking sheet. Make topping in a bowl: mix 2 tbsp. orange juice concentrate, the almond extract and orange honey; brush onto scones and sprinkle with sliced almonds. Bake for 15 minutes. Makes 8 servings.

Nutrition per serving:	Vitamin C --------- 30 mg.	Fat ----------------- 8 g.	Magnesium ------- 21 mg.
Calories ----------- 288	Vitamin E --------- 3 IU	Cholesterol ------- 0	Potassium --------- 195 mg.
Protein ----------- 5 g.	Carbohydrates ---- 50 g.	Calcium ----------- 135 mg.	Sodium----------- 240 mg.
Vitamin A --------- 5 IU	Fiber ------------- 2 g.	Iron -------------- 2 mg.	

Avocado Cream

Rich, creamy, good and nutritious. Don't miss it.

1 pint vanilla RICE DREAM frozen dessert	1 avocado, peeled and cut into chunks	2 tbsp. orange juice concentrate mint leaves

In a blender, mix the RICE DREAM, avocado, and orange juice concentrate until smooth. Spoon into dessert glasses. Top with a mint leaf and freeze. Remove 5 minutes before you want to serve. Makes 4 servings.

Chocolate Cherry Pistachio Fruitcake

½ cup unbleached flour
¼ cup unsweetened cocoa
½ cup date sugar or turbinado sugar
¼ tsp. baking soda
¼ tsp. baking powder
1 cup raisins

3 cups dried cherries
½ cup walnuts, chopped
½ cup dried cranberries
1 cup pistachios, chopped
¼ cup arrowroot powder
2 tsp. vanilla
⅓ cup sherry

2 lbs. fresh apricots
12 oz. fresh pineapple, cut into cubes
½ tsp. grated orange peel
2 tbsp. lemon juice
¾ cup honey
½ cup maple syrup

Preheat oven to 300°F. Lightly oil 2 cake loaf pans. In a large bowl, combine the flour, cocoa, date sugar, baking soda and baking powder. Stir in the raisins, cherries, walnuts, cranberries and pistachios. Set aside.

In a small bowl, mix the arrowroot powder, vanilla and sherry until smooth. Add to dry ingredients, mixing well with hands until fruit and nut pieces are completely coated. Press mixture into loaf pans and bake until batter is set, 45 – 50 minutes. Cool completely before removing from pans.

Serve with Apricot Pineapple Honey Butter: Purée the fresh apricots in the blender. Add the fresh pineapple. Turn into a bowl and mix with the orange peel, lemon juice, honey and maple syrup. Simmer uncovered, stirring occasionally until thick, about 2 hours. Spoon onto fruitcake. Makes 2 loaves (about 16 servings).

Nutrition per serving:			
Calories ----------- 340	Vitamin C--------- 13 mg.	Fat----------------- 6 g.	Magnesium ------- 57 mg.
Protein ------------ 6 g.	Vitamin E --------- 2 IU	Cholesterol------- 0	Potassium --------- 495 mg.
Vitamin A --------- 317 IU	Carbohydrates ---- 77 g.	Calcium ----------- 79 mg.	Sodium------------ 43 mg.
	Fiber ------------- 5 g.	Iron -------------- 2 mg.	

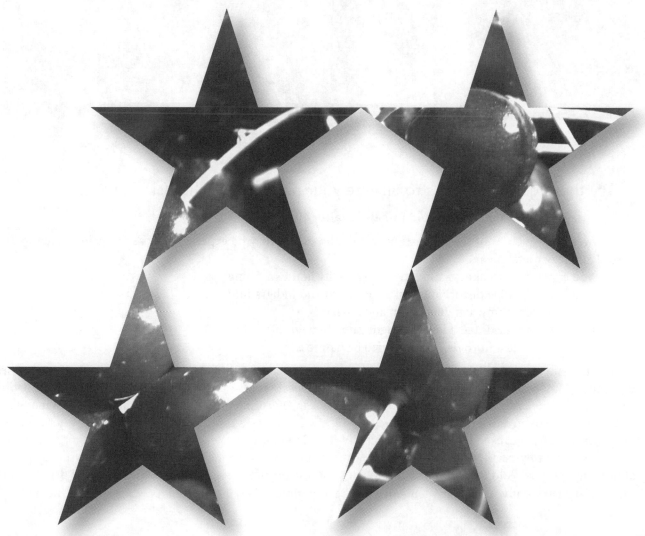

Weight Loss, Weight Control, Fat Management

The latest statistics are shocking. One out of every three Americans is overweight! This doesn't count kids who are rapidly becoming an overweight generation. Right now, two-thirds of Americans are trying to lose weight. Amazingly, of those, only 20% are actually reducing their calories or exercising. Next to smoking, obesity is a leading preventable cause of death in the United States, contributing to in excess of 320,000 deaths each year.

It's all up to you. First, decide you want to be thin.

Once you make the decision to be a thin person, analyze what your weight loss block really is. I've identified three of the most common and developed comprehensive programs to address them. Each of the three plans has years of observed success behind it. Identify your most prominent weight control problem, especially if there seems to be more than one. As improvement is realized in the primary area, secondary problems are often overcome in the process. If lingering problem spots still exist, address them with additional supplements after the first program is underway and producing noticeable results.

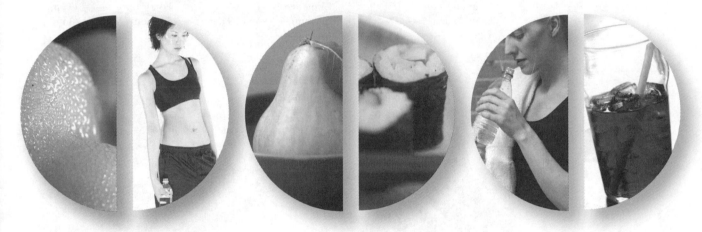

Try these quick self-tests to analyze your personal weight loss challenge:

1. **Lazy Metabolism and Thyroid Imbalance after 40:**

Answering "yes" to 3 of the 5 questions below shows you may be experiencing weight gain related to low thyroid and lazy metabolism.
- Do you experience weakness and fatigue, especially in the morning?
- Do you have digestive disturbances like heartburn and indigestion?
- Do you experience unusual depression and anxiety?
- Have you experienced unexplained weight gain after age 40?
- Have you had breast fibroids, accompanied by hair loss?

Weight gain after 40 or after menopause usually means lowered thyroid and metabolic activity. Huge studies reveal that 1 in 10 women over 65 have early stages of hypothyroidism! Boosting metabolism and supporting your thyroid is easy. Add sea vegetables to your diet like kelp, dulse and nori, rich in natural iodine, as a mainstay. Or take sea greens in capsules, like CRYSTAL STAR® OCEAN MINERALS™ caps. Herbal formulas show good results for weight problems caused by low thyroid activity. Try CRYSTAL STAR® THYROID META MAX™ caps or GAIA HERBS THYROID SUPPORT phytocaps. Add thermogenic spices like cinnamon, cayenne, mustard and ginger to speed up your fat burning process. Add ice to your drinks to boost calorie burning… up to 25 more calories per drink! Avoid breads and pastries; if you have any tendency to wheat or gluten allergies you'll bloat when you eat them.

2. Overeating Fat, and Sugar = Excess Calories:

Answering "yes" to 3 of the 5 questions below shows you may be experiencing weight gain related to overeating fat and sugar calories.
- Do you binge on junk foods, especially fatty and sugary foods?
- Do you eat all of your calories at one meal?
- Do you have second and third helpings at a meal but still feel hungry?
- Do you experience a wired feeling that is only relieved by eating sweets?
- Are you easily frustrated, and moody with frequent crying spells?

Overeating is a big reason why it's so hard to lose weight. Our lifestyles don't help. 45% of every food dollar is spent on eating out, and restaurant portions are bigger than ever as consumers demand more food for their money. Control your portions so you don't overeat. Reduce fats to 20% of your food intake. (Don't replace fats with fat substitutes like Olestra.) Take your time eating to prevent overeating. An herbal appetite suppressant with St. John's wort is appetite will power against cravings for fatty foods. CRYSTAL STAR® WILL POWER™ caps with St. John's wort are great to reduce appetite surges and overeating binges. Target excess sugar in the blood with herbs for weight loss. CRYSTAL STAR® SUGAR CONTROL™ formulas for high or low blood sugar reactions. Increase healthy essential fatty acids (EFAs) from sources like seafood, sea greens, flax seed oil to cut cravings for fat. HEALTH FROM THE SUN CLA is the best weight control EFA source, 3000 mg. daily. Use enzyme therapy to improve fat metabolism. CRYSTAL STAR® DR. ENZYME II: FAT & STARCH BUSTER™ or TRANSFORMATION LIPOZYME.

3. Liver Malfunction, Cellulite Formation, Stress-Related Weight Gain:

Answering "yes" to 3 of the 5 questions below shows your weight gain may be related to stress, liver malfunction and cellulite.
- Do you have chronic daily stress, daytime fatigue and/or nighttime sleeplessness?
- Do you have bulgy, dimply skin on hips, buttocks, thighs, knees (women) torso, stomach (men)?
- Do you have poor digestion that worsens after fatty meals or chronic constipation or heartburn?
- Do you have a thick waist that doesn't go away even with exercise and diet improvements?
- Do you have frequent overeating binges that are triggered by stress reactions?

Today, most of us have a liver overloaded with toxic build-up, and it can be responsible for weight gain and cellulite formation. Detox your liver with CRYSTAL STAR® LIVER RENEW™ caps or PLANETARY BUPLEURUM LIVER CLEANSE. Add B complex to assist with liver detox and fat metabolism. For cellulite control, use HEALTH FROM THE SUN LEAN FOR LESS program or CRYSTAL STAR® CELLULITE RELEASE™ caps (they work).

Cellulite Tip: Seaweed body wraps are especially good because they squeeze cellulitic waste back into the working areas of the body so it can be eliminated. Check out a nearby day spa or take a CRYSTAL STAR® HOT SEAWEED BATH™. New research shows high stress may make you gain weight in the tummy area. CRYSTAL STAR® TUMMY BULGE CORTISOL CONTROL™ caps fight stress reactions and maximize fat burning.

Watchwords:

Everybody knows yo-yo dieting doesn't work. Did you know it increases the risk of gallstones, too? For the best results, start slowly on your weight loss program and stick with it. The five keys to an effective weight control diet: low fat, high fiber, stress control, regular exercise, lots of water.

Fat isn't all bad. It's your body's chief energy source. Most overweight people have too high blood sugar and too *low* fat levels. This causes constant hunger; the delicate balance between fat storage and fat utilization is upset; and your ability to use fat for energy decreases. Eating fast, fried, or junk foods aggravates this imbalance. You wind up with empty calories and more cravings. Fat becomes non-moving energy; fat cells become fat storage depots. But don't replace fats with fat substitutes like Olestra. Fake fats fool your tastebuds, not your stomach. In one study, people who replaced 20% of their fat with fake fats were still hungry at the end of the day and they ate twice as much food as normal! Fake fats are nutrition thieves. Eating a one ounce portion of olestra potato chips on a daily basis reduces blood carotene levels by 50%!

Changing fat composition in your diet is the key. The importance of cutting back on saturated fat cannot be overstated. Saturated fats are hard for the liver to metabolize. Focus on healthy fats from seafood, sea greens, nuts and seeds which curb cravings by initiating a satiety response levels.

Water can get you over diet plateaus. Dehydration slows resting metabolic rate (RMR), so waste products like ketones build up in tissues. Drink juices or green tea each morning to wash out wastes.

A little caffeine after a meal raises thermogenesis (calorie burning) and boosts metabolic rate. Fat burning spices like ginger, cinnamon, garlic, mustard and cayenne in your recipes work, too.

High fiber fruits and veggies are a key to successful body toning. Have an apple every day!

Choose 2 or 3 supplements to help the good fats burn bad fats:

Good fats burn bad fats, help stop binging: CLA (conjugated linoleic acid) 2000 mg. daily; BARLEANS OMEGA-3 FLAX OIL or UDO'S PERFECTED OIL BLEND; RICHARDSON LABS CHROMA-SLIM lipotropic-carnitine.

Stimulate BAT thermogenesis: Evening Primrose oil 3000 mg. daily; Carnitine 3000 mg. daily; CRYSTAL STAR® THERMO THINNER caps (women) or SPARE TIRE REPAIR™ (men); GAIA DIET SLIM phytocaps; ESTEEM TRIM & FIRM AM & PM; NATURE'S SECRET ULTIMATE WEIGHT LOSS; HERPANACINE DIAMOND TRIM.

Nutrient deficiencies lead to food binges: B-complex with extra B6 200 mg. boosts serotonin, metabolizes carbs; low minerals lead to sugar craving: Try CRYSTAL STAR® OCEAN MINERALS™; EIDON ZINC LIQUID.

Control food cravings: CRYSTAL STAR® WILL POWER™ caps with St. John's Wort; 5-HTP as directed; chromium picolinate (400 mcg.); L-glutamine 2000 mg., spirulina and bee pollen for sugar cravings; PINNACLE ESTROLEAN; NADH 5 mg. in the morning for an energy lift and to help drop those last five pounds. Ginkgo biloba extract 2 – 3 times a day to help reduce stress linked to weight gain around the middle (not if you are taking Warfarin).

Natural fat blockers: Fat digesting enzymes, CRYSTAL STAR® DR. ENZYME II: FAT & STARCH BUSTER™ or TRANSFORMATION LYPOZYME; garcinia cambogia in formulas like NOW'S CITRI-MAX or PLANETARY TRIPHALA GARCINIA program; Pyruvate aids in transforming blood sugar into energy, 5 g. daily; try TWIN LAB PYRUVATE FUEL; Chitosan reduces absorption of fats; ESTEEM CHITOSAN HERBAL SLIM or NATURAL BALANCE FAT MAGNET. Note: Gastrointestinal problems may result from excessive use of pyruvate or chitosan.

Boost metabolism: Jump start your weight loss program with calcium, about 1600 mg. daily or LANE LABS ADVACAL ULTRA. ENZYMATIC THERAPY THYROID/TYROSINE caps, or for compulsive eating, tyrosine 1000 mg. with zinc 30 mg. daily. Ayurvedic guggulsterone, like SOLARAY GUGGUL caps; CRYSTAL STAR® THYROID META MAX caps.

Regular exercise almost ensures weight loss

Daily exercise is the key to permanent, painless weight control. Exercise releases fat from the cells. (Exercising early in the day can raise metabolism as much as 25%! Exercising before breakfast is best because the body dips into its fat stores for quick energy.) Even if eating habits are just slightly changed, you can still lose weight with a brisk hour's walk, or 15 minutes of aerobic exercise. One pound of fat represents 3500 calories. A 3 mile walk burns up 250 calories. In less than 2 weeks, you'll lose a pound of real extra fat. That's 3 pounds a month and 30 pounds a year without changing your diet. It's easy to see how cutting down even moderately on fatty, sugary foods in combination with exercise can still provide the look and body tone you want.

Exercise promotes an afterburn effect, raising metabolic rate from 1.00 to 1.05-1.15 per minute up to 24 hours afterwards. Calories are used up at an even faster rate after exercise.

Weight training exercise increases lean muscle mass, replacing fat-marbled muscle tissue with lean muscle. Muscle tissue burns calories; the greater the amount of muscle tissue you have, the more calories you can burn. This is very important because aging decreases muscle mass. Exercise before a meal raises blood sugar levels and thus decreases appetite, often for several hours afterward.

Deep breathing exercises increase metabolic rate.

Intense Fat and Sugar Cleanse

Is your body showing signs that it needs a fat and sugar cleanse?

- Is cellulite collecting on your hips, thighs or tummy? Cellulite is a mixture of fat, water and wastes trapped beneath the skin.
- Are your upper arms slightly flabby? Is your waistline, wrists and ankles noticeably thicker?
- Does your face look jowl-y or puffy?

If your diet problem is eating too much fat and sugars, try my light detox from fats and sugars for 1 – 3 days. It makes you feel terrific and it's so easy. Sugary foods and highly processed foods like fast foods are so devoid of digestive enzymes that they collect as excess fat. If you are congested, your body tries to dump its metabolic wastes to get them out of the way. One of the places that receives metabolic wastes is excess fat.

Start the night before with a green leafy salad to sweep your intestines. Dry brush your skin all over for five minutes before you go to bed to open your pores for the night's cleansing eliminations.

Upon rising: have a cup of green tea to cut through and eliminate fatty wastes. For maximum results, add drops of ginseng extract to control sugar cravings, or licorice extract for sugar stabilizing.

Breakfast: have a Fat Melt Down Juice: juice 2 apples, 2 pears, 1 slice of fresh ginger to help reduce fat from places where it is stored in cellulite. The ginger stimulates better blood circulation.

Mid-morning: a green superfood drink once a day helps cleanse your body of fatty build-up.

Lunch: enjoy a mixed vegetable juice, like KNUDSEN'S VERY VEGGIE. Regular V-8 juice works fine.

Mid-afternoon: Take a glass of papaya-pineapple juice, or a cup of green tea to enhance enzyme production. Enzymes are a dieter's best friend!

Dinner: Have miso soup with snipped sea greens. Sea veggies add minerals and improve sluggish metabolism. Add spices like cayenne, mustard and ginger to speed up fat burning.

Before bed: have a cup of apple juice, licorice or peppermint tea to restore normal body pH.

Watchwords:

- **Focus on reducing fats and sugars in your diet.** Add more fiber to get rid of excess sugar, especially from whole grains, legumes like peas, and vegetables. High fiber foods improve glucose metabolism, help promote weight loss and reduce cravings for sugar.
- **Take a 15 minute dry sauna several days a week for a month.** Raising your body temperature with dry heat really helps balance sugar levels. When I worked at a European spa, we used this technique for weight loss and blood sugar problems with great results!
- **Expert dieters drink 8 glasses of water a day.** Water naturally suppresses appetite and helps maintain a high metabolic rate. In fact, water is the most important catalyst for increased fat burning. It enhances the liver's ability to detox and metabolize so it can process more fats. Don't worry about fluid retention; high water intake actually *decreases* bloating, because it flushes out sodium and toxins.

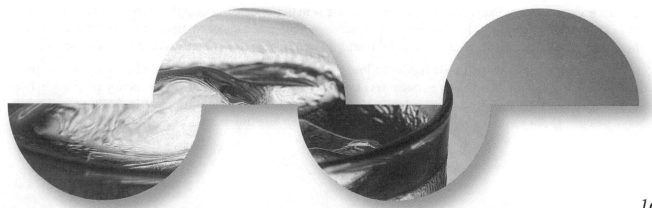

Choose 2 or 3 supplements to keep your diet plan working:

- **Special tips for sugar cravers:** Source Naturals Gluco Science, 1-2 tablets, 3x daily before meals. Also, try acupressure for will power against sugar cravings. Pinch the little bud of cartilage directly above your ear canal for 1 minute to short-circuit nerve impulses that cause cravings.
- **Appetite suppressant help:** Crystal Star Will Power™ caps help control appetite and speed fat burning; Gaia Herbs Diet Slim; Source Naturals Diet-Phen.
- **Essential fatty acids:** If you're on a very low fat diet, you may be missing the good fats. Without essential fatty acids (EFAs), appetite increases and poor fat metabolism is certain. Excess fluid retention is also controlled by EFAs. Add Flax Oil, 1 or 2 tbsp. over a salad; Crystal Star® Evening Primrose Oil, 1000 – 2000 mg. daily; CLA—an Omega-6 fatty acid with fat-burning properties, 1800 mg. daily.
- **Capillary strengthening:** you must tighten capillary walls in order to keep extra fat and cellulite from returning. Bioflavonoids are important: Pure Planet Amla C Plus.
- **Enzyme support:** Crystal Star® Dr. Enzyme II: Fat & Starch Buster (releases trapped fats and starches - highly recommended).
- **Electrolytes dramatically boost energy levels:** Alacer Emergen-C drink mix; Arise & Shine Alkalizer; Nature's Path Trace-Lyte Liquid Minerals.

Regular exercise almost ensures weight loss regardless of the problem

- **Exercise:** Exercise promotes an "afterburn" effect, raising metabolic rates for up to 24 hours. Exercise before a meal raises blood sugar levels and decreases appetite for several hours. Are you a woman with a little menopause tummy bulge? Do 100 hard tummy sucks each morning. It works!
- **Dry brushing:** Fatty wastes can get trapped beneath the skin's surface easily (especially in women) when the liver or lymphatic systems are sluggish. Use a natural bristle brush — brush vigorously in a rotary motion and massage every part of your body in this order: feet and legs, hands and arms, back and abdomen, chest and neck. Five to fifteen minutes is the average time.
- **Massage:** Have a massage therapy treatment at the end of your cleanse to move excess fluid wastes and unattached fats into elimination systems, and to stimulate skin circulation.
- **Enema:** Take an enema the first day of your fat cleanse to help release toxins from the body.
- **Bathe away excess fats:** Crystal Star® Hot Seaweed Bath™; or try this sea salt bath: add 1 cup Dead Sea salts, 1 cup Epsom salts, ½ cup regular sea salt and ¼ cup baking soda to a tub; swish in 3 drops lavender oil, 2 geranium drops oil, 2 drops sandalwood oil and 1 drop neroli oil.

Weight Control After 40

There's no doubt about it. Weight loss gets more difficult after 40. The latest figures show that body fat typically doubles between the ages of 20 and 50. Everybody goes through a change of life, and those middle years affect our body shapes, too… for both men and women. One of the worst problems America's fitness oriented population faces in their 40s and 50s is a disconcerting body thickening and a slow, steady rise in weight. It seems to happen with everybody, even people who have always been slim, who have a good diet, and who regularly exercise.

For women, a major calorie-burning process grinds to a halt after menopause. A woman's menstrual cycle consumes extra calories. Experts say that the metabolic rise in the last two weeks of the menstrual cycle accounts for up to 20,000 calories a year! Those calories really start to add up when menstruation ceases. Women also develop more deep abdominal fat (but less fat around their hips and thighs) as estrogen levels drop with menopause.

A woman needs to work a little harder to lose that extra fat later in life, but once her body adjusts to new hormone levels, weight gain stabilizes, becomes manageable, and, often falls back to premenopausal levels. Lower testosterone levels in andropausal men mean a decrease in muscle mass and increase in fat storage. But, most men, by cutting back on fat and adding fiber to their diets can lose the spare tire.

Add calcium (and magnesium) to your weight loss program after 40! New large studies reveal an entirely new diet fact. People over 40 on weight control diets lost weight if they had enough calcium but did not lose weight if they were calcium deficient... magnesium works with calcium on a weight control diet because serotonin (a natural appetite suppressant) needs magnesium and Vitamin B6 to activate. I prefer herbal calcium combinations like CRYSTAL STAR® CALCIUM MAGNESIUM SOURCE™ caps or FLORA CALCIUM LIQUID with high absorbability and natural calcium-magnesium balance; for regular calcium sources, take at least 1600 mg. a day and 800 mg. magnesium or take LANE LABS ADVACAL ULTRA (high absorbability).

For weight loss after 40, begin with two starting points:

1. Improve body chemistry at the gland and hormone level
2. Re-establish better, long-lasting metabolic rates.

1. Love your liver The liver is your body's chemical plant responsible for fat metabolism. It is intricately involved with hormone functions, so it is the prime target to optimize for weight loss after 40. Weight gain and energy loss signal a liver that has enlarged through overwork, alcohol exhaustion and congestion. A good calorie-burning herbal formula with ginseng works extremely well. Try CRYSTAL STAR® THERMO THINNER™ caps along with CELLULITE RELEASE™ caps; HERBS, ETC. GINSENG SEVEN SOURCE; or add liver tonics: fresh vegetable juices, dandelion greens, milk thistle seed extract (accelerates liver regeneration by a factor of four); or a liver tonic tea: 4 oz. hawthorn berries, 2 oz. red sage, and 1 oz. cardamom seeds. Steep 24 hours in 2 qts. water. Add honey. Take 2 cups daily.

2. Consciously eat less. As metabolism slows, you don't need to fuel it up as much, because your body doesn't use up nutrients like it once did. If you eat like you did in your 20s and 30s, your body will store too much, mostly as fat. Moderate food intake may extend lifespan by as much as ten years!

Make sure you eat a low fat diet. Even with all the fat-conscious foods on the market today, Americans still consume one-third of their calories as fat. Your fat intake should be about 20% for weight control, 15% or less for weight loss. But remember: no-fat is not good for weight loss, either. Your body goes into a survival mode if you eliminate all fat, shedding its highly active lean muscle tissue to reduce your body's need for food. When lean muscle tissue decreases, fat burning slows or stops. Use CRYSTAL STAR® DR. ENZYME II: FAT & STARCH BUSTER™ enzymes to keep food from depositing as fat storage.

Control your food portions. Portion control is a cornerstone of weight control. Even if your diet is healthy and reasonably low in fat, there's no way you can eat all you want of anything. Eat smaller meals every 2 to 3 hours to keep your appetite hole from gnawing, and to keep metabolic rate high. Small meals virtually prevent carbohydrates and proteins from being converted to fat.

Control hunger with safe herbal appetite suppressants. Serotonin is the brain chemical linked to mood and appetite. Serotonin balancers like St. John's wort, and evening primrose oil help reduce food cravings. Try an herbal weight loss compounds like Crystal Star TUMMY BULGE CORTISOL CONTROL™ caps with St. John's wort. Superfoods - barley grass, spirulina, sea greens and alfalfa can be keys to controlling appetite. Take a green drink with these low-calorie foods in mid-afternoon to rapidly decrease a craving for high-calorie foods. Crystal Star's ENERGY GREEN RENEWAL™ drink can raise both metabolic rate and activity levels.

Control your cravings. The herb gymnema sylvestre helps control sugar cravings. Gymnema binds with sugar receptors in the mouth, causing sugary foods to lose their appealing sweet flavor, an effect that lasts up to 2 hours. Seven different clinical studies show garcinia cambogia or HCA *(hydroxycitric acid)* reduces food intake an amazing 46% when taken orally. Gaia Herbs DIET SLIM combines gymnema and HCA. Crystal Star SUGAR CONTROL formulas help reduce high or low blood sugar reactions that contribute to food cravings and weight gain.

3.   **Raise your metabolism.** A high metabolic rate means you burn more fat, lose weight easier, maintain your ideal body weight more comfortably. Crystal Star Thyroid Meta Max™ and guggul 1500 – 3000 mg. a day help.

Don't skip meals, especially breakfast. Breakfast is the worst meal to skip if you want to raise metabolism. It sends a temporary fasting signal to the brain that food is going to be scarce. So stress hormones increase, and the body begins shedding lean muscle tissue in order to decrease its need for food. By the time you eat again, your pancreas is so sensitized to a lack of food, that it sharply increases blood insulin levels, your body's signal to make fat. Eating early in the day, when your metabolism is at its best, and hours of activity ahead in which to burn fats is the best for weight loss. Reduce both sugars and fats - they slow metabolism. Fats have twice the calories, gram for gram, as protein and complex carbohydrates. They also use only 2% of their calories before the fat storage process begins. Protein and carbohydrates burn almost 25% of their calories before storing them as fat. Limit alcohol consumption, even wine, to two glasses or less a day. With seven calories per gram, alcohol sugars shift metabolism in favor of fat depositing; too much alcohol burdens the liver and stimulates the appetite.

Eat fat-burning foods. Foods that raise metabolism are fresh fruits and vegetables (full of enzymes), whole grains and legumes. Eat fruits for breakfast or between meals. If you eat them with or after meals, the fructose is likely to be converted to fat by the liver. Sea greens work especially well for women to recharge metabolism and balance thyroid activity. Sea greens are also a rich source of fat-soluble vitamins like D, and K which help balance estrogen, and DHEA. Two tablespoons a day are a therapeutic dose. Add them chopped and dried to any salad, soup, rice dish or omelet. Or, add 6 pieces of sushi daily to your diet.

Re-activate your fat-burning systems with herbs. Herbal adaptogens like panax and eleuthero ginsengs, suma, gotu kola, and licorice root normalize body homeostasis; ginkgo biloba and hawthorn boost circulation; bee pollen, alfalfa, sarsaparilla and black cohosh support the liver; spices and sea greens like cayenne, ginger, kelp and spirulina help the thyroid. Crystal Star® Thyroid Meta Max™ caps greatly enhance fat burning.

Amino acids boost metabolism and keep lean muscle. L-Phenylalanine (LPA), suppresses appetite, boosts energy and reduces food craving. (Avoid phenylalanine if you take anti-depressants, have high blood pressure, or are pregnant.) L-Tyrosine is a thyroid precursor and reduces appetite. L-Carnitine suppresses appetite, accelerates fat metabolism and helps control sugar levels. Ornithine (1000 mg. daily) helps boost metabolism and curb appetite. Amino acids combined in a formula like Anabol Naturals Amino Balance work extremely well.

Drink plenty of water. Drink at least six 8 oz. glasses of water daily, even if you're not thirsty. Water naturally suppresses appetite, helps maintain a high metabolic rate, promotes good digestion and regular bowel movements, and actually reduces fat deposits. Water may be the most important catalyst for fat burning, because it increases the liver's detoxification and fat metabolism activity. Don't worry about fluid retention. High water intake actually decreases bloating, because it flushes out sodium and toxins. Low water intake causes <u>more</u> fat deposits. Expert dieters know each pound of fat burned releases 22 ounces of water which must be flushed away along with the metabolic by-products of fat breakdown. Try Penta water. It tastes great and rehydrates fast.

4.   **Exercise for sure.** The newest studies find that regular exercise extends life-span and cuts the risk for heart attack in half! Unfortunately other new statistics from the National Institutes of Health find that 58% of adult Americans get no or little exercise. Daily exercise is the key to permanent, painless weight control. No diet will work without exercise; with it, almost every diet will. Exercise before a meal raises blood sugar levels, increases metabolism and decreases appetite. Even if you just slightly change your eating habits, you can still lose weight with a brisk hour's walk. Calories continue burning at a greater pace for several hours after you exercise! Exercise also improves your mood through endorphin release in the brain. Exercise also transports oxygen and nutrients through the body, and helps eliminate carbon dioxide and toxins from the tissues. Exercise not only helps you look better, it helps you feel better.

Get a little sunshine. The sun receives a lot of criticism today, but sunlight in moderation boosts metabolism and digestion. Eat outdoors when you can. Sunlight can produce metabolic effects in the body similar to that of physical training.

Thermogenesis is critical to weight loss after 40.

Thermogenesis is about fat burning. About 75% of the calories you eat work to keep you alive and support your resting metabolic rate. The rest are stored as white fat, or burned up by brown adipose tissue, (BAT), your fat-burning factory. Brown fat is the body's chief regulator of thermogenesis, so the more active your brown fat is, the easier it is to maintain a desirable weight. Dieters who rely solely on restricting their calorie intake usually end up disappointed, because extreme calorie restriction lowers the rate of thermogenesis. Your body actually burns *less* fat than it did before you started dieting. People who yo-yo on and off low calorie diets have even more problems. When a yo-yo dieter begins to increase calorie intake after dieting, their metabolic rate does not return to pre-diet levels, so they store more calories as fat than they did before they started!

Middle-aged spread means you're not burning enough calories after you eat. Everybody increases metabolism after eating, but the amounts of heat (thermogenesis) vary widely. Lean people experience a 40% increase in heat production after a meal. Overweight people may have only an increase of 10%. Obesity occurs primarily when brown fat isn't working properly, only a little thermogenesis takes place, and the body deals with the excess calories by storing them as fat. During mid-life years, starting in our early 40s, a genetic timer shuts down the thermogenic mechanism. Turning this timer back on is the secret to re-activating thermogenesis and a more youthful metabolism.

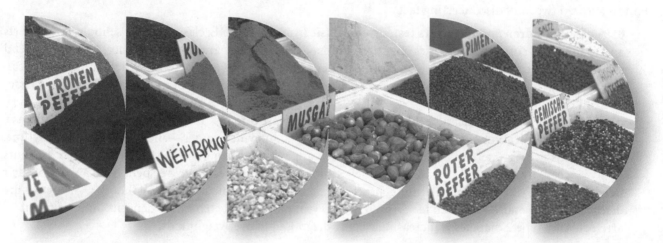

Here's how brown fat works to stimulate thermogenesis: A protein, called uncoupling protein, breaks down, or uncouples, the train of biochemical events that the cells use to turn calories into energy. Brown fat cells continue to convert calories into heat as long as they are stimulated, and as long as there is white fat for them to work on. Brown fat activity is also self-perpetuating, because it energizes more uncoupling proteins, produces more brown fat cells, and results in substantially more excess calories being burned off as heat through thermogenesis.

Research into the genetics of obesity shows that some people are not born with enough brown fat. People who eat lightly but still can't lose weight, gain more weight in middle age because the little brown fat they did have is reduced even further. Thermogenesis research demonstrates that it is possible to reverse this aberration. Thermogenic herbs have been successful at reactivating brown fat in middle age. They can increase calorie burning without additional diet changes or exercise, although these things offer added benefits.

1. Thermogenic herbs increase blood flow to lean muscle tissue, so it works faster and longer.

2. Thermogenic herbs suppress appetite. You eat less with less effort.

3. The longer you take thermogenic herb formulas, the more effective they tend to become, because they help your body produce enough thermogenic activity to make a difference.

CRYSTAL STAR® THIN AFTER 40™ caps contain liver support herbs, appetite control herbs, thermogenic herbs and metabolism boosters. If you put on pounds from fats and starches, add CRYSTAL STAR® DR. ENZYME II: FAT & STARCH BUSTER™.

Weight Control for Kids

Today's children are becoming an overweight generation. America's adults may be paying more attention to *their* diets, but statistics show that U.S. kids are the heaviest they've ever been. Today one in five school children are overweight. In fact, the incidence of childhood obesity has doubled in just the past two decades! Until the 1960s, weight control wasn't much of a problem for kids. But the fifties ushered in the fast food era - refined, chemicalized foods that changed people's metabolism and cell structure. As the fifties kids became parents, they passed on immune defense depletions and digestion problems to their kids who are now the parents of the over-weight, undernourished kids of today. It's only the beginning. T.V. food advertising especially targets kids who are eating an ever widening array of chemical-laced, genetically altered foods, and junky foods with too much fat, salt, sugar and calories. Some kids eat out of a box most of the time!

Overweight children face early diseases, low self-esteem, depression and rejection by peers. If a child's extra weight is still hanging on by their teenage years, there's a 77% likelihood they will be overweight as adults. But, crash diets are not the solution for kids (or adults). Changing the focus to health, to having a *fit* body instead of a *thin* body can make all the difference in a weight management program. Kids need mineral-rich building foods, fiber-rich energy foods, and protein-rich growth foods.

U.S. schools have dropped the ball for children's health. A 10-year study by the President's Council on Physical Fitness showed two very disconcerting facts:

- **85% of the children and teenagers tested failed basic fitness tests.** P.E. classes in U.S. schools, most sports and many extra-curricular activities have been dropped, and our kids are paying the price. Most kids attend only 1 or 2 physical education classes a week. Forty percent of boys ages 6 – 12 can't touch their toes; American girls actually run slower today than they did 10 years ago. P.E. teachers have been reassigned to other classes in a full 75% of U.S. schools.
- **As many as 90% of American children already have at least one risk factor for a degenerating disease.** The telecommunications age brought kids computers, TVs, and video games—and a lot less active playtime. Today's kids get less exercise and outdoor play than any previous generation. Most watch up to 28 hours of TV a week. By the time U.S. kids reach their senior high school year, they've spent over 3 years of their lives watching TV. Even more alarming, heart disease is now traceable to early childhood. U.S. doctors are discovering that many American teens (even some 3 year olds) already have fatty deposits on their coronary arteries. And, type 2 diabetes is increasingly being diagnosed in overweight kids.

2-Day Junk Food Detox for Kids

Today's kids rely on junk foods. Children are rewarded with food for good behavior or denied food for punishment from an early age. As they grow older, kids tend to continue that cycle by rewarding themselves with salty, sugary, fatty snacks, soft drinks, and nitrate-loaded lunch meats before parents even come home from work.

Try a light detox to start a good weight control program for an overweight child, who usually has "toxic overload" from too many chemical-laced foods. A gentle detox normalizes body chemistry. Avoid all highly processed, junky foods, red meats and dairy foods, except yogurt during this detox.

On rising: give citrus juice with 1 tsp. acidophilus liquid, or lemon juice and water with maple syrup.

Breakfast: offer apples, pineapple, papaya or oranges. Add vanilla yogurt, or rice or soy milk.

Mid-morning: give fresh carrot juice. Add ¼ tsp. Ester C crystals to neutralize body toxins.

Lunch: give fresh crunchy veggies with a yogurt dip; or a fresh veggie salad with yogurt dressing.

Mid-afternoon: offer a refreshing herb tea, like licorice or peppermint tea with maple syrup.

Dinner: give a salad, with avocados, carrots, kiwi, romaine, other high vitamin A foods; and a miso soup.

Before bed: offer a relaxing chamomile tea, add ¼ tsp. Ester C crystals; or a cup of miso soup.

Light-Right Diet for Kids

Breakfast is a key to weight loss for kids. A high fiber breakfast cuts a child's calorie intake by up to 200 calories a day and holds a child's energy and hunger until lunchtime. Add plenty of fresh enzyme-rich foods. Many of today's diets don't work because they rely on microwaved foods—a process that kills the enzymes. Enzyme dead foods create a nutritional gap for our kids. For children, this also means weight gain and constipation, a major problem for kids that eat a lot of dairy foods like milk, cheese and ice cream. 20% of Caucasian children and 80% of black children don't produce lactase, the enzyme necessary to digest milk.

Two enzyme-rich juice recipes that even the pickiest of kids will ask for again and again.

1. **Green Drink for Kids:** Make it in a juicer. Make it easy. Use any fresh veggies that your child likes most. Include green leafy vegetables like spinach, sunflower greens and lettuces. I find that kids like baby veggies - baby bok choy, baby carrots and sprouts. Don't forget sweet-tasting veggies like cucumbers, celery and tomatoes. *Note:* If you don't have a juicer, give your child a plant enzyme supplement to keep his metabolism going strong, like TRANSFORMATION'S DIGESTZYME.

2. **Energizing Fruit Smoothie:** Use fresh fruit, not canned or frozen. Blend 1 banana and 1 orange with apple juice. Add half a papaya or one-quarter of a fresh pineapple.

Changing the *type* of food a child eats without restricting the amount can result in easy, spontaneous weight loss. Plenty of fresh fruit, un-buttered spicy popcorn, and sandwich fixings are good defenses against junk foods. Snacks can be satisfying and delicious without adding significant amounts of sugar or fat. Young children need two or three snacks daily to have a nutritious diet, because their stomachs don't hold all they need in three meals. The following diet serves as an easy weight control guideline for kids. It has passed many tests on both overweight and "couch potato" kids for foods that they will eat. Rely on your health food store for good ingredients.

On rising: give a vitamin/mineral drink like ALL ONE MULTIPLE VITAMINS & MINERALS or NATURE'S PLUS SPIRUTEIN (lots of flavors), or 1 teaspoon liquid multi-vitamin in juice (like FLORADIX CHILDREN'S MULTI-VITAMIN/MINERAL).

Breakfast: have a whole grain cereal with apple juice or a little yogurt and fresh fruit; if more is desired, whole grain toast or muffins, with a little butter, kefir cheese or nut butter; add eggs, scrambled or baked (no fried eggs); or have some hot oatmeal or kashi cereal with maple syrup, and yogurt.

Mid-morning: snacks can be whole grain crackers with kefir cheese or low-fat cheese and a sugarless juice or sparkling fruit water; or apples with yogurt or kefir cheese; or dried fruit, or fruit leather; or celery with peanut butter; or a no-sugar dried fruit, nut and seed candy bar (easy to make) or trail mix stirred into yogurt.

Lunch: have a fresh veggie, turkey, chicken or shrimp salad sandwich on whole grain bread, with low-fat or soy cheese and mayonnaise. Add whole grain or corn chips with a low-fat veggie or cheese dip; or a hearty bean soup with whole grain toast or crackers, and crunchy veggies with garbanzo spread; or a baked potato with a little butter, kefir cheese, or soy cheese, and a green salad with light dressing; or a vegetarian pizza on a chapati or pita crust; or whole grain spaghetti or pasta with a light sauce and Parmesan cheese; or a Mexican bean and veggie, or rice or whole wheat burrito with a natural no-sugar salsa.

Mid-afternoon: have sparkling juice and a dried fruit candy bar, or fruit juice-sweetened cookies; or some fresh fruit or fruit juice, or an amazake protein drink with whole grain muffins; or a hard boiled egg, and some whole grain chips with a veggie or low-fat cheese dip; or some whole grain toast and peanut butter.

Dinner: have a light pizza on a whole grain, chapati or egg crust, with veggies, shrimp, and soy or low-fat mozzarella cheese topping; or whole grain or egg pasta with vegetables and a light tomato and cheese sauce; or a baked Mexican quesadilla with soy or low-fat cheese and some steamed vegetables or a salad; or a stir-fry with crunchy noodles, brown rice, baked egg rolls and a light soup; or some roast turkey with corn bread dressing and a salad; or a tuna casserole with rice, peas and water chestnuts, and toasted chapatis with a little butter.

Before bed: a glass of apple juice or vanilla soy milk or flavored kefir. A snack of unbuttered, spicy, savory popcorn is good and nutritious anytime.

Maintenance Recipes for a Weight Control Diet

Use these recipes on an ongoing basis once your initial healing diet is producing good results.

Breakfast

Breakfast Rice with Fresh Tomatoes

6 cups organic chicken or vegetable stock

1 cup fresh tomatoes, chopped

½ tsp. lemon-pepper seasoning

2 cups jasmine rice

3 tbsp. bottled teriyaki sauce

2 tbsp. parmesan cheese

In a large soup pot, bring the chicken stock, chopped fresh tomatoes and lemon-pepper seasoning to a boil. Add the jasmine rice, bring to a boil, cover and simmer until water is absorbed. Stir in teriyaki sauce and parmesan cheese. Serve hot. Makes 4 servings.

Nutrition per serving:
Calories ----------- 373
Protein ----------- 10 g.
Vitamin C--------- 9 mg.
Vitamin E --------- 2 IU
Carbohydrates ---- 77 g.
Fiber -------------- 2 g.
Fat ---------------- 2 g.
Cholesterol-------- 2 mg.
Calcium ----------- 74 mg.
Iron -------------- 5 mg.
Magnesium ------- 34 mg.
Potassium --------- 235 mg.
Sodium------------ 702 mg.

Scrambled Eggs Special

6 eggs

6 parsley sprigs (or 2 tsp. parsley flakes)

½ tsp. sesame salt

⅓ cup low-fat cottage cheese

¼ tsp. lemon-pepper seasoning

1 tsp. dijon mustard

¼ cup minced onion

2 tbsp. vegetable broth

2 tbsp. white wine

In the blender, mix the eggs, parsley, sesame salt, cottage cheese, lemon-pepper and dijon mustard. Set aside. In a skillet, braise the onion in the vegetable broth and white wine until brown and aromatic. Pour the egg mixture into hot onion sauté and cook slowly, stirring frequently but gently until eggs are set. Makes 4 servings.

Nutrition per serving:
Calories ----------- 139
Protein ----------- 14 g.
Vitamin C--------- 3 mg.
Vitamin E --------- 1 IU
Carbohydrates ---- 2 g.
Fiber -------------- 1 g.
Fat ---------------- 8 g.
Cholesterol-------- 320 mg.
Calcium ----------- 56 mg.
Iron -------------- 1 mg.
Magnesium ------- 11 mg.
Potassium --------- 144 mg.
Sodium------------ 397 mg.

Tofu Scramble

Freeze and thaw tofu first for tastiest results.

1 lb. low-fat tofu

1 tbsp. olive oil

1 small onion, sliced

¼ cup fresh shiitake mushrooms, sliced

½ cup yellow bell pepper, diced

1 tsp. soy sauce

1 tsp. sesame salt

In a bowl, crumble the tofu and drain well. Set aside. In a skillet, heat the olive oil and sauté the onion, shiitake mushrooms, and bell pepper for 5 minutes. Add the tofu, soy sauce, sesame salt and sauté for more 5 minutes, until peppers are just tender and tofu is golden. Serve hot as is or on whole grain toast. Makes 4 servings.

Tropical Fruit Platter with Strawberry Sauce

2 cups strawberries, chopped
1 tbsp. honey
2 tbsp. orange juice

1 large pineapple, peeled, cored, quartered lengthwise, and cut crosswise into ¼" slices

1 large ripe papaya, peeled, quartered, and cut into ¼" slices
6 medium kiwi, peeled, and cut into thin slices
extra whole strawberries

In a blender, mix the chopped strawberries, honey and orange juice. Set aside. On a large platter, overlap slices of each fruit. Drizzle strawberry sauce over fruit. Garnish with whole strawberries. Cut each berry into 5 slices from tip to base, (but not all the way through) and flare slightly. Makes 12 servings.

Healing drinks

Morning & Evening Fiber Drink

For daily regularity; use as needed with confidence in its efficiency, without concern about dependency.

4 oz. oat bran or rice bran
1 oz. acidophilus powder

2 oz. flax seed
½ oz. fennel seed

½ oz. apple pectin powder
1 oz. psyllium husk powder

In a blender, combine all ingredients. Take 1 tablespoon in 8 oz. apple juice, morning and bedtime.

Nutrition per serving:			
Calories ----------- 49	Vitamin E --- trace quantities	Cholesterol -------- 0	Potassium --------- 161 mg.
Protein ----------- 3 g.	Carbohydrates ---- 10 g.	Calcium ----------- 75 mg.	Sodium------------ 13 mg.
Vitamin C--------- 3 mg.	Fiber ------------- 4 g.	Iron -------------- 2 mg.	
	Fat---------------- 2 g.	Magnesium ------- 46 mg.	

Dieter's Mid-day Meal Replacement Drink

This drink is good-tasting and satisfying. It is full of foods that help raise metabolism, cleanse and flush out wastes, balance body pH, and stimulate enzyme production.

6 tbsp. rice protein powder
4 tbsp. oat bran
2 tbsp. bee pollen granules
2 tbsp. flax seed

2 tsp. fructose
1 tsp. acidophilus powder
½ tsp. lemon peel powder
½ tsp. ginger powder

2 tsp. spirulina powder (or green superfood blend of your choice)

In a blender, combine all ingredients. Take 1 tablespoon in 8 oz. juice or water. Makes enough for 10 drinks. Drink slowly.

Nutrition per serving:			
Calories ----------- 46	Vitamin E --- trace quantities	Cholesterol -------- 0	Potassium --------- 68 mg.
Protein ----------- 4 g.	Carbohydrates ---- 6 g.	Calcium ----------- 48 mg.	Sodium------------ 47 mg.
Vitamin C --- trace quantities	Fiber ------------- 1 g.	Iron -------------- 3 mg.	
	Fat---------------- 1 g.	Magnesium ------- 15 mg.	

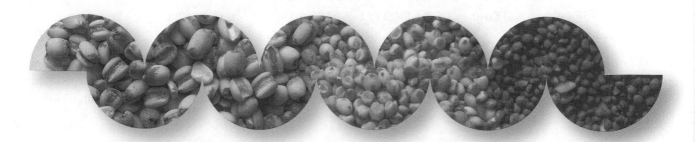

Sweet, Low-Fat Protein Drink

Rich in vitamin C, potassium, antioxidants.

1 cup vanilla soymilk or rice dream
2 bananas

3 ripe kiwis
1 cup pineapple-coconut juice

1 cup seedless grapes
2 tbsp. honey

In a blender, combine all ingredients. Makes enough for 2 large drinks.

Nutrition per serving:			
Calories ----------- 471	Vitamin E --------- 3 IU	Cholesterol-------- 0	Potassium --------- 1202 mg.
Protein ------------ 8 g.	Carbohydrates ---- 99 g.	Calcium ----------- 267 mg.	Sodium------------ 27 mg.
Vitamin C--------- 143 mg.	Fiber ------------- 6 g.	Iron -------------- 4 mg.	
	Fat---------------- 8 g.	Magnesium ------- 96 mg.	

Soups, salads, appetizers

Light, Crunchy, Crisp Salad

2½ lbs. fresh green beans, French-cut
¼ cup fresh lemon juice
2 tbsp. balsamic vinegar

4 tsp. Dijon mustard
½ cup olive oil
½ cup fat-free, organic chicken broth

1 bunch watercress, chopped
1 jicama, diced
1½ cups radishes, thinly sliced
lemon-pepper seasoning

In a large pot of salted water, boil the green beans until crisp-tender, about 5 minutes. Drain beans; rinse in cold water. Drain again; pat dry. In a large bowl, mix the fresh lemon juice, balsamic vinegar, Dijon mustard, olive oil and chicken broth. Add the chopped watercress, jicama, and radishes. Toss with beans. Season with lemon-pepper. Makes 10 appetizer salads.

Rose Petal Fruit Salad

1½ cup blueberries, rinsed
3½ cups nectarines, sliced
½ cup rose petals

¼ cup violets or nasturtiums
2 tbsp. raspberry vinegar
1½ tsp. rose flower water

2 pinches fructose

Arrange the blueberries and nectarines on a platter. Sprinkle fruit with the rose petals and violets. In a small bowl, mix the raspberry vinegar, rose flower water and fructose. Pour over fruit. Serve immediately. Makes 6 servings.

Nutrition per serving:			
Calories ----------- 62	Vitamin C--------- 10 mg.	Fat---------------- 1 g.	Magnesium ------- 9 mg.
Protein ------------ 1 g.	Vitamin E --------- 1 IU	Cholesterol-------- 0	Potassium --------- 210 mg.
Vitamin A--------- 71 IU	Carbohydrates ---- 15 g.	Calcium ----------- 8 mg.	Sodium------------ 2 mg.
	Fiber ------------- 3 g.	Iron -------------- 1 mg.	

Very Light Popovers

Healthy little "carriers" for almost anything.

1 cup unbleached flour
pinch sea salt

3 large eggs
½ cup plain low-fat yogurt

½ cup water

Preheat oven to 425°F. Preheat popover pan, or individual small pyrex custard cups that can take and hold high heat. Leave in the oven until just before use. In a blender, combine all ingredients and mix to the consistency of cream. Fill hot popover cups half full. Bake 2 minutes. Reduce heat to 325°F and bake 15 – 20 minutes more until golden and fully puffed. Makes 6 popovers.

Red & Green Salad

1 cup walnut pieces	1 head of lettuce, shredded	2 tbsp. honey
2 tsp. grapeseed oil	2 ribs celery, sliced	¼ tsp. sesame salt
1 Fuji apple and 1 Granny	2 green onions, sliced	¼ tsp. pepper
Smith apple, chopped	⅓ cup low-fat yogurt	

Pan roast the walnut pieces in the grapeseed oil until fragrant. Set aside. In a large bowl, mix the chopped apple, shredded lettuce, celery, and green onions. Make the Honey-Yogurt Dressing: Mix the low-fat yogurt, honey, sesame salt and pepper, and top salad. Sprinkle with roasted walnuts. Makes 6 servings.

Nutrition per serving:	Vitamin C --------- 10 mg.	Fat ----------------- 14 g.	Magnesium ------- 59 mg.
Calories ----------- 221	Vitamin E --------- 3 IU	Cholesterol -------- 0	Potassium --------- 405 mg.
Protein ------------ 7 g.	Carbohydrates ----- 19 g.	Calcium ----------- 70 mg.	Sodium------------ 74 mg.
Vitamin A --------- 46 mg.	Fiber ------------- 3 g.	Iron -------------- 1 mg.	

Morocco Salad

1½ cup dry couscous	1 diced bell pepper (any	4 tbsp. lemon juice
1 tsp. sesame salt	color)	3 tbsp. orange juice
a pinch of saffron (or 4 tbsp.	1 cup frozen French-cut	½ tsp. lemon-pepper
fresh mint, chopped)	green beans	¼ tsp. cinnamon
½ cup slivered almonds	⅓ cup red onion, diced	¼ tsp. paprika
1 cup carrots, diced	⅓ cup currants	
	6 tbsp. olive oil	

Bring 1¼ cups water to a boil and pour over the dry couscous. Cover; let sit for 10 –15 minutes until water is absorbed. Remove cover and fluff. Add the sesame salt and saffron. Set aside. Toast the slivered almonds in the oven until golden. Set aside. Steam the carrots, diced bell pepper, frozen French cut green beans, and red onion. Drain when done; toss with the almonds and the currants. Mix with couscous and set aside. To make the dressing, mix the olive oil, lemon juice, orange juice, lemon-pepper, cinnamon, and paprika. Toss with the salad ingredients and couscous; chill to blend. Makes 4 salads.

Low-Fat Jalapeño Poppers

4 oz. low-fat cream cheese	3 tbsp. low-fat cheddar	2 large eggs
2 tsp. lemon-garlic seasoning	cheese, shredded	1 cup crumbled dry cornbread
¼ cup scallions, minced	1 tbsp. lime juice	
2 tbsp. green olives, minced	14 fresh jalapeño chiles	

Prepare a 12" x 15" baking sheet. In a bowl, blend the cream cheese with the lemon-garlic seasoning, scallions, olives, cheddar cheese and lime juice. Set aside. Wearing rubber gloves, cut the jalapeños in half lengthwise. With a knife, cut seed pod from beneath the stem inside, leaving stem end in place to form a cup. Remove veins. Fill halves with cream cheese mixture, spreading smooth. In a different bowl, separate the egg whites and whisk until slightly frothy. Place the dry crumbled cornbread in another bowl. Dip filled chile halves, 1 at a time, in the egg whites, and then roll in the cornbread crumbs. Set the chiles slightly apart on a baking sheet, and bake at 350°F until crumbs are brown and crisp, about 20 minutes. Serve hot or warm. Makes 28 appetizers.

Nutrition per serving:	Vitamin C--------- 6 mg.	Fat----------------- 1 g.	Magnesium ------- 2 mg.
Calories ----------- 19	Vitamin E --- trace quantities	Cholesterol-------- 3 mg	Potassium --------- 17 mg.
Protein ------------ 1 g.	Carbohydrates ---- 1 g.	Calcium ----------- 15 mg.	Sodium------------ 33 mg.
Vitamin A --------- 27 mg.	Fiber ------------- 1 g.	Iron -------------- 0	

Two Delicious Tofu Dips

Tofu Dip #1:
2 (8 oz.) cakes tofu
¼ cup plain low-fat yogurt

1 tsp. soy sauce
⅓ cup celery, diced
½ tsp. herbal seasoning

2 green onions, chopped
¼ cup toasted sunflower seeds

Tofu Dip #2:
2 (8 oz.) cakes tofu
⅓ cup plain, low fat yogurt
2 tsp. mustard

⅓ cup sweet pickle relish
½ tsp. sesame salt
¼ cup tomato, diced
¼ cup celery, diced

2 tbsp. chives, chopped
1 hard boiled egg

Mash together all ingredients in a bowl and serve as a healthy dip. Makes about 8 servings.

Nutrition per serving:			
Calories ----------- 49	Vitamin C--------- 2 mg.	Fat----------------- 2 g.	Magnesium ------- 35 mg.
Protein ----------- 4 g.	Vitamin E --- trace quantities	Cholesterol-------- 4 mg	Potassium --------- 110 mg.
Vitamin A--------- 21 mg.	Carbohydrates ---- 4 g.	Calcium ----------- 65 mg.	Sodium------------ 160 mg.
	Fiber ------------- 1 g.	Iron -------------- 2 mg.	

Entrées

Ginger Crab In Wine Broth

2 tbsp. olive oil
2 tbsp. butter
4 cups organic low-fat
   chicken broth

2 cups white wine
¼ cup scallions, minced
6 slices fresh ginger, peeled
1 tbsp. soy sauce

1 tbsp. lemon juice
the meat from 3 Dungeness crabs,
   cooked & cleaned

In a large soup pot, melt the olive oil and butter. Add the chicken broth, white wine, scallions, ginger, soy sauce and lemon juice. Simmer for 10 minutes until fragrant. Add the crab meat and cook on a low simmer for 3-5 minutes. Ladle into soup bowls. Serve hot. Makes 4 servings.

Tunisian Pasta Salad

1 cup European cucumber,
   diced
½ cup black olives, pitted &
   sliced
2 scallions, sliced

1 lb. ripe roma tomatoes,
   chopped
2 tbsp. fresh parsley, chopped
2 tbsp. olive oil
5 tbsp. fresh lemon juice
½ tsp. ground cumin

1 tsp. black sesame seeds
a pinch cayenne
black pepper
1 tbsp. olive oil
1 tsp. sea salt
8 oz. dried penne pasta

In a bowl, toss the cucumber, olives, scallions, tomatoes, and parsley.

To prepare the dressing, combine 2 tbsp. olive oil, fresh lemon juice, ground cumin, black sesame seeds, a pinch of cayenne, and black pepper to taste.

Bring a large saucepan of water to a boil. Add 1 tbsp. olive oil, the salt and the penne pasta. Cook 10 minutes, stirring occasionally, until al dente. Drain the pasta in a colander, run under cold water and drain again. Pour into a serving bowl, and toss with the dressing and the veggie mix. Serve at room temperature. Makes 4 servings.

Nutrition per serving:			
Calories ----------- 264	Vitamin C--------- 21 mg.	Fat----------------- 9 g.	Magnesium ------- 39 mg.
Protein ----------- 7 g.	Vitamin E --------- 3 IU	Cholesterol-------- 0	Potassium --------- 260 mg.
Vitamin A--------- 47 IU	Carbohydrates ---- 38 g.	Calcium ----------- 56 mg.	Sodium------------ 265 mg.
	Fiber ------------- 3 g.	Iron -------------- 3 mg.	

Fettuccine & Fresh Ahi Tuna

Melts in your mouth.

3 cloves garlic	¾ tsp. sea salt	½ cup fresh mint, chopped
1 large onion, diced	½ tsp. cracked black pepper	1 tsp. lemon juice
2 tbsp. olive oil	2 tbsp. olive oil	3 scallions, diced
2 lbs. roma tomatoes, diced	1 lb. fresh tuna steak, cubed	1 lb. fettuccine
1 tbsp. fresh basil, chopped	lemon-pepper seasoning	

Using a heavy skillet, sauté the onion in 2 tbsp. olive oil until soft, about 10 minutes. Add the tomatoes and basil. Season with the sea salt and cracked pepper. Cook, partially covered until juices thicken to form a sauce, about 5 minutes. Remove vegetables from the skillet and set aside in a bowl. Heat 2 tbsp. olive oil in the skillet. Season fresh tuna steak with lemon-pepper. Add tuna to the hot skillet, tossing for 4 minutes <u>only</u>. Add the tomato sauce back to the skillet. Add in the mint, lemon juice and scallions. Cook for 2 – 3 minutes <u>only</u>. Do not overcook. Remove from heat. Set aside.

Bring a pot of salted water to boil. Add 3 cloves garlic to the water to season the pasta. Cook the fettuccine in the boiling water to al dente, about 9 minutes. Drain, and transfer to a shallow serving bowl. Add the ahi tuna and tomato sauce; toss quickly to mix. Serve hot, topping with more chopped basil. Makes 4 servings.

Nutrition per serving:	Vitamin C--------- 30 mg.	Fat---------------- 8 g.	Magnesium ------- 146 mg.
Calories ----------- 367	Vitamin E --------- 1 IU	Cholesterol-------- 21 mg.	Potassium --------- 693 mg.
Protein ------------ 22 g.	Carbohydrates ---- 50 g.	Calcium ----------- 61 mg.	Sodium------------ 190 mg.
Vitamin A --------- 493 IU	Fiber ------------- 8 g.	Iron -------------- 3 mg.	

Crusted Salmon with Citrus-Mint Sauce

3 slices whole grain	1 red grapefruit	½ cup low-fat cream cheese
sourdough bread	1 lemon	¼ cup low-fat plain yogurt
⅓ cup pumpkin seeds	2 egg whites	3 tbsp. capers, drained
⅓ cup chopped almonds	6 thick salmon steaks	2 tbsp. fresh mint leaves, chopped
⅓ cup sunflower seeds	1 tbsp. olive oil	
1 large orange	1 cup grapefruit juice	

Preheat oven to 325°. In a blender, mix the whole grain sourdough bread, pumpkin seeds, almonds and sunflower seeds. Spread this mixture on a baking sheet and bake until browned, about 12 minutes. Move into a shallow bowl. Peel and section the orange, grapefruit and lemon. Set aside.

In a bowl, beat 2 egg whites until frothy. Dip the salmon fillets in the whites. Then roll fillets in the crumb mixture to coat. Lay fillets on wax paper. Heat a large skillet to medium-high heat with 1 tbsp. olive oil. Sear the salmon steaks about 2 minutes each side. Repeat until each piece is seared. Place fillets on the baking sheet and bake for about 6 – 8 minutes.

Make the sauce while salmon is baking: in a saucepan, simmer the grapefruit juice until reduced to ⅓ cup. Remove from heat and stir in the cream cheese and yogurt. Mix in the capers and mint. Spoon sauce over warm salmon fillets. Garnish each plate with the citrus sections. Makes 8 servings.

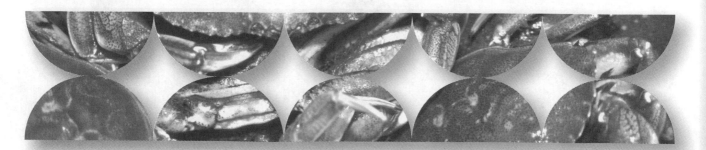

Low-Fat Classic Veggie Pie

½ cup rolled oats
½ cup buckwheat flour
½ cup unbleached flour
¼ tsp. sea salt
⅛ tsp. baking powder
grapeseed oil
2 tbsp. lemon juice
2 tsp. honey
2 tsp. sesame seeds

1 cup onion, diced
1 clove garlic, minced
1 tbsp. white wine
3 cups small broccoli florets
3 eggs
10 oz. package soft, silken tofu
1 tbsp. Dijon mustard
1 tsp. dry basil

¼ tsp. nutmeg
¼ tsp. sea salt
¼ tsp. white pepper
2 tbsp. grated parmesan cheese
red bell pepper strips
black olives

Preheat oven to 375°F. Prepare a large quiche pan. To make the crust: in a bowl, mix the rolled oats, buckwheat flour, unbleached flour, sea salt, and baking powder. Mix while drizzling with 4 – 5 tbsp. grapeseed oil one tablespoon at a time until mixture looks like wet sand. Stir in the lemon juice, honey and 2 tbsp. cold water. Mix lightly with a fork until dough forms a ball. Sprinkle the sesame seeds over bottom of the quiche pan, then pat in dough to cover bottom and sides. Prick sides and bottom of crust with a fork. Crimp edges. Bake at 375°F for 10 minutes or until the edges are slightly colored, remove from oven and reduce temperature to 350°F.

To make the filling: in a skillet, sauté the onions and garlic in 1 tbsp. grapeseed oil and the white wine for 5 minutes. Add the broccoli and 3 tbsp. water; cover and steam until broccoli is bright green and slightly tender (but not soft), about 2 minutes. Drain vegetables and spread evenly over crust.

To make the sauce: in a blender, mix the eggs until frothy. Add the tofu, mustard, basil, nutmeg, sea salt, white pepper and parmesan. Blend until very smooth. Pour mixture over vegetables in pie crust. Arrange red bell pepper strips and black olives in an attractive alternating pattern on top. Bake 40 minutes, until slightly puffy. Allow to cool 5 – 10 minutes before slicing. Makes 8 servings. For leftovers, reheat in a 325°F oven.

Easy Sole Rollatini

Tilapia fillets work well, too. Delicious served with asparagus and brown rice.

½ cup grated parmesan cheese or soy parmesan
1 tbsp. fresh basil, chopped
½ cup toasted almonds, chopped

½ cup fresh parsley, chopped
2 (16 oz.) sole or flounder fillets
3 tbsp. lemon juice

½ tsp. lemon-pepper seasoning
3 tbsp. melted butter

Preheat oven to 375°F. To make the filling: mix the parmesan, basil, almonds and parsley. Place the sole or flounder fillets on a flat surface; spoon some filling on one end. Roll up. Place seam side down in an oiled baking dish. Mix the lemon juice, lemon-pepper seasoning and melted butter; pour this over the fish. Spread the remaining filling on top. Cover the fish with foil and bake for 30 minutes or until fish is opaque throughout. Makes 6 servings.

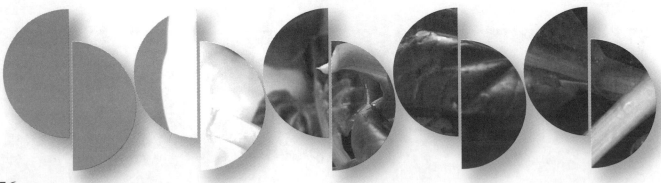

Healthy dessert options

Fruit Juice Bars

1 cup chopped dates
½ cup apple juice
½ cup orange juice
3 tbsp. grated orange zest

1 tsp. vanilla
2 cups rolled oats
2 cups whole wheat pastry
    flour

1 tbsp. cinnamon
1½ cups pear juice
grapeseed oil spray

Preheat oven to 350°F. In the blender, mix dates, apple juice, orange juice, orange zest and vanilla to a purée consistency; set aside. To make the dough: in a blender, grind 2 cups rolled oats to a coarse meal. Stir oats in a bowl with the pastry flour and cinnamon. Stir in the pear juice. Press the dough into a grapeseed oil-sprayed 8" square pan. Spread date purée on top. Bake for 35 – 45 minutes until crust is firm. Cool completely and cut in squares. Makes 16 bars.

Nutrition per serving:			
Calories ----------- 144	Vitamin C--------- 6 mg.	Fat ---------------- 1 g.	Magnesium ------- 43 mg.
Protein ----------- 4 g.	Vitamin E --------- 1 IU	Cholesterol-------- 0	Potassium --------- 221 mg.
Vitamin A --------- 4 IU	Carbohydrates ---- 31 g.	Calcium ----------- 24 mg.	Sodium----------- 3 mg.
	Fiber ------------- 4 g.	Iron -------------- 1 mg.	

Almond Scented Cheesecake Bites

12 oz. low-fat cottage cheese
3 eggs
¼ cup frozen apple juice
    concentrate

¼ cup pineapple juice
    concentrate
3 tbsp. almonds, chopped
1 tsp. almond extract

1 tsp. vanilla
⅓ cup low fat vanilla yogurt
3 tbsp. maple syrup

Preheat oven to 300°F. To make the batter, place the cottage cheese in a strainer over the sink and drain for 30 minutes. Put drained cottage cheese in a blender and mix until smooth, adding the eggs, apple juice concentrate, pineapple juice concentrate, almonds, almond extract and vanilla. Fill paper-lined muffin tins ⅔ full with batter. Bake for 35 minutes or until a toothpick inserted in the center comes out clean. Cool on rack, and then chill. The make the topping, combine the vanilla yogurt and maple syrup and drizzle on the cooling cakes. Makes 24 individual cakes.

Sugar-Free Lemon Caramel Flan

fresh lemon peel, cut into
    thin slices
½ cup honey
2 tbsp. lemon juice

2 tbsp. water
2 cups vanilla rice milk
1 tbsp. grated lemon zest
4 whole cloves

1 whole cinnamon stick
3 eggs
4 tbsp. maple syrup
1 tsp. vanilla

Preheat oven to 325°F. Use 6 oven-ready custard cups in a baking pan. To make the caramel, place 3 or 4 of the lemon slices in the bottom of each custard cup. In a sauce pan, heat the honey and lemon juice and stir until bubbly. Add 2 tbsp. water, stir to blend and divide over lemon slices. To make the custard, simmer the vanilla rice milk, grated lemon zest, cloves and cinnamon stick in a sauce pan. Remove from heat and let steep for 15 minutes covered. Remove cinnamon and cloves. Set aside. In a bowl, mix the eggs, maple syrup and vanilla. Mix in the rice milk mixture, and pour over caramel in cups. Place cups in baking pan; place on center oven rack and pour water around the cups to come halfway up sides. Bake for an hour or until a knife inserted in the center comes out clean. Remove, let cool, then cover cups with plastic and chill overnight. Loosen edges, invert on dessert plates and sprinkle with nutmeg. Makes 6 servings.

Women's Imbalances: Menopause, Fibroids, Endometriosis

A healthy female system works in an incredibly complex balance. It is an individual model of the creative universe. A woman is usually a marvelous thing to be, but the intricacies of her body are delicately tuned; they can become unbalanced or obstructed easily, causing pain and poor function. From child-bearing age to pre-menopause, and menopause, to post-menopause, many women are affected by hormone imbalances and fluctuations that rattle their lives. Fibroids, endometriosis, headaches, PMS, depression, low libido and infertility all reflect hormones out of sync. Hormones help regulate everything from energy flow, to inflammation, to a woman's monthly cycle. Maintaining hormonal balance in today's world is not easy. Every day, we are bombarded with man-made hormones, widespread hormone-mimicking pollutants, hormone drugs and hormones injected in our foods. A high stress lifestyle which depletes the adrenal glands is another major factor in hormonal problems.

A hormone balancing lifestyle plan, like those detailed in this section, gently harmonizes your body, rather than regulating hormones by injection which sometimes stops your own natural hormone production entirely. I find natural, hormone balancing therapies after trauma, stress or serious illness, or after a hysterectomy, childbirth, a D & C, or an abortion allow your body to achieve its own hormone levels and bring itself to its own balance.

Drugs, chemicals and synthetic medicines, standing as they do outside the natural cycle of things, often do not bring positive results for women. These substances usually try to add something to the body, or act directly on a specific problem area. The gentle, but effective nutrients in whole foods and herbs are identified and used by our body's own enzyme action. Nutritional therapy nourishes in a broad spectrum, like the female essence itself. A woman's body responds to it easily without side effects. I find that most women know their own bodies better than anyone else, and can instinctively pinpoint foods within a diet range that are right for her personal renewal. Relief and response time are often quite gratifying. Hormones, incredibly potent substances, seem to be at the root of most women's problems. Even in tiny amounts they have, as any woman can tell you, dramatic effects. Many female ailments are caused by too much estrogen production; fibrocystic breasts, endometriosis, PMS, and heavy, painful menstrual periods reflect this imbalance. The growth and function of the breasts and uterus are controlled by estrogens and prolactin which are produced by the ovaries and pituitary gland. A high fat diet raises these hormones to disease-forming levels.

Are you suffering from estrogen disruption?

Estrogen disrupters are so commonplace in modern society that there is no way to completely avoid them. All of the Earth's waterways are connected, so chemical pollutants containing environmental hormones reach your food supply wherever you live. The problem is so huge that in 1996 the Environmental Protection Agency began implementing a congressionally mandated plan through EDSTAC (Endocrine Disrupter Screening and Testing Advisory Committee) to test 87,000 compounds to determine their effect on the reproductive systems of humans and animals. However, due to the enormous scope of the project, a lack of funding and strong opposition from the chemical industry, very little real progress has been made.

Estrogen disrupters are in pollutants, drugs, hormone-injected meats and dairy products, plastics and pesticides. Nearly 40% of pesticides used in commercial agriculture are suspected hormone disrupters! Man-made estrogens can stack the deck against women by increasing their estrogen hundreds of times over normal levels. Scientists may believe there is no significant difference between man-made and natural hormones, but thousands of women say that even if a lab test can't tell the difference, their bodies can. Women aren't the only ones endangered by the estrogen-mimics. Substantial evidence shows that man-made estrogens threaten male reproductive health, too. The most alarming statistics relate to sperm count and hormone driven cancers.

Are designer estrogens, the SERMs, (selective estrogen receptor modulators) estrogen disrupters? SERMs, under the brand name Evista, are the new generation of estrogen replacement drugs, developed to address the serious health concerns of menopausal women. Preliminary reports suggest these drugs, like traditional HRT drugs (Premarin and PremPro), still disrupt a woman's delicate hormone balance.

Signs and symptoms that you may have estrogen disruption:

- Heavy, painful periods. Breast inflammation and pain that worsens before menstrual periods
- Weight gain (especially in the hips). Head hair loss—facial hair growth
- Hot flashes (a sign of estrogen disruption in the brain)
- Endometriosis and pelvic inflammatory disease
- Breast and uterine fibroid development; ovarian cysts
- Early puberty (nearly half of African-American girls and 15% of Caucasian girls now begin to develop sexually by age 8, a clear indicator of estrogen disruption.)
- Breast, uterine and reproductive organ cancer (A 1992 study shows up to 60% more DDE, DDT and PCBs, known estrogen disrupters, in women with breast cancer.)

Is there any way to reduce your exposure to estrogen disrupting chemicals?

1.   Cut back on fat! Hormone disrupters accumulate in body fat. This is why a high fat diet is a major risk for long term exposure to them, and why it may lead to increased risk for hormone-driven cancers.

2.   Eat sea greens like arame, nori and dulse regularly. Algin, a gel substance in sea greens, protects against chemical overload, often involved in breast cancer, by binding to chemical wastes so to eliminate them safely.

3.   Avoid hormone-injected commercial meats, especially beef and pork. Choose hormone-free dairy.

4.   Limit hormone-disrupting drugs like HRT drugs for menopause and birth control pills. Use only when all other options have been ruled out. Avoid hormone-mimics in hair treatment placenta products.

I believe herbs are still a better choice for hormone balance.

Many of the phytoestrogen containing herbs, like black cohosh for instance, are not just natural (instead of chemical) direct estrogens. As living medicines, they can work intelligently with your body. In many cases, these herbs don't compete for receptor sites or have a direct estrogenic activity in the body. In fact, they work mainly as adaptogens which balance glandular activity and normalize body temperature fluctuations. They do what herbs always do best no matter what the problem is… they are body normalizers.

Is hormone replacement therapy always necessary after a hysterectomy?

More than a half million American women have hysterectomies every year. 50% will have a hysterectomy in their lifetime. The surgery is major, requiring a month or more of recovery time. 1 in 1,000 women actually die as a result. Endometriosis, uterine fibroids, or heavy periods are common reasons for a hysterectomy, but just 10 percent of hysterectomies are medically necessary. According to one UCLA-Rand study, 14% of women who have a hysterectomy have no symptoms that warrant the surgery. The surgical removal of a woman's uterus or ovaries (or both) can mean major disruptions in hormonal health throughout her life, and a lifelong prescription of hormone replacement drugs. Natural therapies can help a woman avert surgery and help her body normalize naturally. Vitex extract and natural progesterone creams for example, help manage heavy, abnormal bleeding.

Herbs can help boost hormone production by the adrenal glands if surgery has already been done. The rainforest herb Maca for instance, can control hysterectomy-induced symptoms like depression, low libido, constipation and hot flashes. A bonus: Maca is rich in absorbable calcium, magnesium and silica, important for bone strength. MACA MAGIC HRT FORMULA has herbs like wild yam, vitex and maca to balance hormones and increase libido.

Fibroids and Endometriosis

An astounding 40% of American women 35 and older have fibroids. Uterine fibroids are actually more common than blue eyes! A hysterectomy is the common medical solution, but most women tell me they would rather deal with the fibroids! Uterine fibroids are benign growths between the size of a walnut and orange that appear on uterine walls. Their symptoms can be mild to severe with excessive menstrual bleeding, abdominal pain, bladder infections, painful intercourse and infertility topping the list.

Most fibroids are not cancerous, and have less than ½ of 1% chance of becoming cancerous before menopause. Most fibroids go away on their own after menopause.

Breast fibroids are also common. They feel like moveable, rubbery nodules near the breast surface. Women complain they swell, so that even getting a hug is too painful. In a small number of cases, breast fibroids can be fast-growing and may require medical diagnosis. Even then, false cancer positives are reported in 30% of cases.

How is endometriosis different?

Endometriosis is specifically caused by excess growth of endometrial tissue that is not shed during menstruation. The tissue escapes the uterus and spreads, attaching to other areas of the body—ovaries, lymph nodes, fallopian tubes, bladder, rectum, even kidneys and lungs. It grows abnormally, bleeding severely during the menstrual cycle, from the vagina or rectum, or bladder or back through the fallopian tubes, instead of normally through the vagina.

Endometriosis means heavy periods and pain all month long, and it increases risk for benign uterine and breast fibroids. It's credited with up to 50% of infertility cases in American women.

Even in advanced cases, fibroids and endometriosis can be reduced, even eliminated entirely by making simple diet changes and following specific herb and supplement protocols.

Do you have warning signs of fibroids or endometriosis?

A visit to your holistic physician will give you a definitive diagnosis, but two or more yes answers to the symptoms below should alert you to a potential problem.
- severe abdominal cramping and shooting pain; and abdominal-rectal pain
- excessive, painful menstruation; passing large clots; prolonged abnormal menstrual cycles
- chronic fluid retention, bloating
- irregular bowel movements or diarrhea during menses

What causes endometriosis and fibroids?

Scientists are still not entirely certain why endometriosis and fibroids develop, but here are major risk factors:

Excess estrogen levels / Low progesterone levels: Excess estrogen fuels abnormal tissue growth and is a direct cause of both fibroids and endometriosis for the majority of women. And, as I mentioned, when estrogen production declines during menopause, fibroids normally go away on their own. However, quite understandably, this isn't nearly soon enough for women who are suffering from the problem.

X-Ray consequences: Even low dose radiation may mean increased risk for fibroids. Breast tissue is so sensitive that the time between a mammogram and fibroid growth is sometimes as little as three months.

High fat diet with too much caffeine and commercial meat: This is especially a problem for breast fibroids. Eliminating caffeine and hormone-injected meats dramatically reduces fibrocystic breasts for many women.

Oral contraceptives may play a role: Your physician will tell you that newer pills are much better, and they are. Still, feedback I've had from birth control users has me convinced that even the newest low dose oral contraceptives can cause breast swelling, and aggravate fibroid problems and endometriosis for susceptible women.

Do you need a gland cleanse?

A healthy endocrine system is a must for solving female problems because the glands are the deepest level of the body processes. Glands are critical to good health, especially as you age. The comment "you're as young as your glands" has merit. Good nutrition for the glands can "change the world" for a woman. Many hormones are protein based, so a diet high in vegetable proteins and whole grains, with some lecithin and nutritional yeast on a regular basis, can be important to effective gland health and overcoming fibroids and endometriosis.

Hormones, like adrenaline, insulin, and thyroxine, are chemical messengers exerting wide-ranging effects. Hormones affect our moods, energy levels, mental alertness and metabolism. Glands, hormones and the brain are affected first by nutritional deficiencies, pollutants, chemicalized foods and synthetic hormone mimics. Lack of minerals, for instance, something most Americans live with today, undermines the health of almost every gland and organ. The chronic stress loads that most Americans live under have a direct effect on hormone balance. We can see this easily in low levels of steroidal hormones produced by our "stressed-out" adrenals.

Is your body showing signs that it needs a gland cleanse?
- unexplained bloating or weight gain caused by sluggish metabolism (impaired thyroid activity)
- unstable blood sugar reactions like unexplained moodiness or hyperactivity (unbalanced insulin levels)
- chronic poor digestion (low enzyme output from a congested pancreas)
- sallow skin color; poor skin texture (often means a sluggish liver and poor gallbladder activity)
- chronic fatigue yet the inability to sleep through the night (adrenal exhaustion or pineal imbalance)
- mental fuzziness, dizziness when you get up quickly, heart palpitations (adrenal exhaustion)
- cold hands and feet; hair, skin and nails problems; or menstrual problems (thyroid malfunction)
- constant colds or flu bouts, even out of season (glands are always affected by respiratory infections)
- PMS, fibroids and endometriosis (hormone imbalance disorders)

Get the best results from your gland cleanse:
- Trace minerals and protein are important. Add green superfoods to your diet for the most rapid results.
- Herbal adaptogens like ginseng noticeably improve the way your body handles stress. Add herbs like panax ginseng, suma, jiaogulan, Siberian eleuthero, gotu kola, dong quai and ashwagandha to your program.
- Eat smaller meals. Overeating can suppress hormone production.
- Limit dairy foods and meats (especially beef and pork), notoriously high in hormone-disrupting chemicals. Chicken is also an offender. I hear from women who have an immediate reaction with breast swelling from eating chicken injected with hormones. Look for hormone-free poultry at health food stores—Petaluma Poultry Rosie the Organic Chicken, Diestel and Coleman Natural Products.
- Wash produce to reduce hormone disrupting pollutant residues; Healthy Harvest Fruit, Vegetable Rinse.
- Add fermented soy foods (tofu, tempeh, miso, etc.) to your diet for hormone normalizing isoflavones.
- Drink green tea to flush out fats that harbor estrogen-disrupting chemicals.
- Eat cruciferous veggies like steamed broccoli and cauliflower to help flush excess estrogens out.

A Woman's Fresh Foods Gland Cleanse

A fresh foods cleansing diet is recommended to clear your body of toxins and allow it a brief rest before beginning a new way of eating to nourish your glands. A cleanse of this type for women also generates clearer skin, a more even temperament, fewer allergies, sweeter breath, softer hair and brighter eyes as clogging toxins and congestion leave the body. Hormone imbalance disorders like PMS, fibroids and endometriosis can be overcome or reduced as congestive wastes leave the body. Note: Glands are affected first by dehydration. Drink 8 glasses of water each day of your cleanse. Eliminate caffeine during your cleansing diet for the best improvement of female problems; limit caffeine after your cleanse for preventive health. Avoid red meats, hard alcohol (too much sugar), sodas and tobacco.

The night before a gland cleanse... Take a gentle herbal laxative: CRYSTAL STAR® LAXA-TEA™; YOGI DETOX TEA; NATURE'S SECRET SUPERCLEANSE.

The next day: if in season, for the first day of your juice cleanse, go on a watermelon juice-only cleanse. Drink throughout the day to rapidly flush and alkalize. If watermelon is not available, start with the following:

On rising: take lemon juice in water with 1 tsp. maple syrup; or a glass of aloe vera juice with herbs and 1 tsp. RED STAR nutritional yeast flakes; or green tea, or CRYSTAL STAR® CLEANSING & PURIFYING TEA™.

Breakfast: take 2 tsp. of cranberry concentrate in water with 1 tsp. honey; or JARROW FERMENTED SOY ESSENCE drink for estrogen balancing; or fresh fruit with yogurt and toasted wheat germ.

Mid-morning: apple or carrot juice with 1 tbsp. green superfood, like WAKUNAGA HARVEST GREENS, or 1 tsp. sea greens; or V-8 juice (page 18), or KNUDSEN'S VERY VEGGIE JUICE with 1 tsp. BRAGG'S LIQUID AMINOS; and some raw celery or cucumber sticks with kefir cheese or yogurt cheese, and a small bottle of mineral water.

Lunch: have a bowl of miso soup with sea greens snipped on top. Sprinkle with 1 tsp. nutritional yeast for B vitamins; or have a green salad with sprouts, carrots and lemon/oil dressing and sea greens snipped on top.

Mid-afternoon: have a green drink, with 1 tsp. BRAGG'S LIQUID AMINOS; or a mixed veggie juice, or a high vitamin/mineral drink like ALL ONE for balance; have some raw crunchy veggies (especially broccoli and cauliflower) with a vegetable dip or soy spread; and a balancing herb tea, like CRYSTAL STAR® FEMALE HARMONY TEA™.

Dinner: have a Mineral Rich Broth: Simmer 30 minutes: 3 carrots, 1 cup parsley, 1 onion, 2 potatoes, & 2 stalks celery. Strain and add 1 tbsp. BRAGG'S LIQUID AMINOS; or a green salad with yogurt dressing and green tea.

Before Bed: have an apple-alfalfa sprout juice; or a glass of papaya-pineapple juice to enhance enzyme activity; or 1 tsp. cranberry concentrate in chamomile tea; or a cup of miso broth for B vitamins; or CRYSTAL STAR® STRESS ARREST™ tea for easier sleep.

Choose 2 or 3 supplements especially for women's bodies:

For female hormone balance: CRYSTAL STAR® FEM-SUPPORT CFS STAMINA™ extract, or FEMALE HARMONY™ caps or tea, or CRYSTAL STAR® PRO-EST BALANCE™ herbal progesterone roll-on (rapidly effective). Add Vitex or black cohosh extract; or take ESTEEM WOMEN'S COMFORT formula.

For women with abnormal periods: Vitex extract or RAINBOW LIGHT VITEX-BLACK COHOSH COMPLEX; Una de Gato caps; MOON MAID BOTANICALS PRO-MENO wild yam cream, or CRYSTAL STAR® PRO-EST BALANCE™ wild yam cream; HERBAL MAGIC FEMSTRUATION. Note: New Research shows taking standardized St. John's wort with oral contraceptives can increase intracyclic bleeding (J. Clin Pharmacol 2003; 56:683-90).

For breast fibroids: CRYSTAL STAR® BREAST & UTERINE FIBRO DEFENSE™ caps for 3 months, then Vitex extract 2x daily with Burdock tea 2 cups daily for one month. Evening Primrose Oil 3000 mg. daily, or vitamin E 800IU with folic acid 800 mcg. daily. Nature's Way DIM-PLUS.

For uterine fibroids and endometriosis: CRYSTAL STAR® WOMEN'S BEST FRIEND™ 6 daily for 3 months, then BREAST & UTERINE FIBRO DEFENSE™ for 3 months (highly recommended); or CRYSTAL STAR® PRO-EST™ BALANCE roll-on for fibrous areas; or Cordyceps 750 mg.; or PACIFIC BIOLOGIC GYNOEASE. Protease enzyme therapy shows excellent results. Consider CRYSTAL STAR® DR. ENZYME™ WITH PROTEASE & BROMELAIN. Note: Protease may thin the blood. Ask your natural health practitioner if protease enzyme therapy is right for you.

Hormone tonics for more energy: CRYSTAL STAR® FEEL GREAT NOW™ and ADRENAL ENERGY BOOST™ formula; PLANETARY SCHIZANDRA ADRENAL SUPPORT; CRYSTAL STAR® TOXIN DETOX™ if you are regularly exposed to pollutants.

Essential fatty acids normalize hormone production: Evening primrose oil, 3000 – 4000 mg. daily; BARLEANS ESSENTIAL WOMAN; NATURE'S SECRET ULTIMATE OIL; UDO'S PERFECTED OIL BLEND.

For hormone boosting after hysterectomy or during menopause: PRINCE OF PEACE ROYAL JELLY-RED GINSENG combo; Rainforest herb Maca; SOURCE NATURALS TRIBULUS TERRESTRIS.

Hormone support nutrients: Calcium-magnesium 2000 mg. daily, iron 20 mg.; B-complex 100 mg.; Iodine, potassium and silica from sea veggies are key to endocrine health: CRYSTAL STAR® OCEAN MINERALS™ or GREEN FOODS ION KELP tabs (highly recommended). Note: If you are taking synthetic hormones, they can destroy vitamin E in the body, increasing risk for heart disease. Add natural vitamin E 400IU daily to counteract this.

For adult acne or facial hair growth: Saw palmetto extract. (Not if pregnant or on HRT.)

These bodywork techniques can accelerate and maximize your cleanse

- **Exercise:** Exercise is a cleansing nutrient in itself because it changes body chemistry.
  1. Take a regular 20 minute "gland health" walk every day.
  2. Do yoga stretches every morning.
  3. Get morning sunlight on the body every day possible, on the arms for women.
  4. Do deep breathing.
- **Acupressure points:** Stroke the tops of both feet for 5 minutes each to stimulate hormone secretions.
- **Massage therapy:** reestablishes unblocked meridians of energy and increases circulation.
- **Bathe/Sauna:** A relaxing mineral bath—add 1 cup Dead Sea salts, 1 cup Epsom salts, ½ cup regular sea salt and ¼ cup baking soda to a tub; swish in 3 drops lavender oil, 2 drops chamomile oil, 2 drops marjoram oil and 1 drop ylang-ylang; or CRYSTAL STAR® HOT SEAWEED BATH™ for pH balance.

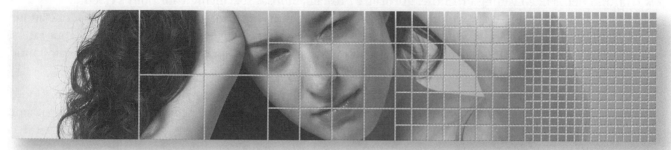

Preventing PMS Naturally

PMS is by far the most common women's health complaint.

Experts say a whopping 90% of all women between the ages of 20 and 50 experience some degree of PMS. Symptoms like headaches, acne, food cravings, bloating, constipation or diarrhea, and mood swings can last anywhere from 2 days to as long as 2 weeks! Some women say their cycles make them feel out of control all month! Over 150 symptoms have been documented. The hormone shift in estrogen/progesterone ratios during the menstrual cycle is the major factor in PMS symptoms. (Women report the most symptoms in the two week period before menstruation, when the ratios are the most elevated.) The modern woman's lifestyle seems almost made-to-order for stress and imbalance. Low brain serotonin, low or no exercise, excess estrogen, prostaglandin imbalance, and a diet loaded with sugar, salt, food chemicals and caffeine are all implicated in PMS.

Still, PMS seems to be partially a consequence of the modern woman's emancipation. In times past, women were a silent, long-suffering lot, who felt that female disorders were just part of being a woman. Women were not out in the high profile workplace with men; they could go to bed and suffer alone. In addition, our diets consisted of more fresh foods than they do today.

While most women try to "grin and bear" the aggravation of PMS, up to 10% have symptoms serious enough for them to seek professional help. But drugs and chemical medicines, standing as they do outside a woman's natural cycle, usually do not bring positive results for women. Indeed the medical establishment, with its highly focused "one-treatment-for-one-symptom" protocols has not been successful in addressing PMS. For example, contraceptive drugs, regularly given to reduce symptoms, make PMS worse for some women. Antidepressant drugs like Prozac, the new rage for PMS treatment, mean insomnia and shakiness for many.

Natural treatment is much more gratifying. It emphasizes a highly nutritious diet, herbal tonifiers, and naturally-derived vitamins to encourage the body to provide its own balance for relief.

PMS symptoms tend to get worse for most women in their late thirties and beyond. They are often magnified after taking birth control pills, after pregnancy, and just before menopause because of hormone imbalances. But, with such a broad spectrum of symptoms affecting every system of the body, there is clearly no one cause and no one treatment. A holistic approach is far more beneficial, and self care allows a woman to tailor treatment to her own needs.

The Natural Keys To Controlling PMS:

Menstruation is a natural part of our lives. PMS is not. Women can take control of PMS naturally and effectively. Natural therapies work well for most women because they address the full spectrum of factors involved. A woman can expect a natural therapy program for PMS to take at least two months, as the body works through both ovary cycles with nutritional support. The first month, there is a noticeable decrease in PMS symptoms; the second month finds them dramatically reduced. Don't be discouraged if you need 6 months or more to gently coax your system into balance. Even after many of the symptoms are gone, continuing the diet recommendations, and smaller doses of the herb and vitamin choices makes sense toward preventing PMS return.

1.   **Essential fatty acids balance prostaglandins.** Prostaglandins are vital hormone-type compounds that act as transient hormones, regulating body functions almost like an electrical current. Foods like ocean fish, olive oil, and herbs like Evening Primrose, normalize prostaglandins by balancing your body's essential fatty acid supply. Too much saturated fat from meats and dairy foods inhibits prostaglandin balance and proper hormone flow. Arachidonic acid in animal fats tends to deplete progesterone levels and strain estrogen/progesterone ratios. Evening Primrose oil 3000 – 4000 mg. daily, especially along with a broad spectrum herbal balancing compound like CRYSTAL STAR® FEMALE HARMONY™, shows excellent results for many women.

2.   **Love your liver to balance estrogen and progesterone levels.** Lower your fat intake and reduce dairy foods to help your liver do its job. A high-fat diet hampers liver function. Many dairy foods are a source of synthetic estrogen from hormones injected into cows. At the very least, switch to non-fat dairy products. Estrogen is stored in fat; non-fat foods don't contribute to estrogen stores. Focus on high quality vegetarian protein to improve estrogen metabolism. On PMS days, avoid dairy products altogether. A cup of green tea, or CRYSTAL STAR® DR. VITALITY™ each morning can go a long way toward relieving organ congestion and detoxifying the liver. Non-fat yogurt is a good choice because it also contains digestive lactobacillus. Reduce caffeine to one cup of coffee or less a day. Caffeine tends to deplete the liver and lowers B vitamin levels, contributing to anxiety, mood swings, and irritability. Fifteen to 30% of women with breast tenderness during PMS find relief by stopping caffeine use. A little wine is fine, but avoid hard liquor to control PMS. Strong alcohol compromises liver function by lowering B vitamin levels, reducing its ability to break down excess estrogen. Consider Milk Thistle Seed extract, CRYSTAL STAR® LIVER CLEANSE FLUSHING TEA™ or a dandelion tea daily.

4.   **Enhance your thyroid to reduce PMS.** Estrogen levels are controlled by thyroid hormones. If the thyroid does not have enough iodine, insufficient thyroxine is produced and too much estrogen builds up. Sea greens are a good choice for thyroid balance because they are rich in potassium and iodine. Two tablespoons daily in a soup or salad, or over rice, or six pieces of sushi a day, are a therapeutic dose. Or, try sea veggies in capsules, like CRYSTAL STAR® OCEAN MINERALS™, GAIA HERBS THYROID SUPPORT phytocaps, or GREEN FOODS ION KELP.

4.   **Phytohormone-rich herbal compounds help balance body estrogen.** Phyto-estrogens are remarkably similar to human hormones. They help raise body estrogen levels that are too low by stimulating the body's own hormone production, or by attaching to estrogen receptor sites. Remarkably enough, when the plant estrogens bind to a woman's receptor sites, they block the uptake of strong environmental estrogens, or even too much of a woman's own estrogen. The net effect is a lowering of body estrogen levels, thus reducing the risk of excess estrogen-driven diseases and related PMS symptoms. Phytohormone-rich plants like soybeans and wild yams, and hormone-rich herbs like black cohosh, panax ginseng, licorice root and dong quai, have a safety record of centuries. Take an herbal combination like CRYSTAL STAR FEMALE HARMONY™ tea or capsules, or ESTEEM WOMEN'S COMFORT as a stabilizing resource for keeping the female system female, naturally. Whole wild yam creams also show success against PMS as transdermal sources for estrogen/progesterone balance.

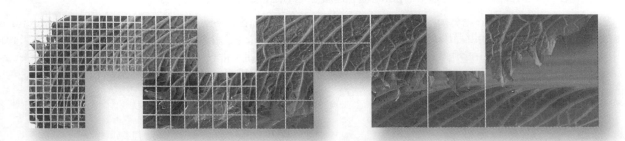

A Woman's PMS Prevention Diet

Improve your diet to control PMS. Women with severe PMS symptoms eat 60% more refined carbs, 280% more sugars, 85% more dairy products, and 80% more sodium than women who don't get PMS. The right diet can help alleviate even your worst symptoms, like water weight, cramping and mood swings. Avoid highly processed (fast and junk) foods, and dairy foods during PMS. A low fat, vegetarian diet with regular seafood clearly diminishes symptoms. Add soy foods like miso and tofu, and cruciferous veggies like broccoli to reduce excess estrogen linked to PMS. The diet below focuses on nourishing adrenals for balanced hormone secretions. Keep the diet low in salt and sugar. Eat plenty of cultured foods, like yogurt and kefir for friendly flora. Eat brown rice often for B vitamins. Eat smaller meals often for blood glucose balance. If you're like most women, you'll thrive on fresh fruits and vegetables and brown rice, with limited yeasted breads and beans. Caffeine foods should be limited; red meats, tobacco and hard alcohol should be avoided. Drink 6 glasses of water daily to keep the system flowing and fats flushed out. Have a small bottle of water with any of the meals in the following diet.

On rising: take ALL ONE VITAMIN/MINERAL drink or METABOLIC RESPONSE MODIFIERS WHEY PUMPED protein; or a fruit smoothie with 1 tsp. spirulina added.

Breakfast: make a mix of *2 tbsp. each* lecithin granules, nutritional yeast, flax seeds, and wheat germ. Sprinkle on whole grain cereal, fresh fruit or yogurt, poached or baked eggs, or oatmeal with a little maple syrup; or have a fresh fruit smoothie with prunes and apples; or some tofu scrambled "eggs," with toasted pita bread; or rice pilaf with soy sauce.

Mid-morning: try a mood swing, anti-constipation blender drink: 2 cups fresh peaches, chopped; 2 frozen bananas, chopped and 1 cup apple juice; or alfalfa/mint tea; or a cup of miso or ramen noodle soup with sea greens and rice cakes.

Lunch: have some steamed veggies with rice, tofu and a light tamari dressing; or a salad with baked, marinated tofu and greens, and a lemon-oil vinaigrette; or a seafood salad with brown rice or veggie pasta; or a light oriental soup and salad, with sea greens and crunchy noodles; or a baked potato with yogurt or kefir cheese, a green salad and green tea; or hot soup.

Mid-afternoon: have a green drink, WAKUNAGA HARVEST BLEND, GREEN FOODS GREEN MAGMA, or CRYSTAL STAR® ENERGY GREEN RENEWAL™ with 1 tsp. Bragg's LIQUID AMINOS; or a refreshing herb tea like CRYSTAL STAR® FEMALE HARMONY™ or STRESS ARREST™; or whole grain crackers with kefir cheese, or soy spread; or have celery with a little low-fat cheese dip; or a hard boiled egg with a little sesame salt, some whole grain crackers and mineral water.

Dinner: have baked or grilled fish with a light sauce, brown rice, and sautéed veggies; or an oriental meal, with miso soup and sea greens, rice pasta, and Chinese greens; or have an oriental vegetable stir-fry with miso soup and brown rice; or a veggie or seafood quiche with a whole grain crust; or a small omelet with a low-fat filling; or a light Italian meal with spinach or artichoke veggie pasta and baked vegetables; or a baked potato or steamed broccoli or cauliflower with low-fat cheese. A light white wine at dinner is fine for digestion and relaxation.

Before bed: have a glass of water or an herb tea like peppermint or CRYSTAL STAR® STRESS ARREST™ TEA.

Choose 2 or 3 supplements especially for PMS relief and prevention

• **Normalize hormone fluctuations:** CRYSTAL STAR's 2-month program is highly successful: FEMALE HARMONY™ capsules 2 daily each month, with Evening Primrose oil 6 daily the 1st month, 4 daily the 2nd month. Before your period, drink green tea or CRYSTAL STAR® GREEN TEA CLEANSER™ each morning as a mini detox. Take TINKLE TEA™ for 5 days for pre-period edema. Use PRO-EST BALANCE™ roll-on or MUSCLE RELAXER™ caps, 4 at a time for cramping (very effective). During your period use CRYSTAL STAR® PMS RELIEF CRAMP BARK COMPLEX™ extract as needed. (CRYSTAL STAR® HERPEX™ Lysine/licorice gel for PMS mouth sores.)

• **Relieve estrogen build-up:** CRYSTAL STAR® OCEAN MINERALS™ caps; or NATURE'S WAY DIM PLUS; MOOD MAID PRO-MENO wild yam cream; vitamin E 400 IU daily. Rebalance hormone levels with burdock tea 2 cups daily. Add fiber: NATURE'S SECRET ULTIMATE FIBER tabs; , or JARROW GENTLE FIBERS; Saw palmetto extract caps 320 mg. for testosterone balance (especially if you have excess facial hair or acne).

- **Relieve cramping:** Chamomile tea; Ginger tea or NEW CHAPTER DAILY GINGER extract drops in water; PURE ESSENCE LABS FEM CREME - rub on abdomen; Homeopathic magnesium phosphate; Calcium/magnesium caps to relax the uterus and for mood management. Vitex extract for breast tenderness and pain.
    - **Pelvic applications for cramps:** Ice packs; Ginger compresses; NEW CHAPTER ARNICA GINGER gel.
- **Ease mood swings:** 5-HTP, 50 mg.; CRYSTAL STAR® DEPRESS-EX™ or RELAX™ caps; Now SAMe caps. Nature's Secret ULTIMATE B; GABA 2000 mg. daily; Vitamin C up to 5000 mg. daily to neutralize heavy metal toxins.
- **Relieve excessive flow:** Bayberry caps 4 daily; Cranesbill/red raspberry tea; Vit. C 3000 mg. with bioflavonoids or Bilberry extract (bioflavonoids); vitamin K 100 mcg.
- **Relieve lower back pain:** Barleans Omega-3 rich flax oil 3 daily; quercetin 1000 mg. and bromelain 1500 mg.; CRYSTAL STAR® DR. ENZYME™ WITH PROTEASE & BROMELAIN.

These bodywork techniques can maximize your program

- **A good massage or shiatsu session** before your period releases clogging mucous and fatty formations. Massage breasts and ovary areas to relax reproductive organs.
- **Exercise** is a must for female balance. Exercise improves the way your body assimilates and metabolizes hormones. It changes food habits, and decreases craving for alcohol or tobacco. It boosts beta endorphin levels in the brain. It improves circulation to relieve congestion. It encourages regularity for rapid elimination of toxins.
- **Stretching-relaxation exercises:** yoga with deep breathing and tai chi help. Acupuncture and reflexology are also effective.
- **End your daily shower with a cool rinse** to stimulate circulation and relieve lymph congestion.
- **Meditate to banish PMS.** Harvard studies show 57% improvement for women with PMS who meditate twice daily for 15 – 20 minutes.
- **Light is linked to PMS.** Get out in the sunshine at least 20 minutes a day.
- **Stop smoking,** and avoid second-hand smoke. Nicotine inhibits hormone function.

Menopause: Updating your Choices

There is a big difference between just surviving menopause and being prepared for it—knowing what to expect and what can help you adjust. Menopause is intended by nature to be a gradual reduction of estrogen by the ovaries with few side effects. In a well-nourished, vibrant woman, the adrenals and other glands pick up the job of estrogen secretion to keep her active and attractive after menopause. This phenomenon increases with age as nature compensates for menopause... as well as for hysterectomy side effects.

Over 40 million women in the U.S. are going through "the change" today. By 2010, that number is expected to grow to 60 million women. By the year 2015, *almost half* of all American women will be in menopause. As of this writing, synthetic hormones are the most prescribed drugs in the U.S., of any kind. Science tells women that menopause increases the risk of heart disease and osteoporosis as estrogen and progesterone levels change.

But is this really true? Certainly, menopause does effect the balance of important minerals, like calcium and magnesium, and vitamins like E and B complex. These pressures are some of the reasons so many physicians prescribe Hormone Replacement Therapy, or HRT, for menopausal women.

Prempro, an estrogen replacement drug for menopausal women made from pregnant mare's urine, is one of the top selling drug of any kind in the U.S. But there is a firestorm of controversy about synthetic hormone replacement. The threat of breast and uterine cancer is dramatically increased with HRT drugs, and the risk increases as a woman ages. In an action that received wide media attention, U.S. government scientists halted a study on hormone replacement in July 2002 because it was such a threat to the health of the participants. Increased risk of invasive breast cancer, heart disease, stroke and pulmonary embolism (blood clots in the lungs) were all cited as reasons for halting the study. The drugs being tested—Premarin, Prempro and Provera.

Truth be told, scientists have known since the late 1980s that HRT could increase the risk of breast cancer. Studies released within the last few years have drawn the connection between HRT and breast cancer as well. A 2000 study showed women taking HRT for just five years have a 40% greater risk of developing breast cancer. A more recent study found that long term HRT may boost the odds of one of the most dangerous types of breast cancer as much as 85%. The good news is that some research finds that the higher risk for breast cancer diminishes and largely disappears when a woman has been off HRT treatment for five years.

Drug companies and much of the medical community, for whom synthetic hormones are an incredibly profitable business, continue to justify the risks because of the perceived advantages to osteoporosis and estrogen management. Yet, the newest research reveals that benefits for these diseases are not validated over the long-term.

Menopause may actually be Nature's way of lessening hormone production to *protect* women from hormone-driven cancers like breast and uterine cancer. There is a general misconception that estrogen is lost at menopause. But estrogen is not lost - production is simply reduced by 50 – 60%. Nature, in its wisdom, curtails estrogen enough to preclude pregnancy and menstruation, but not enough to stop estrogen protections, or the female essence. Women continue to manufacture estrogen after menopause, supplying it from steroidal substances in the body. Adrenal and pituitary glands help pick up estrogen production to keep the female system female.

If you are in your 40s or 50s, and are about to be confronted with the great Hormone Replacement Therapy choice, consider carefully before you agree. Of the women in menopause today, about half start synthetic hormone replacement, but only half of those stick with it because of the side effects or fear of cancer risk.

I don't believe hormone replacement is the right course for most women. In fact, 80 percent of postmenopausal women in the U.S. do not use any form of HRT at all! I listen to thousands of women around the country as I speak about menopause. The overwhelming vote is that there are numerous problems, side effects and unknowns about hormone replacement drugs. Unless you have specific, extenuating circumstances, a natural menopause with herbal support, is the best way. Even women who don't have a symptom-free menopause, say they feel younger and more energetic when they address their menopausal changes the gentle, natural way. If you do decide to try HRT, ask your physician about plant derived estrogen. The newest studies show women who take estrogen derived from plant sources instead of animal or synthetic sources experience all the benefits, have less side effects and require about half the dose!

Does HRT really protect against menopausal heart disease?

Using hormone replacement therapy or ERT to protect against heart disease is highly debatable. There is no conclusive evidence that estrogen protects against heart disease. A 1997 review concluded that the heart protective benefits attributed to estrogen may result from population selection bias or even changes towards healthier lifestyles during the course of the studies. A more recent report shows that HRT does not help treat or prevent heart disease in menopausal women. In addition, HRT drugs can deplete folic acid, raising homocysteine levels, a known risk factor for heart disease, and destroy vitamin E, a heart protective antioxidant. With its links to uterine and breast cancer, HRT should never even be considered as a long-term preventive for heart disease. There are better solutions for preventing heart disease that don't carry these risks.

What's the HRT connection to osteoporosis?

Long considered a woman's problem because of its female hormone involvement, osteoporosis affects from 35 to 50 percent of women in the first five years after menopause. HRT is still strongly promoted for osteoporosis prevention. Many menopausal women are so afraid of osteoporosis that with a little coaxing from their physicians they begin taking hormone drugs right away. Of those, about 60% discontinue the therapy because of side effects or fear of cancer! There is no question that hormones are involved in bone-building and bone loss, but declining estrogen levels after menopause do not by themselves cause osteoporosis. Although some studies show estrogen inhibits bone cell death, the newest tests reveal that as many as 15% of women on estrogen therapy continue to lose bone. Moreover, estrogen isn't the only hormone involved in bone building. The hormone progesterone actually increases bone density in clinical tests. Low androgen levels of DHEA and testosterone also play a role in bone loss, particularly in men's osteoporosis. Osteoporosis prevention is a program not a pill.

Understanding Estrogen

There are three major kinds of estrogen: estradiol, estrone and estriol.

1. Estradiol is the primary estrogen produced in the ovaries and is the most powerful natural estrogen.

2. Estrone is formed by the conversions of estradiol. Scores of studies show estradiol is the cancer-inducing form of estrogen. Therapy with estradiol-containing drugs is known to deplete other hormones produced by the ovaries like DHEA and testosterone.

3. Estriol is formed in large amounts during pregnancy and is protective against breast cancer. Estriol is found in many plants; high levels of cancer-protecting estriol are found in Asian women and vegetarians. Estriol is widely used in Europe as a breast cancer protective, but not in the U.S. because the HRT lobby is too powerful. Estriol is a natural substance which cannot be patent-protected. Bottom line: we don't hear much about estriol in the U.S. because the pharmaceutical giants can't profit from it.

The female body naturally produces about 10% estrone, 10% estradiol, and 80% estriol. The natural reduction of estradiol and estrone later in life is thought to help protect a woman from breast cancer and other kinds of postmenopausal cancers. Both estrone and estradiol have pro-carcinogenic activity. Estriol is the only type of estrogen which has anti-carcinogenic activity. A major problem with Premarin and other drugs and synthetic estrogens is that these drugs are largely formed of estradiol and estrone. Medical scientists are aware of this and add progestin as a balancing factor, as in the drug Provera.

Yet combination HRT drugs with synthetic progestin have proven to be even more dangerous than taking estrogen alone. According to the National Cancer Institute, women taking combination HRT actually have a 40% greater breast cancer risk after five years than women taking estrogen alone, who have just a 5% breast cancer risk increase (currently only women who have had hysterectomies take estrogen alone).

The latest on Hormone Replacement Therapy?

No drawbacks have been reduced. Many have increased. Drug companies who added Alzheimer's prevention as a benefit of HRT drug, have seen this claim discredited. In a group of 120 women with mild to moderate Alzheimer's, those taking estrogen actually had a higher level of dementia than those who didn't.

There are still more studies and more bad news:

*   HRT can increase a woman's risk of developing insulin resistance and Type II diabetes after menopause.
*   HRT artificially continues menstruation, spotting and bleeding, because it deters complete shedding of the uterine lining. Persistent bleeding has been linked to increased risk of endometrial cancer. Endometrial cancer may be a risk with HRT, although some studies show decreased risk when progesterone is added to estrogen.
*   HRT increases risk for gallbladder disease and blood clots.
*   HRT can destroy Vitamin B-6, potentially increasing homocysteine levels to risk heart disease.
*   HRT increases appetite, fluid retention and dry eye syndrome (DES), aggravates mood swings and localizes fat deposits on the hips and thighs. Many women get PMS symptoms, like depression or migraines.
*   HRT can increase growth of uterine and breast fibroids. Estrogen-dependent fibroids stay active.
*   HRT should not be used by women with high blood pressure, high cholesterol, chronic migraines, or endometriosis. Avoid HRT if you have a history of breast, bone or uterine cancer, or blood vessel clots (thrombosis). Many physicians advise against its use if you have diabetes, or are pregnant.

Note: Studies don't reflect the different ways that HRT acts in individual women. Women have widely different diets, weight, liver function, enzyme activity, age, alcohol sensitivity, estrogen levels and metabolism. Some women feel better on HRT, some don't see any effects and some are worse with the drug.

Do women have credible hormone replacement alternative to drugs? Yes, they do.

Plant hormones can be a better answer. A 1996 Cambridge University Medical School study says that plant-derived estrogen (estriol) "is an effective, economical, acceptable alternative to equine estrogen." Many doctors agree.

The best option, in my opinion, is a combination of phytohormone (estriol) rich herbs that can help a broad spectrum of a woman's needs during menopause. Plant hormones provide ample support with fewer long-term risks for women. My experience has been that none of the man-made hormones work as well as natural, plant-derived hormones from herbal combinations, especially over the long term.

Plant hormones offer a gentle, effective way to stimulate a woman's own body to produce amounts of estrogen and progesterone that are in the right proportion for her needs as menopause progresses. They can help control hot flashes, tighten sagging tissue, lubricate a dry vagina and normalize circulation. In addition, phytohormone-rich herbs help uterine and organ tone by improving circulation, acting as system tonics for women.

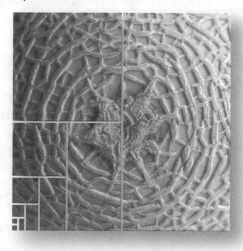

We know that plant hormones are remarkably similar to human hormones. Phytoestrogens and phytosterols have hormonal effects and behave like hormones as they lock into human cell receptors. Yet, plants are taken in naturally by the body as foods, through the enzyme system, not as drugs working outside the system. Plant estrogen has very mild estrogenic activity. At only $1/400^{th}$ to $1/1000^{th}$ of the potency of circulating estrogen, plant estrogens do not have the unpleasant side effects of increased appetite, fluid retention, heavy periods or cellulite deposits caused by synthetic hormones. Yet they offer menopause symptom control for a woman who is not producing enough estrogen on her own. Naturally-occurring flavonoids in many phytohormone rich herbs also exert a similar balancing effect on hormone secretions. Much like the body's own estrogen and progesterone hormones, plant flavonoids help elevate good cholesterol HDLs and keep arterial pathways clear.

The full medicinal value of herbs for hormone activity is in their complexity and balance, not in their concentration or strength. A single herb contains dozens of natural chemical constituents working together with little danger of toxicity.

A balanced combination of plant hormone-rich herbs works even better—addressing a broader range of needs, yet still with whole plant gentleness and absorbability. Phytohormone-rich herbal compounds are effective, yet safe and gentle. Research experts in Europe involved with medicinal plants say the benefits of a medicinal plant cannot be explained by one constituent, but involve a synergistic effect from diverse compounds. The American Cancer Society even advises that food sources (don't forget that herbs *are* foods) are the best sources of nutrients, providing potential cancer protection benefits not offered by synthetic or isolated supplements.

Focus on these four areas to sail through menopause naturally:

1. Adrenal gland health is the key to an easy menopause.

Adrenal stress symptoms are similar to menopausal symptoms—nervous tension, mild to severe depression, irritability, fatigue, and unpredictable mood swings. Stressful living and poor eating habits mean many women reach their menopausal years with prematurely worn out adrenals. Depleted adrenals cannot help a woman achieve her new hormone balance after menopause.

As I travel around the country, talking to women about more natural ways to deal with menopausal symptoms, it's almost the first question I ask when a woman complains of dramatic symptoms. Excessive hot flashes, and extreme fatigue are the first two things I hear, so it's a pretty safe bet that she has swollen, exhausted adrenals. Results are quick for many women. Changing your habits to support long term adrenal health will almost certainly result in eliminating unpleasant menopausal symptoms.

Are your adrenals exhausted? Three or more yes answers should alert you.

- Lack of energy or alertness? Unexplained moodiness, unusual crying spells, unfounded guilt?
- Severely cracked, painful heels? Nervous moistness of hands and soles of feet?
- Brittle, peeling nails or extremely dry skin?
- Frequent heart palpitations or panic attacks?
- Chronic heartburn and poor digestion?
- Chronic lower back pain (adrenal swelling)?
- Hypoglycemia and cravings for salt or sweets?
- High incidence of yeast or fungal infections? Severe reactions to odors, or to certain foods?

A. Stress is toxic to the adrenal glands. Adrenal exhaustion can keep you locked in a low-energy/high-stress loop. Herbs are some of the best therapy I know for revitalizing swollen, exhausted adrenal glands.
- Stress reactions: herbal nervines like scullcap, St. John's wort, kava, passionflower, valerian, chamomile.
- Chronic stress: herbs like black cohosh, ashwagandha, Siberian eleuthero, sarsaparilla and gotu kola.
- For adrenal integrity, try Vitamin C 5000 mg daily to help convert cholesterol to adrenal hormones.

B. Revitalize your adrenal health with sea greens.
- Sea vegetables act as total body tonics to restore female vitality during menopause. Add sea greens to your diet like nori, wakame, dulse, arame and kelp (2 tbsp. daily, chopped into salads and soups). Sea vegetables are a rich source of fat-soluble vitamins like D, K which assist with production of steroidal hormones like estrogen, and DHEA that support the female body during menopause. New studies indicate that up to 40% of the U.S. population is deficient in Vitamin D. Eating sea veggies is a great way to shore up a Vitamin D deficiency.

2. Keep your thyroid healthy.

Is your thyroid low? Do you suffer from Hashimoto's disease?

Low thyroid symptoms aggravate menopausal problems like depression, head hair loss, slow weight gain and loss of energy. Underactive thyroid, or hypothyroidism, is common in the U.S. Since the 1940s, the number of people with thyroid problems has increased. Researchers speculate that the enormous amount of chemicals that came into our culture after World War II (some only marginally tested for safety) affected thyroid health.

HRT prescriptions can depress thyroid health and worsen hypothyroidism. Thyroid disease affects nearly 15 million women. Among women over 65, almost one of ten has early-stage hypothyroidism. In 1999, Synthroid, a synthetic thyroid drug, overtook the HRT drug Premarin as the top-selling prescription drug in the U.S.

Hashimoto's disease, an autoimmune disorder where the immune system suddenly attacks healthy tissue, is the most frequent cause of poor thyroid performance in these women and the most common cause of enlarged thyroid, or goiter, in America. A prime factor in low thyroid may be iodine depletion from X-rays or low dose radiation like mammograms. For this reason, many natural health experts advise against mammograms unless a woman is at elevated risk of breast cancer. Sluggish thyroid is also related to diabetes, adrenal exhaustion, Grave's disease and vitiligo (milk white skin patches).

Many women suffer from sub-clinical hypothyroidism called Wilson's syndrome, a condition with the symptoms of hypothyroidism, but not detected by laboratory tests. Unlike true hypothyroidism, Wilson's syndrome is not caused by a thyroid hormone deficiency, but is caused by irregular processing of thyroid hormones. A stressful event like childbirth, a death, or divorce usually precedes Wilson's. A *chronically* low body temperature (below 98.6) is a major warning sign. A physician knowledgeable in natural therapies can diagnose this syndrome.

Signs of low thyroid, Hashimoto's, Wilson's? Three or more 'yes' answers should alert you.

- Great fatigue and muscular weakness, especially in the morning?
- Hormonal imbalances like PMS, delayed or absent menstruation?
- Bloating, gas and indigestion after eating? Unusually high LDL "bad" cholesterol levels?
- Unexplained depression, usually with markedly reduced libido and/or noticeable memory loss?

• Unexplained hair loss in women, often accompanied by breast fibroids?
• Unexplained obesity, with frequent constipation; puffy face and eyelids, unhealthy nails, dry or itchy skin?
• Chronically low body temperature (below 98.6)? Unusual sensitivity to cold or heat?
• Appearance of goiter (swelling of the thyroid gland)?

A. Boost your thyroid levels safely and naturally.

- Avoid table salt (use an herb salt instead), but eat plenty of iodine-rich foods. Sea greens because of their high minerals, especially iodine, are the fastest way to nourish an underactive thyroid. I recommend 2 tbsp. daily over rice, soup or a salad. Also consider sea foods, fish, mushrooms, garlic, onions and watercress.
- An immune-boosting diet full of fruits and vegetables should be your mainstay diet. Avoid fried foods, saturated fats, sugars, white flour and red meats.
- Avoid "goitrogen" foods that prevent your body's use of iodine, like cabbage, turnips, peanuts, mustard, pine nuts, millet, tempeh and tofu. (Cooking these foods inactivates the goitrogens.)
- Eat vitamin A-rich foods: yellow vegetables, eggs, carrots, dark greens, raw dairy.

3. Bladder control problems during menopause are a big problem.

People may not want to talk about it, but the numbers don't lie. Over 15 million menopausal women suffer from bladder control problems, who spend nearly $30 billion on adult diapers and medical treatments for incontinence every year! Stress incontinence and urge incontinence are the two most common types of bladder control problems. Causes include weakened pelvic muscles from childbirths, hormone imbalances related to menopause, overactive bladder, urinary tract infection, drug side effects, nutrient deficiencies, and excessive caffeine.

- Do you experience the sudden, but uncontrollable urge to urinate? (urge incontinence)
- Do you experience urine leakage when you exercise, laugh, cough, sneeze? (stress incontinence)
- Do you experience dribbling after urination? (weak or damaged pubococcygeus muscles)

A. Regain bladder control with natural therapies.

- What you eat and drink makes a difference. Caffeine foods, like coffee, tea, cola, or chocolate make urine control difficult because they act as a powerful diuretic. Avoid alcoholic beverages which over-relax bladder muscles and cause leakage. Eat small meals more frequently, rather than large meals.
- Drink lots of water. Dehydrated women have *more* incontinence than women who drink enough fluids. Highly concentrated urine irritates the bladder causing muscle spasms. Do simple toning Kegel exercises daily, to reduce stress incontinence. Tighten pelvic-floor muscles for 10 seconds, then relax for ten seconds.
- Herbal therapy shows promise for bladder control problems. A bladder control, tissue strengthening and toning formula like CRYSTAL STAR® BLADDER KIDNEY CONTROL™ is highly recommended. I personally know many people who have reduced or reversed "stress incontinence," by using this combination.
- Biofeedback or acupuncture both show success for bladder control problems. Both biofeedback and acupuncture have been successful for women's incontinence regardless of cause. Medicare coverage for biofeedback for incontinence is now mandated by the Health Care Financing Administration (HCFA).

To find a biofeedback practitioner visit: Association for Applied Psychophysiology and Biofeedback website, www.aapb.org.

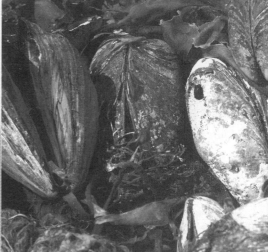
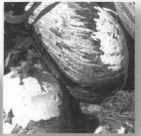
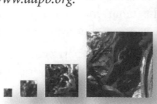

3. Have you grown facial hair but lost head hair since menopause?

Extremely common for menopausal women, female pattern baldness is a disconcerting problem. The slow-down in estrogen production affects the functioning of hair follicles, resulting in the head hair loss and facial hair growth women hate. Excess dihydrotestosterone (DHT) in women can cause hair follicles to become dormant as in men. Balanced thyroid hormone production is critical to normal hair growth. *Hypo*thyroidism leads to coarse, lifeless hair which easily falls out. *Hyper*thyroidism causes soft, thinning hair and hair loss.

1. Sea greens make a big difference: Women notice improved hair growth and texture in 3 – 4 weeks. Take 2 tbsp. daily of dry chopped sea greens, and eat lots of sushi. Reduce animal fats to unclog hair follicles; add cultured soy foods for plant protein (hair is 97% protein!).

2. So do supplements: Take Evening Primrose Oil 4000 mg. daily; and Crystal Star® Calcium Magnesium Source™ or a cal/mag/zinc combination with high magnesium daily. Take B-complex 100 mg. with extra B-6 daily and sublingual B-12, 2500 mcg. every other day.

3. Apply herbs to hair: Blend fresh ground ginger with aloe vera gel and apply; leave on 15 minutes. Apply rosemary or nettles tea for falling hair. Apply hot olive and wheat germ oils for 30 minutes for hair growth.

Women's Hormone Balancing Menopause Diet

If you're on a raging hormone roller coaster, with hot flashes, mood swings, vaginal dryness and low libido, this diet can help you "keep the change!" Compose your diet of 50% fresh foods for the best enzyme benefits. Limit dairy foods and meats, especially beef and pork, high in hormone disrupting chemicals. Reduce sugars and alcohol. (A little wine with dinner is fine.) Avoid caffeine. It taxes the adrenal glands, and upsets hormone levels. Steam and bake foods—never fry. Especially eat cold water fish like salmon and tuna for EFAs and to cut heart disease risk. To reduce hot flashes, add soy foods like miso and tofu, and avoid spicy foods.

Balance estrogen levels by boosting boron foods, like green leafy veggies, fruits, nuts, and legumes. (Boron also helps harden bones.) Whole grain fiber, fresh fruits and veggies regulate estrogen levels and reduce mood swings. Eat calcium-rich vegetables and soy foods. Eliminate carbonated drinks loaded with phosphates that deplete calcium.

On rising: take a protein drink like Nutricology Progreens; or lemon juice in water with 1 tsp. maple syrup. Add 1 tsp. Red Star nutritional yeast for best results.

Breakfast: add a ginseng-royal jelly-honey blend (Prince of Peace) to hot tea water; make a mix of 2 tbsp. each: toasted sesame seeds, sunflower seeds, wheat germ and lecithin granules. Sprinkle some each morning on yogurt and/or fresh fruit, or oatmeal, a whole grain cereal or rice pilaf. Top with apple juice and maple syrup.

Mid-morning: have a superfood green drink, Fit For You, Intl. Miracle Greens or Crystal Star® Energy Green Renewal™ with sea greens, and/or a cup of miso or noodle ramen soup with sea veggies sprinkled on top.

Lunch: have an onion or black bean soup with a carrot and raisin salad; or baked or broiled seafood with a green leafy salad; or a baked yam with a low-fat yogurt dressing and a small green salad; or some steamed veggies with rice, tofu and light tamari dressing; or a salad with baked, marinated tofu and greens, and lemon-oil vinaigrette; or a seafood salad with brown rice; or soup and salad, with sea greens and crunchy noodles.

Mid-afternoon: have low-fat cottage cheese with nuts and seeds and rice cakes; or a dried fruit and nut mix with a bottle of mineral water; or a hard boiled egg with a refreshing herb tea like spearmint or hibiscus tea.

Dinner: a broccoli or asparagus quiche with a chapati crust; or a stir-fry with Chinese greens, shiitake mushrooms and tofu, or miso soup with sea greens; baked or grilled fish with a light salsa, brown rice, and sautéed veggies; or a baked rice and veggie casserole with yogurt sauce; or a light Italian meal with spinach or artichoke pasta, baked veggies and low-fat cheese. A little wine at dinner helps relaxation, digestion, and stress release.

Before bed: have papaya-pineapple juice to enhance enzyme activity; or 1 tsp. cranberry concentrate in chamomile tea; or miso soup for B vitamins; or Crystal Star® Stress Arrest™ tea for easier sleep; or a mint tea.

Choose 2 or 3 supplements especially for menopausal relief and balance:

Most women need 6 – 8 weeks to gradually wean off of HRT. Women who have been using HRT drugs for a very long time may take longer. Start by adding the whole herb formulas in this section as you gradually decrease your HRT dosage. Some women begin by cutting their daily HRT dosage in half. Working with a holistic physician produces the best results.

- **For hot flashes:** CRYSTAL STAR's highly successful program: 1. EST-AID™ caps 4-6 daily the first month, 2 daily for 2 months, to control hormone imbalances; 2. CALCIUM MAGNESIUM SOURCE™ caps or LANE LABS ADVACAL ULTRA for bone weakness accompanying estrogen changes; 3-Evening primrose oil caps 4000 mg. daily for mood swings. 4. EASY CHANGE™ caps; 5. ADRENAL ENERGY BOOST™ or FEMALE HARMONY™ caps for a feeling of well-being. 6. Add FEEL GREAT NOW™ caps for energy; and Milk Thistle Seed extract to help normalize estrogen levels.
- **- More suggestions:** PURE ESSENCE LABS PRO FEMA and FEM CREME as directed; TRANSITIONS FOR WOMEN HOT FLASH FORMULA, or MOON MAID PRO-MENO WILD YAM CREAM; IMPERIAL ELIXIR DONG QUAI 3000; Vitex extract.
- **Normalize body fluctuations:** Bioflavonoids, similar to body estrogen, 500 mg. daily or Ester C with bioflavs 4x daily; CoQ10 300 mg. daily.
- **For sleep disturbances:** NATURAL BALANCE RHODIOLA ROSEA; 5-HTP, 100 mg. or CRYSTAL STAR® NIGHT CAPS™.
- **Elevate mood - increase energy:** Ginkgo biloba extract; Siberian eleuthero extract; PLANETARY GINSENG REVITALIZER TABS; NATURE'S SECRET ULTIMATE B; Stress B-complex 100 mg.; JAGULANA WOMEN'S RELIEF with jiaogulan.
- **Iodine therapy for thyroid-metabolism:** Sea greens, 2 tbsp. daily or 6 pcs. sushi daily to your diet; CRYSTAL STAR® OCEAN MINERALS™, GREEN FOODS ION KELP or BERNARD JENSEN LIQUI-DULS; or NATURE'S PATH TRACE-MIN-LYTE.

These bodywork techniques can help you sail through menopause

- **Exercise regularly** like a brisk daily walk outdoors to get natural vitamin D for bone health.
- **Do Yoga for body toning.** Deep stretches on rising and each evening before bed.
- **Weight training 3 times a week,** along with aerobic exercise is a perfect way to keep skin from sagging. Weight training helps you keep the muscle while you lose the fat. In a natural menopause, when estrogen levels drop naturally, so does some body fat and excess fluids.
- **Get a massage therapy treatment once a month** for energy restoration, and a feeling of well-being.
- **Smoking contributes to breast cancer, emphysema, osteoporosis, wrinkling.** Now is the time to quit!
- **Twenty minutes in a sauna daily** significantly cuts night sweats for menopausal women.

Resource used with permission: Page, Linda, N.D., Ph.D. "Look and Feel Your Best: Go Through Menopause The Natural Way Without Hormone Replacement," Institute of Health Sciences, Copyright 2002, www.hsibaltimore.com.

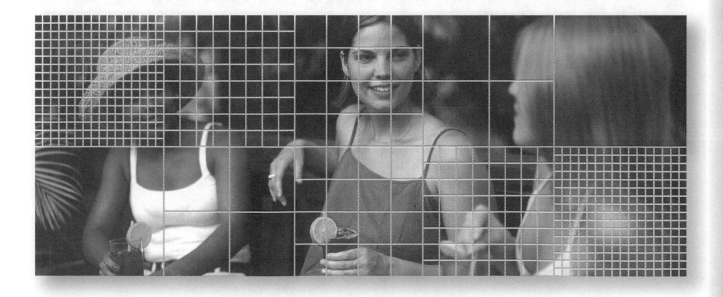

Maintenance Recipes for a Women's Health Diet

Use these recipes on an ongoing basis once your initial healing diet is producing good results.

Breakfast

Yogurt Cheese Topping for Fruit or Granola

Delicious dairy substitute to use on fresh fruits, granola or hot cereal, toast or bagels.

1 pint plain yogurt	1 tbsp. lemon juice	grated zest of 1 fresh lemon
1 tbsp. honey		

Make the fresh yogurt cheese the night before. Simply spoon a pint or more of plain yogurt onto a large cheesecloth square. Tie up the ends of the square and loop over your kitchen sink faucet to drain into the sink overnight. Store airtight in the fridge. Then, mix together in a small bowl the yogurt cheese, honey, lemon juice, lemon zest. Store in the refrigerator.

Nutrition per serving:	Vitamin E --- trace quantities	Cholesterol-------- 7 mg.	Potassium --------- 360 mg.
Calories ----------- 187	Carbohydrates ---- 38 g.	Calcium ----------- 252 mg.	Sodium------------ 89 mg.
Protein ----------- 7 g.	Fiber ------------- 2 g.	Iron -------------- 0	
Vitamin C--------- 35 mg.	Fat---------------- 2 g.	Magnesium ------- 26 mg.	

Green Tea Fruit Bowl

granola	apple slices	toasted, slivered almonds
vanilla yogurt	½ pint of fresh raspberries	
toasted sunflower seeds	½ cup green tea	

Build this in layers in a glass bowl. Cover bottom of bowl with granola. Gently spread the yogurt and smooth with the back of a spoon. Cover with toasted sunflower seeds. Top with apple slices. Layer another thin coat of yogurt. In a blender, mix the raspberries with the green tea. Pour over the fruit bowl and sprinkle with toasted slivered almonds. Makes 2 servings.

Scrambled Eggs with Smoked Salmon

12 eggs	3 tbsp. grapeseed oil	8 oz. low-fat cream cheese,
½ tsp. salt	6 oz. thinly-sliced smoked	well-chilled
½ tsp. lemon-pepper seasoning	salmon, cut into ½" wide strips	fresh chives, chopped

Use a non-stick skillet. In a bowl, whisk the eggs, salt and lemon-pepper. Heat the grapeseed oil over medium-high heat, and add egg mixture. Using wooden spoon, stir until eggs are almost set, about 5 minutes. Gently fold in the salmon. Stir just until eggs are set, about 1 minute. Transfer eggs to platter. Dot hot eggs with the cream cheese, cut in small cubes. Sprinkle with chives before serving. Makes 6 brunch servings.

Breakfast Fruit Salad

3 peaches	1 basket of strawberries,	ground cardamom
2 baskets blueberries	sliced	4 tbsp. honey

Peel and slice the peaches. In a bowl, toss with the blueberries and strawberries. Drizzle with honey and sprinkle with cardamom. Eat as is, or top waffles or french toast with a spoonful instead of syrup or butter. Makes 4 servings.

Cottage Cheese Pancakes

1 lb. low-fat cottage cheese	⅓ cup oatmeal	½ tsp. vanilla extract
6 eggs	3 tbsp. honey	¼ tsp. ground cardamom
⅔ cup whole wheat pastry flour	2 tbsp. vanilla rice milk	maple syrup or honey, if desired

To make the batter, mix the cottage cheese, eggs, flour, oatmeal, honey, rice milk, vanilla extract, and cardamom. Heat a non-stick skillet until a drop of water bounces. Spray lightly with a lecithin cooking spray, and ladle in 2 – 3 pancakes at a time. Cook until bubbles burst on the surface. Flip and cook until golden. Oil cooking surface between each batch. Serve with maple syrup or honey. Makes 4 servings.

Healing drinks

Restorative Blood Tonic

An amazingly simple, but effective Chinese medicine restorative for women. This recipe works for: Recovery from Surgery, Female Balance, Healthy Pregnancy.

35 black dates	1 tsp. fresh royal jelly (or 1	1 tbsp. sesame tahini
5 slices fresh ginger, peeled	tbsp. royal jelly mixed with	
8 cups water	honey)	

In a large soup pot, simmer the dates, ginger and water. Stir in the royal jelly and tahini. Cool and serve. Sip throughout the day for several weeks. Makes 8 drinks.

Non-Alcoholic Cranberry Maple Nog

2 cups apple cider	1 (8 oz.) can frozen	½ cup maple syrup
2 cups orange juice	cranberry juice	12 cloves, whole
32 oz. green tea, lemon or	2 cinnamon sticks	a little extra maple syrup
peach flavored	1 lemon, thinly sliced	a few extra cinnamon sticks

In a large soup pot over low-medium heat, stir the apple cider, orange juice, green tea, cranberry juice, cinnamon sticks, lemon slices, maple syrup and cloves. Simmer 1 hour. Remove spices and lemon slices. Serve hot with extra maple syrup and cinnamon sticks. Makes 8 servings.

Nutrition per serving:	Vitamin C --------- 185 mg.	Fat ---------------- 1 g.	Magnesium ------- 16 mg.
Calories ----------- 164	Vitamin E --- trace quantities	Cholesterol-------- 0	Potassium --------- 387 mg.
Protein ----------- 1 g.	Carbohydrates ---- 40 g.	Calcium ----------- 65 mg.	Sodium----------- 22 mg.
Vitamin A --------- 14 IU	Fiber ------------- 2 g.	Iron -------------- 1 mg.	

Soups, salads, appetizers

Carrot Ginger Soup

2 tbsp. olive oil	1 cup carrots, diced	½ cup sliced almonds
2 tbsp. crystallized ginger, minced	1 cup yellow dutch potatoes, diced	2 tbsp. orange juice
1 cup onions, diced	4 cups water	1 tbsp. honey
		½ cup sherry

In a soup pot, sauté the onions and 1 tbsp. of the crystallized ginger in olive oil for 5 minutes. Add the carrots, potatoes and sauté for another 8 minutes. Add the water and bring to a boil. Then, cool and let simmer for 20 minutes. Remove from heat and add the almonds, orange juice and honey. Purée the ingredients in a blender. Pour the mixture in a soup tureen and stir in the remaining ginger, and the sherry. Makes 4 servings.

Quick Potato-Tofu Stew

1 onion, chopped	¼ tsp. pepper	16 oz. tofu, diced
2 cloves garlic, minced	1 (16 oz.) jar tomato sauce	1 tbsp. miso paste
3 red potatoes, diced	1 cup red wine	1¼ cups cheddar cheese, grated
½ tsp. sea salt	3 cups water	

In a large soup pot, sauté the onions and garlic in olive oil for 3 minutes. Add the red potatoes, sea salt, pepper and sauté for another 5 minutes. Add the tomato sauce, red wine, water, tofu, miso paste and bring to a boil. Reduce heat and simmer for 20 minutes until potatoes are tender, but not crumbly. Remove from heat and stir in grated cheddar. Stir in until cheese is just melted. Makes 6 serving.

Asian Turkey Salad with Ginger Dressing

⅓ cup grapeseed oil	½ tsp. ground ginger	3 cups turkey, cooked and cubed
¼ cup brown rice vinegar	1 tsp. NEW CHAPTER'S GINGER WONDER syrup	2 stalks celery, chopped
1 tbsp. honey	4 oz. mung bean threads	4 green onions, diced
1 tbsp. tamari	½ head lettuce, shredded	2 tbsp. toasted almonds
½ tsp. lemon pepper		

Make the ginger dressing first: in a bowl, whisk the grapeseed oil, brown rice vinegar, honey, tamari, lemon pepper, ground ginger and GINGER WONDER syrup. Chill for 2 hours. Place the bean threads in hot water for 2 minutes until soft. Drain and set aside. Into a large bowl, mix the lettuce, turkey, celery and green onions. Pour the ginger dressing over lettuce mix. Toss with half the noodles. Place the remaining noodles on a large platter. Spoon salad over noodles. Sprinkle with the almonds. Makes 6 servings.

Winter-Spring Salad with Cranberry Dressing

¼ cup fresh cilantro	1 tsp. dijon mustard	1 cup red cabbage, shredded
1 shallot, chopped	herb seasoning salt	1 cup radicchio leaves
⅓ cup balsamic vinegar	⅓ cup dried cranberries	⅓ cup red onion, thinly sliced
⅓ cup cranberry juice blend	10 cups baby green salad leaves	1 red bell pepper, thinly sliced
1 tbsp. honey		

Make the cranberry dressing: in a blender, combine the cilantro, shallots, balsamic vinegar, cranberry juice blend, honey, dijon mustard, and herb seasoning salt to taste. Pour the dressing into a bowl and stir in dried cranberries. In a large bowl, toss the baby green salad leaves, red cabbage, radicchio leaves, red onion, red bell pepper and cranberry dressing. Makes 8 servings.

Party Artichoke Quiche

1¼ cups unbleached flour	1 (11 oz.) jar water packed	3 eggs
2 tbsp. grapeseed oil	artichokes, sliced	½ cup low-fat cream cheese
4 tbsp. butter	1 tsp. dijon mustard	¼ cup water
1 egg	6 mushrooms, sliced	2 tbsp. sherry
low-fat cheese, your choice	2 scallions, sliced	½ tsp. Chinese 5-spice powder

Preheat oven to 325°F. Make a simple crust: mix the flour, grapeseed oil, butter, and the egg until crumbly. Press into a quiche pan and bake at 350°F for 5 – 8 minutes. Remove and cool. Grate the cheese onto the crust to 1" thickness. Arrange sliced artichokes on top of the cheese. Set aside. In a small saucepan, sauté the dijon mustard, mushrooms and scallions in butter. Layer on top of artichokes. In a blender, combine the eggs, cream cheese, water, sherry and Chinese 5-spice powder. Pour over quiche. Lightly sprinkle with nutmeg and bake at 325°F until firm. Serve warm. Makes 6 servings.

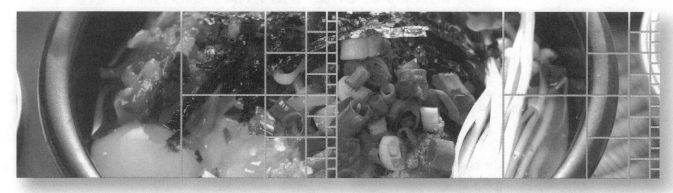

Entrées

Traditional Japanese Stew

1 lb. tofu	1 small head napa cabbage,	4 cups miso soup
8 oz. package dried bean	shredded	2 tbsp. sake
threads	8 large dry shiitake	1 orange
1 lb. organic chicken breast,	mushrooms	tamari sauce
thinly-sliced bite-sized pieces	1 small bag baby spinach,	1 tsp. ground ginger
1 large onion, cut in half	chopped	
lengthwise, then sliced	4 oz. bean sprouts	

Press the tofu between 2 plates with a weight on top. Let stand for 30 minutes to press out excess water. Drain, slice in thin strips and set aside. Soak the dried bean threads in water until soft. Set aside. Soak the dry shiitake mushrooms until soft. Discard woody stems, and slice caps. Set aside and save the mushroom soaking water. Mix the baby spinach with the bean sprouts and set aside.

Make the orange tamari dipping sauce: squeeze the juice of the orange into a measuring cup. Add an equal amount of tamari and the ground ginger.

Assemble the stew. Bring the miso soup to a boil. Add mushroom soaking water, sake, tofu strips and chicken. Cook for 5 minutes. Remove tofu and meat with a slotted spoon and divide in shallow soup bowls. Add the onions to the stew and simmer 5 minutes. Add the cabbage and mushrooms and simmer 5 more minutes. Ladle stew into soup bowls. Add the sprouts and spinach to the stew for 30 seconds just to wilt. Ladle into soup bowls. Add bean threads and heat through. Divide the liquid and threads between bowls. Serve with the orange tamari dipping sauce. Dipping sauce can be put in small individual bowls near each person's plate. Serve with chopsticks so pieces of the stew can be easily picked up and dipped into the sauce. Makes 8 servings.

Nutrition per serving:	Vitamin E --------- 3 IU	Cholesterol-------- 35 mg.	Potassium --------- 494 mg.
Calories ----------- 305	Carbohydrates ---- 7 g.	Calcium ----------- 121 mg.	Sodium------------ 524 mg.
Protein ----------- 21 g.	Fiber ------------- 4 g.	Iron -------------- 5 mg.	
Vitamin C--------- 24 mg.	Fat--------------- 9 g.	Magnesium ------- 112 mg.	

Pasta with Fresh Basil & Tomatoes

3 qts. water	olive oil	½ cup scallions, sliced
1 tsp. sea salt	2 lbs. roma tomatoes,	1½ cups fresh basil leaves, minced
4 cups egg pasta shells, dry	chopped	parmesan-reggiano cheese, grated

In a large soup pot, bring the water and sea salt to a rolling boil. Add the pasta shells and cook 12 – 15 minutes to al dente. (Test for doneness by biting into a piece.) While pasta is cooking, sauté in a skillet until fragrant the 2 tbsp. olive oil, roma tomatoes, scallions, and fresh basil. Drain pasta shells in a colander, run under cold water and then drain again. Toss with 1 tsp. olive oil to separate. Toss vegetable sauté with the cooked pasta. Top with grated parmesan-reggiano cheese. Makes 8 servings.

Sweet & Sour Shrimp

4 tbsp. grapeseed oil	½ cup water chestnuts, sliced	2 tbsp. fructose
2 cups cooked rice	1 small can bamboo shoots,	1 clove garlic, minced
1½ lb shrimp, peeled and	drained	1 tbsp. ginger, freshly grated
deveined	16 oz. fresh, trimmed	4 tbsp. tamari
16 oz. broccoli florets	peapods	½ cup pineapple juice
2 carrots, sliced	2 green onions, sliced	2 tbsp. arrowroot powder
½ cup celery, sliced	2 tsp. toasted sesame oil	2 tbsp. sherry

In a large wok, stir-fry the cooked rice in 2 tbsp. grapeseed oil for 10 minutes or until almost dry. Put stir-fried rice on a serving platter and set aside. Add the shrimp to the wok, and cook until just pink, about 5 minutes. Place cooked shrimp on rice and keep warm. Add 2 tbsp. grapeseed oil to hot wok. Stir fry broccoli florets, carrots, celery, water chestnuts, bamboo shoots, and peapods, until green veggies turn bright green. Sprinkle green onions on stir fried vegetables. Scoop the stir fried vegetables onto the hot rice.

In a small saucepan, make the sweet and sour sauce: sauté the garlic, ginger and fructose in toasted sesame oil until fragrant. Add the tamari, pineapple juice, and arrowroot powder (first dissolved into the sherry). Stir briefly and pour over stir-fry mixture. Makes 8 servings.

Healthy dessert options

Almond Tofu Cream Pie

Make this a day ahead for best results.

2 cups whole wheat graham	16 oz. firm silken tofu	1 tsp. orange zest
cracker crumbs	16 oz. kefir cheese	2 tbsp. orange juice
4 tbsp. honey	4 tbsp. fructose	2 tbsp. arrowroot powder
1 tbsp. grapeseed oil	4 tbsp. almond butter	2 tbsp. sherry
½ tsp. almond extract	½ tsp. sea salt	
3 tbsp. water	1 tsp. almond extract	

Preheat oven to 350°F. Prepare a springform pan or 10" pie plate. Make the crust: mix the whole wheat graham cracker crumbs, honey, grapeseed oil, almond extract and water. Press into grapeseed oil sprayed baking pan and bake for 5 minutes. Remove and cool.

Make the filling: in a blend, mix until smooth, the firm silken tofu, kefir cheese, fructose, almond butter, sea salt, almond extract, orange zest, orange juice, arrowroot powder, sherry. Pour the mixture into the crust. Bake 35 minutes. Remove and chill until ready to serve. Serves 8.

Sweet Yam Muffins

1 large yam	¼ tsp. allspice	1 egg
1 cup unbleached flour	¼ tsp. nutmeg	4 tbsp. butter
⅓ cup whole wheat pastry	¼ tsp. ground cloves	2 tbsp. grapeseed oil
flour	¼ tsp. ground ginger	¼ cup chopped walnuts
2 tsp. baking powder	½ tsp. sea salt	¼ cup raisins
fructose	3 tbsp. maple syrup	¾ tsp. cinnamon
½ cup date sugar	¼ cup plain yogurt	
½ tsp. cinnamon	¼ cup water	

Preheat oven to 350°F. Use paper-lined muffin cups. Bake until soft, then peel and mash 1 large yam. Mix dry ingredients: unbleached flour, whole wheat pastry flour, baking powder, ⅓ cup fructose, date sugar, cinnamon, allspice, nutmeg, cloves, ginger and sea salt. Combine wet ingredients: the mashed yam, maple syrup, plain yogurt, water, egg, butter and grapeseed oil. Stir mixtures together; add the chopped walnuts and the raisins. Spoon into muffin cups. Mix 1 tsp. fructose with ¾ tsp. cinnamon and sprinkle a pinch on each muffin. Bake 25 minutes until muffin tops spring back when touched. Makes 12 muffins.

Nutrition per serving:	Vitamin C --------- 7 mg.	Fat ---------------- 8 g.	Magnesium ------- 25 mg.
Calories ----------- 226	Vitamin E --------- 1 IU	Cholesterol-------- 28 mg.	Potassium --------- 231 mg.
Protein ------------ 4 g.	Carbohydrates ---- 36 g.	Calcium ----------- 95 mg.	Sodium------------ 163 mg.
Vitamin A --------- 664 IU	Fiber ------------- 2 g.	Iron -------------- 1 mg.	

Glazed Pear Cake

This recipe works for: Allergies and Asthma, Women's Health.

3 eggs	4 tbsp. butter	cream of tartar
1 cup oat flour	½ cup maple syrup	grapeseed oil
½ cup barley flour	2 tbsp. orange juice	2 large pears, thinly-sliced
2 tsp. baking powder	concentrate	1 cup frozen apple juice concentrate
½ tsp. baking soda	2 tsp. vanilla	

Preheat oven to 350°F. Separate the eggs. Mix the yolks with the oat flour, barley flour, baking powder, baking soda. In a small sauce pan, melt together the butter, maple syrup, orange juice concentrate and vanilla. Blend mixtures together. Beat egg whites stiff with a pinch of cream of tartar. Fold into batter. Pour into a grapeseed oil-sprayed baking pan. Bake for 20 minutes. Make the pear glaze: simmer the pears with the frozen apple juice concentrate until most juice is cooked off. The remaining pears and glaze should be thick and syrupy. Arrange pears on top of the cake decoratively. Spoon glaze over. Let cool. Makes 10 pieces.

Nutrition per serving:	Vitamin C--------- 4 mg.	Fat ---------------- 7 g.	Magnesium ------- 32 mg.
Calories ----------- 246	Vitamin E --------- 1 IU	Cholesterol-------- 76 mg.	Potassium --------- 293 mg.
Protein ------------ 5 g.	Carbohydrates ---- 42 g.	Calcium ----------- 104 mg.	Sodium------------ 165 mg.
Vitamin A --------- 75 IU	Fiber ------------- 3 g.	Iron -------------- 2 mg.	

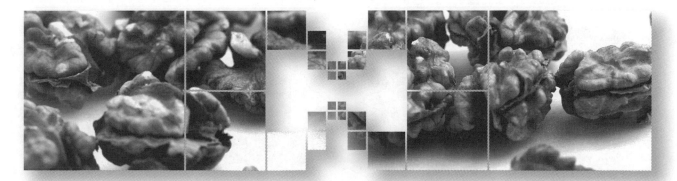

Anti-Aging Lifetime Diet

It's happening to everybody, most of the time faster than we'd like. Still, youth is not a chronological age. It's good health and an optimistic spirit. Even though the hourglass tells us we're older, the passage of time isn't really what ages us. It's the process that reduces the number of healthy cells in our bodies. Today, the concept of anti-aging is gaining momentum as more people realize they can positively affect their own aging process. We can see anti-aging in today's elite athletes who perform at world class levels well into their thirties or even forties. And there are pockets throughout the world of people living healthy lifestyles past the century mark, proving that the downward spiral associated with aging may not be necessary.

Whenever the gold and silver years begin for you, it's when the fun begins. Hectic family life quiets down, financial strains ease, business retirement is here or not far off, and you can do the things you've always wanted to do but never had time for—travel, art, music, a craft, gardening, writing, quiet walks, picnics, more social life… doing what you want to do, not what you have to do. We all look forward to the treasure years of life, and picture ourselves on that tennis court, bike path or cruise ship, healthy and enjoying ourselves. But, there's a catch—our freedom comes in the latter half of life, and many of us don't age gracefully in today's world.

The good news? The longer you live, the longer your expected life span becomes!

Life expectancy lengthens as you age. In 1928, life expectancy in the U.S. was just 57 years, compared to 76 years today. Women's life expectancy is expected to rise to between 92.5 and 101.5 by 2070. Researchers say the human life span is at least 20 to 30 years longer than most of us actually live today, that we are living only two-thirds of the years our bodies are capable of. Scientists have gathered a wealth of clear data that shows living to 100 or even 120 in a disease-free state is entirely possible, indeed may be a natural state of human life. Right now, people 100 or over are the fastest growing segment of the U.S. population. There are 61,000 centenarians living in the U.S. today. Researchers predict that number will grow to 214,000 by 2020!

The Fountain of Youth has been available all along. A balanced life is the key. Good food, pure water, energizing herbs and vitamins, exercise, proper rest, fresh air, sunshine, and optimism about life, really keep you young.

Age is not the enemy… illness is.

Our cells don't age; they're sloughed off as their efficiency diminishes, to be replaced by new ones. Given the right nutrients, cell restoration continues—well past current life expectancy. But in industrialized countries, pollutants, diets full of chemical-laced, refined foods, and overuse of prescription drugs prevent our seniority dreams from becoming a reality.

Today, 80% of citizens of industrialized nations over 65 years old are chronically ill. The average person over 75 has three different chronic diseases and uses at least five prescription drugs, as well as over-the-counter drugs.

Yet, loss of vitality and the onset of disease are usually the result of diet, lifestyle or environment—things we can do something about. Youthfulness is restored from the inside, by strengthening lean body mass, boosting metabolism, increasing immune response with good nutrition, regular exercise and a positive outlook.

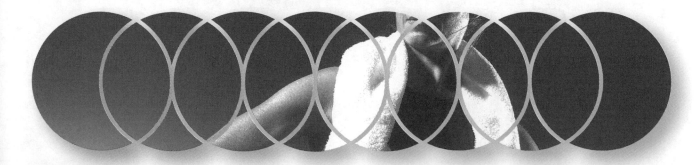

Restore your looks and energy by addressing the factors that affect aging most:

1. Take a look at your prescription drugs: Many drugs lead to serious body imbalances by impairing nutrient uptake, and they can spur a free radical assault that accelerates aging. They also tend to interact, especially hormonal drugs, like Propecia, or HRT drugs, and drugs that affect circulation like Viagra.

2. Take a look at your habits: Smoking for example, greatly increases the body's free radical load, is a clear contributor to premature skin aging, and is by far the #1 cause of preventable deaths in our country.

3. Take another look at your diet: You may have already cut down on fat and fried foods, but chemicals and additives in foods like lunch meats, hot dogs and most prepared foods are real culprits for early aging. They can create an over-acid condition that aggravates arthritis, triggers many allergies, and like drugs, set up a free-radical cascade favorable to disease.

Research into fake fats like olestra (widely popular in snack foods) shows that they rob the body of vitamins like A, D, E, and K, and carotenoids. Even if your diet is good, you may need to take digestive enzymes and HCl with pepsin if digestion has become sluggish with age. Consider CRYSTAL STAR® DR. ENZYME II: FAT & STARCH BUSTER™.

4. Take a look at your sugar intake: A high sugar diet wipes out immunity and reduces tissue elasticity. If you eat a lot of sweets or drink hard alcohol regularly, you're taking in a lot of sugar. Sugar is also a hidden ingredient in most processed foods. Artificial sweeteners with aspartame are linked to degenerative nerve disorders.

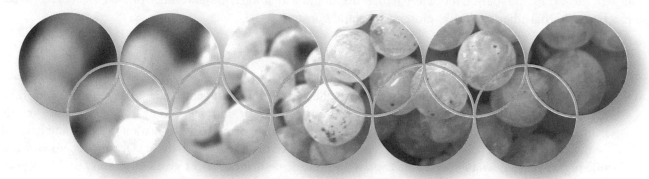

5. Watch your stress levels. A little stress helps motivate us in meeting a goal. But chronic stress can steal your health and your youth. Over time, high levels of the stress hormone cortisol can cause brain cells to age prematurely, or even die off! High levels of cortisol are also linked to middle-aged weight gain around the waist.

6. Interrupted sleep is a major aging trigger. A recent study links a lack of sleep to premature aging and serious illness. During sleep, important anti-aging hormones like growth hormone and melatonin are released which help regulate metabolism, heal tissues and boost immune response.

7. Regular moderate exercise actually reverses the aging process. A sedentary lifestyle paves the way for obesity and chronic disease. A 1994 JAMA study reveals that the bodies of postmenopausal women become up to 20 years more youthful just by lifting weights twice weekly for one year!

8. Take a look at your teeth and gums: Almost nothing shows age faster than discolored teeth, lost teeth or red, receding gums. Take CoQ-10 right away for gum problems, about 200 mg. daily, for the first month. See a holistic dentist for discoloration problems.

9. Take a look in the mirror: Is your neck no longer straight, but at a slight forward angle; are your shoulders looking hunched? You may be losing bone density: start a strengthening exercise program right away. Make sure it includes elongating muscle stretches and stick with it. This is one aging sign that exercise can rapidly reverse.

10. Look at your workplace: Radical early aging happens to people working around chemicals in the automotive, pesticide or household cleaners industry; these chemicals overload your body's natural detox system.

11. As we age, many of us move to southern climates: But 90% of skin cancers and wrinkles are traced to sun exposure. Use SPF 40 for your face, up to SPF 26 for your body and wear a hat, or face those fine lines in your mirror. CRYSTAL STAR® DR. VITALITY™ caps and tea (green and white tea) offer significant sun protection.

Longevity Begins with a Good Diet

A nutrition rich diet is the centerpiece of a vibrant long life. Health experts agree that the food health pyramid needs to be modified as we age. Your diet must become even more nourishing, even higher in antioxidants as the years pass. A good diet improves health, provides a high energy level, maintains harmonious system balance, keeps memory and thinking sharp, staves off disease, and contributes to a youthful appearance. The aging process slows down if your internal environment is good.

Lower your daily calories to reduce the signs of aging. Overeating dramatically hastens the aging process; moderate food intake may extend lifespan by as much as ten years. Your body needs fewer calories and burns calories slower as you age; optimum body weight should be 10 to 15 pounds less than in your 20s and 30s. A low calorie diet protects DNA from damage, and prevents tissue degeneration. An easy way to control a slow upward weight gain is to compose your diet of 50% fresh foods.

Fresh, organically grown foods protect your skin from aging. Your skin is a diet window. Already saturated with chemicals from pesticides, preservatives and additives, today over 70% of our foods are genetically altered. Brown age spots and rough skin texture are signs that our bodies are less able to process our foods correctly.

Keep your glands young! Trace minerals, essential fatty acids and protein are important for youthful gland function. Good gland foods: sea foods and sea greens, fresh figs and raisins, pumpkin and sesame seeds, broccoli, avocados, yams and dark fruits. Herbal digestive tonics with ginger, mineralizers from dark leafy greens like spinach, and herbal adaptogens like ginseng are gland boosters.

The best anti-aging foods:

- **Fresh fruits and vegetables!** Fresh foods gives you the most vitamins, minerals, fiber and enzymes. Plants have the widest array of nutrients and are the easiest for your body to use. Enzyme-rich fruits and vegetables are the essential link to stamina levels. (Increased free radical production, abnormal tissue formation (fibrosis) and reduced digestive capacity are all hallmarks of aging, and directly related to low enzyme activity.) Organically grown foods insure higher nutrient content and aren't sprayed with toxic pesticides. Have a green salad every day! European research reveals the immune cells of vegetarians are twice as effective as meat eaters in killing cancer cells.
  Note: Eat fresh foods whenever you can. Fresh fruit and vegetable juices offer quick absorption of antioxidants, which protect the body against aging, heart disease, cancer, and degenerative conditions.
- **Sea greens are the ocean's superfoods.** They contain all the necessary elements of life and transmute the energies of the ocean to us as proteins, complex carbohydrates, vitamins, minerals, trace minerals, chlorophyll, enzymes and fiber. Sea greens and sea foods stand almost alone as potent sources of natural iodine. By regulating thyroid function, they promote higher energy levels and increased metabolism for faster weight loss after 40.
- **Whole grains, nuts, seeds and beans for protein, fiber, minerals and essential fatty acids.** Sprouted seeds, grains, and legumes are some of the healthiest foods you eat… living nutrients that go directly to your cells.
- **Cultured foods for friendly digestive flora.** Yogurt tops the list, but kefir and kefir cheese, miso, tamari, tofu, tempeh, even a glass of wine at the evening meal also promote better nutrient assimilation. Raw sauerkraut is especially good for boosting friendly bacteria. (Avoid commercial sauerkraut processed with alum) Bonus: Cultured foods act as a mild appetite suppressant for better weight control.
- **Six to eight glasses of bottled water every day** keeps your body hydrated and clean.
- **Green drinks, green foods, miso and brown rice** keep body chemistry balanced for optimum health.
- **Two to three tablespoons of healthy, unsaturated fats and oils** keep your body at its best.
- **Fish and seafoods** 3 times a week enhance thyroid and metabolism for weight control and brain acuity.
- **Eat poultry, other meats, butter, eggs, and dairy in moderation.** Avoid fried foods, excess caffeine, red meats, highly seasoned foods, refined and chemically processed foods altogether.

Day-by-Day Diet:

On rising: take a high nutrient drink, like CRYSTAL STAR® ENERGY GREEN RENEWAL™, or ALL 1 VITAMIN/MINERAL DRINK in orange or apple juice; or an aloe vera juice. Add 2 tsp. CC POLLEN HIGH DESERT BEE POLLEN granules.

Breakfast: make a mix of 2 tbsp. <u>each:</u> nutritional yeast, lecithin granules, toasted wheat germ, bee pollen granules and flax seeds. Sprinkle some on your breakfast choice—fresh fruits, plain or with yogurt; or whole grain granola with apple juice, yogurt, rice milk or almond milk; or whole grain muffins with a little kefir cheese; or a baked or poached egg or omelet.

Mid-morning: have a green drink, or SUN WELLNESS CHLORELLA, GREEN FOODS GREEN MAGMA, or WAKUNAGA HARVEST GREENS drink in apple juice; or a tonifying herb tea, like Siberian eleuthero tea, or CRYSTAL STAR® GREEN TEA CLEANSER™ tea; and more fresh fruit with yogurt.

Lunch: have a leafy green salad with a cup of miso or ramen noodle soup; or a cup of black bean, lentil, or other protein soup with baked potato and kefir cheese or yogurt sauce; or a fresh fruit salad with cottage cheese or yogurt cheese, and veggie baked chips or crackers; or a light seafood or turkey salad; or a hot or cold vegetable pasta salad.

Mid-afternoon: have fresh or dried fruits with low fat yogurt; or crackers or rice cakes with a vegetable, soy or kefir spread, and miso broth; or a cup of ginseng tea, mint tea, and some crunchy veggies with a yogurt or rice or soy cheese dip.

Dinner: a hearty, high protein vegetable, nut and seed salad with soup and whole grain muffins or cornbread; or an Asian stir-fry with brown rice and miso soup; or a baked veggie, tofu and whole grain casserole; or a vegetable quiche with a whole grain crust, and light yogurt-wine sauce; or baked or broiled seafood with a green salad and brown rice or steamed veggies; or roast turkey with cornbread or rice and a salad.

Have a glass of wine for digestion, heart health and relaxation.

Before Bed: have a cup of chamomile tea or apple, pomegranate or papaya juice, or a cup of miso soup; or a glass of aloe vera juice for regularity the next morning.

Choose 2 or 3 anti-aging supplements to really make a difference:

- **Anti-aging superfoods:** My favorites: BARLEANS GREENS, FIT FOR YOU MIRACLE GREENS, ESTEEM PRODUCTS GREEN HARVEST; NUTRICOLOGY PROGREENS; GREEN FOODS VEGGIE MAGMA; PURE PLANET 100% SPIRULINA; NATURE'S SECRET ULTIMATE GREEN tabs.
- **Boost your enzymes:** the length of life is tied to your food enzymes because they decrease your body's rate of metabolic enzyme exhaustion. My favorites: CRYSTAL STAR® DR. ENZYME II: FAT & STARCH BUSTER™, TRANSFORMATION PUREZYME (PROTEASE); HERBAL PRODUCTS & DEVELOPMENT POWER PLUS.
- **Boost antioxidants to stay disease free:** My favorites: Alpha lipoic acid; NAC (N-Acetyl-Cysteine); Bee pollen-Royal Jelly; CoQ-10; Germanium; Carotenes; Vitamin C with bioflavonoids; Vitamin E; Glutathione; (OPCs) Oligomeric Proanthocyanidins; Selenium.
   - Best herbal antioxidants: Ginkgo biloba; Astragalus; Shiitake mushrooms; Reishi mushrooms; Cat's Claw; Arjuna; Pine bark; Garlic; Grapeseed; Alfalfa; Hawthorn.
- **Optimize your nootropic brain nutrients:** My favorites: DIAMOND HERPANANCINE DIAMIND MIND; NADH *(Co-enzyme Nicotinamide Adenine Dinucleotide)*—helps protect against Alzheimer's; Phosphatidylserine; Choline: (Just eating 2 tbsp. of lecithin a day can do the job!) GPC *(L-alpha glycerylphosphorylcholine)*: a precursor to choline which can help repair brain damage caused by aging.
- **Adaptogen herbs keep immune response strong:** My favorites: CRYSTAL STAR® FEEL GREAT NOW™ WITH GINSENG; Panax Ginseng (red, white and American ginsengs); Siberian Ginseng (eleuthero); Jiaogulan (especially for women); Noni; Schizandra; Suma; Gotu Kola; Fo-Ti (Ho-Shou-Wu); Cordyceps; Horsetail; Bilberry.
- **HGH growth hormone:** Liddell VITAL HGH; ALLERGY RESEARCH BIOGEN GH OR BIOGEN PRO (practitioners)

Bodywork keeps you fit... fitness makes you look and feel far more youthful

- **Advantages of regular exercise for anti-aging:**
- Exercise boosts circulation and oxygen use for energy.
- Exercise reduces the risk for heart attacks and cancer.
- Exercise fans the metabolic fires for weight control.
- Exercise reduces stress and tension, and relaxes you.
- Exercise stimulates hormone production.
- Exercise contributes to strength; Inactivity to fatigue.
- Weight bearing exercises trigger bone remineralization.
- Exercise helps agility and joint mobility.
- Exercise lowers insulin levels and promotes regular elimination.
- Exercise releases heavy metals, especially cadmium, lead and nickel, pesticides and other toxic material through increased perspiration.
- Regular exercise helps manage glaucoma by reducing intraocular pressure.
- Regular exercise boosts immunity, especially as you age. Research shows 73-year old women who are fit have immune response comparable to women half their age!

- **Deep breathing is a powerful way to decrease stress and slow the aging process.** Deep diaphragm breathing lowers anxiety, relaxes and loosens muscles, and generates an inner feeling of peace and calm. Diaphragm breathing strengthens heart and lungs, AND encourages more restful sleep.
- Inhale deeply through your nose. Try to fill your lungs.
- Exhale slowly through your mouth.
- Breathe deeply for 30 seconds to calm and center during anxious moments. Breathing deeply for *just one minute* prevents the short breaths which negatively affect the blood's oxygen-carbon dioxide balance.
- Breathe deeply to fill the lower part of your lungs. Notice the pop-pop feeling in your chest as unused lung pockets open up. Slowly exhale; your abdomen tightens.
- As you breathe in, think of oxygen reaching and recharging all the cells of your body. As you exhale, imagine all the stress and tension leaving your body.

And finally… limit your use of microwaves. Microwaving foods, kills enzymes, an important tool for healing, detoxification, glandular functioning and estrogen metabolism. See "Microwaving," on pg. 233 of this book.

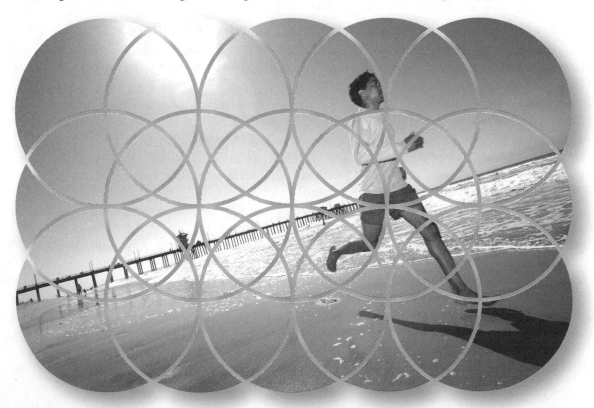

Maintenance Recipes for an Anti-Aging Diet

Use these recipes on an ongoing basis once your initial healing diet is producing good results.

Breakfast
Cranberry-Walnut Bread

3 cups cranberries
¾ cup chopped walnuts, toasted
2 cups unbleached flour

1½ cups whole wheat pastry flour
1½ tsp. baking powder
1 tsp. baking soda
½ tsp. sea salt

¼ cup grapeseed oil
¾ cup date sugar
2 eggs
1 cup orange juice
1 tsp. orange zest

Preheat oven to 350°F. Lightly oil and flour 2 loaf pans. In a bowl, sift together the unbleached flour, whole wheat pastry flour, baking powder, baking soda, and sea salt. In another bowl mix the grapeseed oil, date sugar, eggs, orange juice, and orange zest. Gently combine flour mixture and batter. Fold in walnuts and cranberries. Pour the batter into loaf pans and bake for 40 – 45 minutes, or until a toothpick inserted into the center comes out clean. Remove from pans and let cool. Makes 2 loaves (16 servings).

Nutrition per serving:
Calories ----------- 210
Protein ----------- 6 g.
Vitamin A --------- 18 IU

Vitamin C--------- 11 mg.
Vitamin E --------- 1 IU
Carbohydrates ---- 31 g.
Fiber ------------- 3 g.

Fat ---------------- 7 g.
Cholesterol-------- 26 mg.
Calcium ---------- 51 mg.
Iron -------------- 2 mg.

Magnesium ------- 37 mg.
Potassium --------- 190 mg.
Sodium----------- 189 mg.

Healing drinks

Elliot's Healing Green Smoothie

1 cup cranberry juice
1 cup apple juice
2 tbsp. aloe vera juice concentrate
1 tsp. GREEN FOODS GREEN KAMUT powder

1 tsp. GREEN FOODS GREEN MAGMA powder
1 tsp. GREEN FOODS BETA CARROT powder
1 tsp. royal jelly
1 banana

1 apple
1 orange

In a blender, combine all ingredients and blend until smooth. Add water if necessary. Makes 2 drinks.

Nutrition per serving:
Calories ----------- 262
Protein ----------- 3 g.
Vitamin C--------- 481 mg.

Vitamin E --------- 1 IU
Carbohydrates ---- 63 g.
Fiber ------------- 5 g.
Fat ---------------- 1 g.

Cholesterol-------- 0
Calcium ---------- 83 mg.
Iron -------------- 2 mg.
Magnesium ------- 33 mg.

Potassium --------- 748 mg.
Sodium----------- 30 mg.

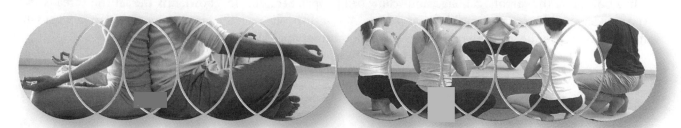

Soups, salads, appetizers

Baby Asian Greens Soup

Simple, delicious, detoxifying.

3 cups organic chicken broth	1 head baby bok choy, sliced	1 scallion, thinly-sliced
6 dry shiitake mushrooms	one 4 oz. cake tofu, diced	
½ cup water	6 drops toasted sesame oil	

In a 1 quart heavy saucepan, gently heat the chicken broth. In a bowl, soak the dry shiitake mushrooms in ½ cup water until soft; then slice thinly, discarding the stems. Add mushrooms and soaking water to broth and simmer 15 minutes. Add the baby bok choy and tofu. Simmer until the bok choy is bright green and tender. Remove from heat. Add the sesame oil and scallion slices. Makes 2 servings.

Nutrition per serving:			
Calories ----------- 144	Vitamin E --------- 1 IU	Cholesterol-------- 0	Potassium --------- 655 mg.
Protein ----------- 13 g.	Carbohydrates ---- 12 g.	Calcium ----------- 28 mg.	Sodium------------ 103 mg.
Vitamin C-------- 26 mg.	Fiber ------------- 3 g.	Iron -------------- 4 mg.	
	Fat---------------- 5 g.	Magnesium ------- 86 mg.	

Enzyme Booster Green Soup

1 tbsp. olive oil	1 tbsp. wheat germ	4 cups miso soup
2 garlic cloves, minced	1 cup leafy greens (spinach,	1 tbsp. lemon juice
¼ cup leeks, minced	chard, endive, romaine,	½ tsp. herb salt
½ cup green onions, minced	etc.), finely chopped	¼ tsp. white pepper
2 tbsp. shallots, minced	¼ cup fresh parsley, minced	daikon white radish, thinly sliced
¼ cup celery, minced	¼ cup watercress, minced	

In a skillet, sauté the garlic, leeks, green onions, shallots, and celery in 2 tbsp. of olive oil. Sprinkle with the wheat germ and toss to coat. Remove from heat and toss in: the leafy greens, fresh parsley, and watercress.

In a soup pot, heat the miso soup briefly. Add the sautéed vegetables, lemon juice, herb salt, and white pepper. Heat just through; top with the daikon white radish. Makes 6 servings.

Fresh Vegetable Salad With Saffron & Ginger

½ lb. carrots, shredded	¼ tsp. saffron threads	4 tbsp. white wine vinegar
1 small head green cabbage, shredded	1 tsp. curry powder	1 jalapeño chile, seeded and minced
1 yellow bell pepper, thinly sliced	1 tbsp. water	½ tsp. sea salt
	4 tbsp. olive oil	¼ tsp. pepper
	3 tbsp. ginger, minced	

In a bowl, mix the carrots, cabbage, and yellow bell pepper. Set aside. In a bowl, mix the saffron threads and curry powder in 1 tbsp. water until it turns orange. Add 4 tbsp. olive oil, the ginger, vinegar, jalapeño, sea salt, and pepper. Pour on the vegetable mix. Toss and chill until serving. Makes 4 salads.

Entrées

Avocado Chicken Salad

2 cups organic chicken, cooked, diced	1 rib celery, diced	lemon pepper seasoning
1 large avocado, diced	2 hard-boiled eggs, crumbled	6 Boston lettuce cups
	4 tbsp. raspberry vinaigrette	

In a large mixing bowl, toss the chicken, avocado and celery. Add the hard-boiled eggs. Mix in 4 tbsp. raspberry vinaigrette and season to taste with lemon-pepper. Serve in Boston lettuce cups. Makes 6 servings.

Nutrition per serving:	Vitamin C --------- 4 mg.	Fat ----------------- 9 g.	Magnesium ------- 48 mg.
Calories ----------- 213	Vitamin E --------- 2 IU	Cholesterol-------- 0	Potassium --------- 465 mg.
Protein ------------ 28 g.	Carbohydrates ---- 5 g.	Calcium ----------- 32 mg.	Sodium------------ 88 mg.
Vitamin A --------- 65 IU	Fiber -------------- 2 g.	Iron -------------- 2 mg.	

Quick Salmon Salad

I love to use left-over barbecued salmon here.

1 pound skinless salmon filet, cooked and cubed	3 tbsp. fresh lemon mint, minced (or lemon balm herb)	1 tsp. olive oil
½ cup white wine	1 cup jicama, peeled and diced	pepper to taste
2 tbsp. lemon juice	1 tbsp. lemon juice	dulse granules
		1 small bag of spinach and endive
		red bell pepper rings

Use a large, lemon-rubbed salad bowl to mix the salmon with the white wine and lemon juice. In a separate bowl, mix the lemon mint, jicama, lemon juice, olive oil, pepper and dulse granules to taste. Mix gently with the salmon. Serve on plates covered with a bed of torn spinach and endive. Top each salad with red bell pepper rings. Makes 4 salads.

Nutrition per serving:	Vitamin E --------- 7 IU	Cholesterol-------- 0	Potassium --------- 778 mg.
Calories ----------- 231	Carbohydrates ---- 6 g.	Calcium ----------- 34 mg.	Sodium------------ 192 mg.
Protein ------------ 25 g.	Fiber -------------- 3 g.	Iron -------------- 3 mg.	
Vitamin C --------- 45 mg.	Fat ----------------- 9 g.	Magnesium ------- 76 mg.	

Baked Turkey Supreme

4 cups turkey, cooked and diced	1 (7 oz.) can sliced water chestnuts	4 tbsp. lemon juice
1 (10 oz.) can cream of mushroom soup	1 cup low-fat Swiss cheese, shredded	½ tsp. lemon-pepper seasoning
1½ cups celery, chopped	1 cup chopped pecans	crunchy Chinese noodles
	4 tbsp. green onions, minced	a handful of toasted, chopped pecans

Preheat oven to 425°F. Have the cooked turkey ready. Mix the cream of mushroom soup with enough water or white wine to make 2 cups sauce. In a bowl, mix the turkey and sauce with the celery, water chestnuts, Swiss cheese, 1 cup pecans, green onions, lemon juice and lemon-pepper seasoning. Pour into a casserole and cover with crunchy Chinese noodles and a scattering of toasted chopped pecans. Bake for about 15 minutes, just to heat through and melt the cheese. Makes 8 servings.

Beauty Diet for Skin, Hair, Nails and Eyes

Today, the media tells us forty is the new twenty, they say fifty is the new thirty. I've talked to renowned facial surgeons who tell me their clients don't want to age at all… they want to maintain their looks at 45!

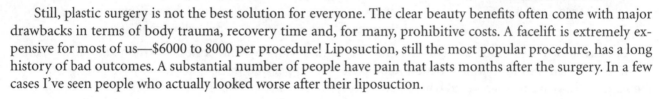

We all want to look our best at every age. Healthy hair and nails, radiant skin and a fit body are signs of health and success. In America, good looks have become almost a matter of self defense, for both men and women. Job competition is fierce and pressure comes at us from every social angle, so we take looking good seriously.

Answers don't come cheap to the "beauty equation." Cosmetic surgery is booming. Technology has advanced enormously just in the last 10 years and Americans are rising to the challenge of reclaiming our youth under the knife. In 2003, over 100,000 face lifts were performed—up from 40,000 in 1990! Over 1 million people used Botox injections, scorning warnings about possible botulism bacteria toxicity to reduce laugh lines and crow's feet. Less invasive therapies like non-surgical facelifts and micro-dermabrasion are rising exponentially.

Still, plastic surgery is not the best solution for everyone. The clear beauty benefits often come with major drawbacks in terms of body trauma, recovery time and, for many, prohibitive costs. A facelift is extremely expensive for most of us—$6000 to 8000 per procedure! Liposuction, still the most popular procedure, has a long history of bad outcomes. A substantial number of people have pain that lasts months after the surgery. In a few cases I've seen people who actually looked worse after their liposuction.

Is there another way? Can the right diet turn back time?

A beautiful body comes from within. Radiant skin, lustrous, lively hair, bright eyes and strong pink nails, all mirror a body in good health. Good dietary care and habits show quickly. If your hair, skin and eyes need help, I find that most people experience noticeable appearance improvement from diet changes in about three weeks.

Beautiful skin, for example, is more than skin deep. Your skin is your body's largest organ. Skin mirrors our emotional state and our hormone balance. The skin's protective acid mantle inhibits the growth of disease-causing bacteria. Skin problems reflect a stressed lifestyle almost immediately. (Allergies show up first on your skin.) Our skin is the essence of renewable nature… it sloughs off old, dying cells every day for a new start. Herbal nutrients are great for skin… they're packed with absorbable minerals, antioxidants, EFAs and bioflavonoids to cleanse, hydrate, heal, alkalize, and balance—improvements that show quickly in skin beauty.

Your hair is another mirror of your health. Changes in hair are often the first indication of nutritional deficiencies. We all want it… thick, gorgeous hair. Your scalp has at least 100,000 hairs so you have a lot to work with. Hair consists of protein layers called keratin. In healthy hair, the cell walls of the hair cuticle lie flat like shingles, leaving hair soft and shiny. In damaged or dry hair, the cuticle shingles are broken and create gaps that make hair porous and dull. Hair problems are never isolated. They are the result of more basic body imbalances.

Your eyes are not only the windows of your soul, but windows to body health as well. Your lifestyle profoundly affects your "eyestyle." No other sense is so prone to poor health conditions. Many drugs, (prescription, recreational and over-the-counter), react with your eyes. The worst offenders are cocaine, excessive use of chemical diuretics, sulfa drugs or tetracycline, erectile dysfunction drugs, aspirin, nicotine, phenylalanine and hydrocortisone. A happy liver is the key to healthy eyes. The most stressful eyesight situations are using a computer for most of your workday, and a sedentary lifestyle. Most eye-improving supplements need 2 – 3 months for effectiveness.

Are your appearance elements showing signs they need some TLC?

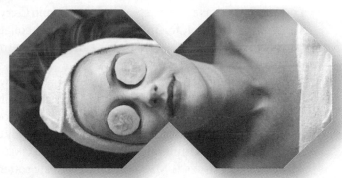

- **Check your hair:** Is it too dry or too oily? Do you have split ends or flaky deposits on your scalp? Does it lack of bounce and elasticity? Do you have lots of falling hair (normal shedding is about 25 to 50 hairs a day)?
- **Check your eyes:** Is your vision degenerating? Do your eyes strain easily? Does your sight become worse as the day goes on? Do you get frequent headaches over your eyes? Do you get spots and floaters before your eyes?
- **Check your skin:** Is your skin and its acid mantle out of balance? with sores or spottiness? Does it look dry and cracked? Is it itching, chapped, always scaling? Is it too dry or too oily? Is it red, rough and rashy? (all signs of an unbalanced acid mantle).

One Week Toxin Elimination Cleanse for Skin, Hair and Eyes

A brown rice cleanse is based on macrobiotic principles for body balance. A brown rice diet is cleansing, yet filling. You don't feel like you're on a cleanse at all, yet it does the trick. It's a diet that uses rice as a nutrient building food, and vegetables and vegetable juices as concentrated cleansing supplements. A brown rice diet is loaded with B-vitamins and essential fatty acids. It's full of potassium, natural iodine, and other minerals, so most people notice improvement in their hair, skin texture and nail growth. Many people experience about a 2 to 5 pound weight drop during this cleanse, as well as almost immediate rises in vitality and energy levels too. It's a great way to transition from an unhealthy diet into a better diet.

The night before your brown rice cleanse....

A green leafy salad for dinner sweeps your bowels. Take an herbal enema the night before your cleanse.

The next day...

On rising: take 2 fresh squeezed lemons, 1 tbsp. maple syrup in 8 oz. of water; or a glass of aloe vera juice, apple juice or pomegranate juice.

Breakfast: watermelon juice (rich in silica); or apple juice with Crystal Star Iodine, Potassium, Silica extract.

Mid-morning: have a skin tonic: juice 1 cucumber, 1 handful fresh parsley, 1 (4 oz.) tub of fresh sprouts and sprigs of fresh mint, or have a green drink, like Sun Wellness Chlorella or Crystal Star® Energy Green Renewal™.

Lunch: have a veggie juice like Personal Best V-8 (page 18); or take Crystal Star® Cleansing & Purifying™ Tea or Detox Tea by Yogi with 2 Crystal Star® Dr. Enzyme II: Fat & Starch Buster caps.

Mid-afternoon: have a carrot juice; or an herb tea like nettles or green tea; or apple juice; or a green drink, like Crystal Star® Energy Green Renewal™ with 1 tsp. nutritional yeast and 1 tsp. wheat germ added.

Dinner: have steamed brown rice and vegetables. Sprinkle with snipped, dry sea greens (like dulse or kelp). Use 1 tbsp. flax or olive oil, and 1 tbsp. Bragg's Liquid Aminos. Or make a high luster skin broth: In 2½ cups water, cook 2 cups chopped fresh mixed vegetables, add 1 tsp. miso and 2 tbsp. chopped dried sea greens. Add 4 tbsp. sunflower or sesame seeds for a protein boost. Vegetable protein aids faster healing for damaged skin.

Before Bed: have Crystal Star® Beautiful Skin™ tea or green or white tea; or a pineapple/papaya, papaya or apple juice; or Red Star nutritional yeast broth for high B vitamins; or a cleansing drink like Crystal Star® Fiber & Herbs Colon Cleanse™ caps or Nature's Secret Ultimate Cleanse to stimulate the body to eliminate wastes.

The next 6 days... Have 2 – 3 glasses of any blend of mixed vegetable juices throughout the day. Don't eat any solid food during the day. Have steamed brown rice and mixed vegetables for an early dinner each evening. Drink at least 6 – 8 glasses of pure bottled or mineral water throughout the day for best results.

Choose 2 or 3 supplements to smooth out and support your cleanse:

- **During detox:** Take ¼ – ½ tsp. ascorbate vitamin C crystals with any drink or juice 3 to 4 times daily throughout the elimination diet, for interstitial tissue and collagen formation. Note: be sure to add liquid acidophilus with any juice or drink—1 tsp. 3 – 4 times daily throughout the elimination diet, for best assimilation and to keep the system alkaline.
- **Skin herbal support:** CRYSTAL STAR® BEAUTIFUL SKIN™ white tea caps, blemishes and skin maintenance; PLANETARY YELLOW DOCK CLEANSE caps, blood purifiers and pH balancers; HERBS ETC. DERMATONIC, waste elimination.
- **Smoothing/hydrating herbs:** NUTRICOLOGY SKIN GLOW (hyaluronic acid softgels); chamomile tea, CAMOCARE FACIAL THERAPY; lavender aromatherapy oil for puffiness; MYCHELLE FRUIT ENZYME mist for inflammation relief.
- **Skin vitamins and minerals:** DIAMOND HERPANACINE; FUTUREBIOTICS HAIR, SKIN & NAILS; MSM *(Methyl Sulfonyl Methane)*, or TRIMEDICA MSM caps, helps create softer & smoother skin and repairs damaged or scarred skin.
- **Essential fatty acids:** helps skin dehydration and wrinkling: Evening Primrose oil 4000 mg. daily.
- **Silica, a mineral for collagen support, reduces dry, wrinkled skin.** EIDON SILICA MINERAL SUPPLEMENT; FLORA VEGESIL; CRYSTAL STAR® IODINE, POTASSIUM, SILICA extract.
- **Antioxidants are important for skin health:** Beta carotene protects against the sun's free radicals; Vitamin E protects against the lipid peroxidation caused by UV rays; Bioflavonoids improve vascularization of the skin; MYCHELLE PERFECT C SERUM; SOURCE NATURALS SKIN ETERNAL caps and serum (Ester-C, Lipoic Acid, DMAE).
- **Protease heals skin:** CRYSTAL STAR® DR. ENZYME™ WITH PROTEASE & BROMELAIN; TRANSFORMATION PUREZYME.

These bodywork techniques add to your beauty quotient right away

- **Get early morning sunlight** on the face and body every day possible, for natural A and D.
- **Rub your face with the inside surface of papaya and cucumber skins** when you peel them. They are excellent for alkalizing acid waste and are a natural AHA treatment.
- **AHAs:** MYCHELLE FRUIT ENZYME CLEANSER, NONI OF BEVERLY HILLS BRILLIANT CREAM with 5% AHA.
- **Make a skin beauty face tea:** chamomile and calendula flowers, lemon juice, rose hips and rosewater. Strain, and apply with cotton balls to the skin, or pour as a rinse through the hair, to add minerals and toning agents.
- **Dry brush for healthy skin:** Use a natural bristle brush. Start with the soles of your feet—brush vigorously making rotary motions and massage every part of your body—starting at the feet and work up to the neck.
- **Bathe:** High mineral bath. Add 1 cup DEAD SEA SALTS, 1 cup EPSOM SALTS, ½ cup regular sea salt and 4 tbsp. baking soda to a tub; swish in 3 drops lavender, 2 drops geranium, 2 drops sandalwood and 1 drop neroli oil.

Good Looks Restoration Diet for Skin, Hair and Eyes

A good diet is the first place to turn when you want to make real improvements in your appearance. Beautiful eyes, skin, hair and nails need a diet rich in fresh fruits and vegetables, and plenty of water. Beautiful skin, hair and eyes all depend on a healthy liver. Too much alcohol, caffeine and drugs put a heavy load on the liver and rob the body of B vitamins. All tissues need a rich, high oxygen blood supply, and plenty of mineral building blocks. Plants are the most absorbable way for the body to get them.

Watchwords for beautiful skin, hair, nails and eyes:

1.   Soft smooth skin depends on vitamin A, vitamin C, mineral-rich foods, and vegetable protein foods for collagen and tissue strength. Eat potassium-rich foods if your skin is dry: leafy greens, spinach, bell peppers, bananas, broccoli, sesame and sunflower seeds, fish and sea greens. Eat cleansing foods if your skin tone is muddy: fresh fruit, vegetable and fruit juices, celery, cucumbers. Eat vitamin C, E, carotene-rich foods for better skin texture: sea foods and fresh greens. Eat cultured foods if your skin is spotty: yogurt, tofu and kefir. Eliminate red meats, fried, fatty and fast foods. Reduce caffeine, dairy foods and salty, sugary foods. They show up on your skin. Eat high fiber foods: fruits, vegetables and whole grains to maintain regularity, and healthy skin.

Sea greens offer a collagen boost for skin health and beauty. Kelp and ulva (sea lettuce) are rich in the collagen-building, amino acid proline. Red Sea Algae, or "Ogo" which grows in Hawaii, also has a very high content of proline, and is widely used in natural skin care products. Collagen replacement drinks made with seaweed show excellent results for anti-aging and wrinkle reduction. I use and recommend LANE LABS TOKI drink mix.

I've seen firsthand the power of using seafood in transforming your looks. Just eating fish or seafood 2 – 3 times a week notably reduces skin dryness or wrinkling. Fish are loaded with EFAs that plump up gaunt or crepey-looking skin. People notice real improvement, sometimes right away.

The safest seafood choices I've researched are Pacific halibut, farmed abalone, Dungeness crab, shrimp and salmon. *(Note: There is expanded information on mercury contamination in fish at www.nrdc.org)*

Wild salmon is a beautifying food especially for lifting for after-40 sags and bags because it contains high amounts of DMAE, *di-methyl-amino-ethanol*, an antioxidant that tightens and tones skin tissue, especially when used with alpha lipoic acid. Farmed salmon usually has a lower nutrient profile and higher contaminate levels.

2.   Turn your hair from drab to fab with vegetable or whole grain protein for maximum growth, and high carotene foods like broccoli, carrots and greens for "permanent" appeal. Eat these foods if your hair is brittle: carrots, green peppers, lettuces, bananas, strawberries, apples, peas, onions, green peppers, cucumbers, sprouts, green tea. Have aloe vera juice in the morning if your hair is dry. Avoid saturated fats, sugars and processed, refined foods. They show up in hair texture. Include healthy fats from seafood, sea greens (use dulse if there is also iron deficiency), cantaloupe, spinach, perilla or flax oil for shine and volume.

3.   Your eyes sparkle when you eat protein from the sea and soy foods (rich in omega-3 fatty acids), whole grains, low fat dairy foods, and eggs (full of zeaxanthin). Good vision vegetables are broccoli, sunflower and sesame seeds, orange and yellow veggies, parsley, leeks, onions, cabbage, cauliflower, corn, barley, blueberries, watercress. Eyes love vitamin A and high mineral foods: leafy greens, sea greens, seafood, loaded with carotenoids and EFAs (2 dry tbsp. daily). Reduce your sugar intake. Avoid chemicalized foods, especially fried and fatty foods, dairy and red meats. These foods metabolize slowly, use sugars poorly, and form crystallized clogs in your eyes.

Liver malfunction is a common cause of eye problems. Keep your liver happy with B-vitamins, high fiber foods that absorb excess bile and increase regularity; potassium-rich sea foods, chlorophyll-rich leafy greens (esp. dandelion) and sea greens, enzyme-rich yogurt and kefir, and sulphur-rich eggs, garlic and onions.

When you're working on the appearance of your eyes, try to have a vision drink twice a week: Mix 1 cup carrot juice, 15 drops of CRYSTAL STAR® EYES RIGHT!™ EXTRACT, 1 egg, 1 tbsp. toasted wheat germ, 1 tsp. rose hips powder, 1 tbsp. honey, 1 tsp. sesame seeds, 1 tsp. RED STAR nutritional yeast, 1 tsp. kelp granules.

The Daily Beauty Diet

On rising: a glass of watermelon juice in summer, apple/cranberry juice in winter; and/or a superfood drink, like WAKUNAGA HARVEST GREENS with sea greens, or CRYSTAL STAR® RESTORE YOUR STRENGTH™ drink. A low fat protein drink each morning has a dramatic effect on dry hair; add 1 tsp. RED STAR nutritional yeast for hair color; a glass of aloe vera juice like HERBAL ANSWERS ALOE FORCE JUICE for cleansing.

Breakfast: have a glass of grapefruit or watermelon juice; make a mix of the following hair and skin foods and take 3 tbsp. daily: wheat germ (oil or flakes), blackstrap molasses, nutritional yeast and sesame seeds. Sprinkle some every morning on your breakfast food—whole grain cereal or granola with yogurt and fresh fruit (especially bananas, strawberries, papaya and peaches); or oatmeal or whole grain pancakes, with maple syrup.

Mid-morning: have a cup of miso soup with sea greens sprinkled on top; or some low fat yogurt with fresh fruit; or a green drink, such as BARLEANS GREENS or CRYSTAL STAR® ENERGY GREEN RENEWAL™ drink.

Lunch: have a green leafy salad, with cucumber, sprouts, bell pepper and lemon-oil dressing; or steamed vegetables with marinated tofu and brown rice or a baked potato; or a fresh fruit salad, with peaches, apricots and cottage cheese or yogurt cheese; or an avocado, low-fat cheese sandwich with lentil, or onion soup.

Mid-afternoon: have a carrot juice or GREEN FOODS CARROT ESSENCE drink; have a cup of refreshing herb tea, like chamomile or red clover tea, or CRYSTAL STAR® BEAUTIFUL SKIN™ tea; or a cup of ramen soup with noodles, or miso soup; and/or crunchy raw veggies with kefir cheese or yogurt cheese.

Dinner: have a dinner salad with red onions, cucumbers and sprouts, and whole grain muffins with kefir cheese; or a light beans and rice dish with a small green salad; or a broccoli, or asparagus quiche with onion soup; or baked or broiled seafood or fish with veggies and brown rice; or a stir-fry with greens, rice and miso soup.

Before bed: have a glass of papaya, cranberry (a specific for rosacea) or apple juice; or RED STAR nutritional yeast broth for relaxation and B vitamins.

Note: Drink plenty of pure bottled water (or filtered water) every day for clear skin. Avoid red meats, refined sugars and flour, caffeine-containing foods, fried or fatty foods, foods with colorings and preservatives. All slow metabolism, use sugars and fats poorly, and encourage clogs to form. NO JUNK FOODS.

Choose 2 or 3 supplements to enhance your beauty elements:

- **Minerals are critical to hair health:** CRYSTAL STAR® BEAUTIFUL HAIR & NAILS™ caps; Horsetail extract; or CRYSTAL STAR® IODINE, POTASSIUM, SILICA SOURCE™ extract daily or FLORA VEGISIL caps. Sea greens minerals are dramatic for hair growth: 2 tbsp. daily dried chopped sea greens or 6 kelp tablets daily; or CRYSTAL STAR® OCEAN MINERALS™ caps 2 daily or GREEN FOODS ION KELP tabs. For premature graying, GREEN NUTRITION INDIUMEASE (excellent results).
- **EFAs for hair shine:** Evening Primrose oil 3000 mg. daily. Rub in Jojoba oil daily; Shampoos rich in EFAs: Hemp or Henna, Neem Oil or Babassu Palm shampoo; LAMAS WHEATGRASS DEEP CLEANSING shampoo for oily hair.
- **Essential fatty acids are critical for skin:** Eat chia, pumpkin and sunflower seeds; Evening primrose oil 4000 mg. daily; NATURE'S SECRET ULTIMATE OIL; Aloe vera gel; BARLEANS FLAX OIL caps 3 daily. ZIA ULTIMATE MOISTURE (nice); Vitamin A & D 25,000/1,000IU; MYCHELLE DEEP REPAIR cream.
- **Smoothing hydrators for skin:** MSM, 1000 mg. daily; Cysteine 1000 mg. Make my sea plant rapid facial: sprinkle 1 tsp. kelp granules in a bowl. Blend with 1 tbsp. aloe vera gel. Apply to face and neck; leave on 10 minutes, rinse. CRYSTAL STAR® RED SKIN RELIEF™ for inflammatory skin reactions like rosacea, eczema and psoriasis.
- **Expand your eye power:** CRYSTAL STAR® EYES RIGHT!™ EXTRACT, 15 drops daily; HERBALIST & ALCHEMIST BLUEBERRY EXTRACT; Ginkgo biloba extract 2x daily; NUTRICOLOGY OCUDYNE 2 (targeted nutrients for vision).
- **Clarifying natural eye treatments** Sea greens caps for blurry vision; Raspberry tea bags or green tea bags for bloodshot eyes; Borage seed tea for sore eyes.
- **For "computer" eyes:** Press points under eyebrows; press points in inner corners of eyes; squeeze eyebrows; look up, down, right and left every half hour. ESTEEM BRIGHT EYES (specific for eye strain); SIMILASAN EYE DROPS #3 (rapid results for computer eyes). Bathe eyes in cool witch hazel, or diluted chamomile or rosemary tea.

These bodywork techniques add to your beauty quotient right away

- **Bodywork for hair:** Massage scalp each morning for 3 minutes to stimulate hair growth. Sunlight helps hair grow, but too much sun dries and damages. Wash hair in warm water. Rinse in cool water for scalp circulation.
- **A super hair tonic:** Mix 8 oz green tea and 8 oz. rosemary tea (fresh sprigs best). Strain; add 1 tbsp. lemon juice, 1 tbsp. white vinegar. Work through hair, leave on 1 minute. Rinse. Chlorine residue? Add 2-3 tbsp. of apple cider vinegar to your regular shampoo for an at-home clarifying treatment.
- **Hot oil treatment:** Mix olive oil with drops of essential lavender and rosemary oils; rub in hair. Leave on 5 minutes; rinse. For dry, limp hair, apply ¼ cup of warm honey from scalp to ends. Leave on 10 minutes (use a shower cap to keep from dripping) for a natural deep conditioning treatment.
- **Beautiful skin secrets:** Swirl 3 tbsp. honey in bath water for silky skin. Apply lotion after your shower before you dry off for the most skin moisture. Dry skin brushing once a week for circulation and to slough dead cells.
- **My own make-up remover:** Mix in a dark bottle, avocado, almond, kukui, jojoba oils; very nourishing.
- **Kitchen cosmetic face lifts:** apply, leave on 30 minutes, rinse off.
   1. Yogurt/lemon juice to balance pH and restore acid mantle.
   2. Honey/almond/oatmeal scrub or MYCHELLE INCREDIBLE PUMPKIN PEEL to exfoliate. Follow with blend of aloe vera gel and vitamin E oil.
   3. Egg whites or ZIA SEAWEED LIFT for skin tightening.
   4. Honey/ red wine mix for AHA wrinkle treatment.

Maintenance Recipes for a Beauty Diet

Use these recipes on an ongoing basis once your initial healing diet is producing good results.

Breakfast

Detox Morning Melon Soup

Loaded with EFAs.

1 cup cantaloupe, cut into chunks

2 cups honeydew melon, cut into chunks

2 cups watermelon, cut into chunks

¼ cup lemon juice

2 tbsp. fresh mint, chopped (reserve sprigs for garnish)

2 cups sparkling water

In a food processor, dice the cantaloupe. Add the orange juice, lemon juice and yogurt; process until smooth. Top each glass with 1 tsp. mint. Makes 4 servings.

Healing drinks

Easy Hawaiian Punch

Naturally good, with all the health benefits.

1½ cups pineapple-coconut juice

1 cup papaya juice

¼ cup orange juice

2 tbsp. lime juice

Pour all ingredients into a large pitcher, stir well and chill. Makes 6 servings.

Soups, salads, appetizers

Sweet Pea & Fresh Mint Soup

2 cups yellow onions, diced

3 tbsp. olive oil

3 cups organic vegetable broth

1 small bag baby spinach, finely chopped

2 cups fresh mint leaves, finely chopped

1 cup plain lowfat yogurt

10 oz. package frozen peas

herbal seasoning salt

white pepper

In a large soup pot, sauté the onions in the olive oil until fragrant. Add the vegetable broth and bring to a boil. Reduce heat and simmer 10 minutes. Remove from heat. Add half of the baby spinach and fresh mint to the soup. Add the soup to a blender and mix with the low-fat yogurt until smooth. Return to soup pot and add the frozen peas. Heat soup until peas turn a bright green. Add the rest of spinach and mint. Season with herbal seasoning and white pepper. Makes 8 servings.

Nutrition per serving:	Vitamin C --------- 24 mg.	Fat ----------------- 4 g.	Magnesium ------- 35 mg.
Calories ----------- 99	Vitamin E --------- 2 IU	Cholesterol -------- 0	Potassium --------- 319 mg.
Protein ----------- 5 g.	Carbohydrates ---- 12 g.	Calcium ----------- 98 mg.	Sodium ----------- 136 mg.
Vitamin A --------- 193 IU	Fiber ------------- 3 g.	Iron --------------- 2 mg.	

Chilled Cucumber-Yogurt Soup

2¼ cups plain low-fat yogurt	2 tsp. garlic-lemon seasoning	2 tsp. crystallized ginger
1¼ pounds lemon cucumbers, peeled and sliced	1½ tsp. ground cumin	thin slices of daikon white radish

In a blender, mix the low fat yogurt, lemon cucumbers, garlic-lemon seasoning, ground cumin, and crystallized ginger until smooth. Strain through fine sieve into large bowl. Chill well, about 2 hours. Top with thin slices of daikon white radish at serving. Makes 6 servings.

Asian Crab-Cucumber Salad

1 red pepper, diced	1 (7 oz.) can crab meat, rinsed and drained	baby Asian greens
1 large European cucumber, diced	4 tbsp. plain, low-fat yogurt	ANNIE'S RASPBERRY VINAIGRETTE
		8 tsp. sesame seeds

Mix the red pepper, European cucumber, crab meat and yogurt. Serve on a bed of baby Asian greens. Pour a little Annie's raspberry vinaigrette (from your health food store) on each salad. Sprinkle each salad with 2 tsp. sesame seeds. Chill. Makes 4 servings.

California Fruit Salad

Make in a large bowl. Serve in individual bowls.

¼ cup pine nuts (or slivered almonds)	2 avocados, peeled and cubed	¼ cup raspberry vinegar
2 large navel oranges	1 firm-ripe papaya, peeled and sliced	1½ tbsp. Dijon mustard
2 kiwi fruit, peeled and sliced	large lettuce leaf cups	1½ tbsp. lemon juice
2 ruby grapefruit, peeled and sectioned	¼ cup grapeseed oil	1½ tbsp. honey
	¼ cup olive oil	2 tsp. poppy seeds
		½ tsp. lemon pepper seasoning

In a skillet, pan roast the pine nuts over medium heat until golden, about 3 – 5 minutes. Remove the nuts from the skillet and set aside. In a large mixing bowl, mix the oranges, kiwi fruit, and grapefruit. Add the avocado and papaya. Toss fruit to coat slices with the citrus juice from the bowl. Line 8 salad bowls with large lettuce leaf cups. Spoon in the fruit. Top with roasted nuts. Make the poppy seed dressing: mix the grapeseed oil, olive oil, raspberry vinegar, Dijon mustard, lemon juice, honey, poppy seeds, and lemon pepper seasoning. Pour over the salad to taste. Makes 8 servings.

Nutrition per serving:	Vitamin C --------- 100 mg.	Fat ----------------- 22 g.	Magnesium ------- 49 mg.
Calories ----------- 295	Vitamin E --------- 7 IU	Cholesterol-------- 0	Potassium --------- 785 mg.
Protein ----------- 4 g.	Carbohydrates ---- 26 g.	Calcium ----------- 78 mg.	Sodium------------ 33 mg.
Vitamin A --------- 125 IU	Fiber -------------- 6 g.	Iron -------------- 1 mg.	

Entrées

Grilled Salmon Steaks Asian Style

¼ cup olive oil	1 tbsp. dried sea vegetables (any kind), chopped	1 tbsp. ginger, peeled and minced
3 tbsp. soy sauce		4 fresh, skinless salmon steaks
2 scallions, chopped		

Make a quick fresh marinade: mix the olive oil, soy sauce, scallions, sea vegetables, and ginger. Rub onto 4 fresh, skinless salmon steaks; marinate for 1 hour in the fridge. Grill steaks about 4 minutes per side, basting often with marinade. Makes 4 servings.

Sizzling Ginger Stir-Fry

1 tbsp. grapeseed oil	1 package firm tofu, drained	2 tbsp. hoisin sauce
3 tbsp. fresh ginger, peeled	and cut into ½" pieces	2 tbsp. chives, chopped
and minced	6 drops toasted sesame oil	2 tbsp. toasted sesame seeds
4 cloves garlic, minced	1 tsp. honey	

In a wok, heat 1 tbsp. grapeseed oil over medium heat. Add the ginger and garlic and sauté for 10 minutes. Add the tofu, toasted sesame oil, honey and hoisin sauce; gently cook through while stirring, about 10 more minutes. Top with chives and toasted sesame seeds and serve. Makes 4 servings.

Nutrition per serving:	Vitamin C --------- 3 mg.	Fat ----------------- 12 g.	Magnesium ------- 86 mg.
Calories ----------- 190	Vitamin E --------- 1 IU	Cholesterol-------- 0	Potassium --------- 223 mg.
Protein ------------ 14 g.	Carbohydrates ---- 10 g.	Calcium ----------- 159 mg.	Sodium------------ 138 mg.
Vitamin A --------- 95 IU	Fiber ------------- 1 g.	Iron -------------- 8 mg.	

Sushi Salad

1 cup short-grain sushi rice	2 carrots, diced	2 sheets toasted nori, sliced into
1 cup mixed brown and wild	1 rib celery, diced	small squares
rice	4 scallions, thinly sliced	½ cup brown rice vinegar
4 cups cold water	2 tbsp. pickled ginger,	2 tbsp. soy sauce
2 cups broccoli, diced	minced	2 tsp. wasabi paste
1 red bell pepper, diced	½ cup almonds, slivered	

In a saucepan with a tight-fitting lid, combine the sushi rice, mixed brown and wild rice, and 4 cups of cold water. Bring to a boil, stirring occasionally. Reduce heat to low, stir, then cover and cook for 15 minutes, lifting the lid to stir only once. Remove pan from heat, stir, cover again, and set aside for 20 minutes. Brown and wild rices should be chewy in texture. Cool in a large bowl.

In a soup pot, blanch the broccoli, red bell pepper and carrots in boiling water for 1 minute. Drain and rinse with cold water to stop cooking; set aside. When rice is cool, toss with blanched vegetables, celery, scallions, ginger, almonds, and toasted nori. Make the dressing: whisk together the brown rice vinegar, soy sauce, and wasabi paste to make a dressing. Toss with salad and serve. Makes 6 servings.

Nutrition per serving:	Vitamin C--------- 57 mg.	Fat ----------------- 5 g.	Magnesium ------- 86 mg.
Calories ----------- 195	Vitamin E --------- 5 IU	Cholesterol-------- 0	Potassium --------- 390 mg.
Protein ------------ 7 g.	Carbohydrates ---- 32 g.	Calcium ----------- 68 mg.	Sodium------------ 308 mg.
Vitamin A --------- 792 mg.	Fiber ------------- 4 g.	Iron -------------- 2 mg.	

Orange, Fennel & Arugula Salad

2 tbsp. balsamic vinegar	4 navel oranges, peeled and	2 tbsp. fresh basil, chopped
2 tsp. Dijon mustard	sectioned	4 bunches arugula (8 cups), washed
2 tbsp. olive oil	2 cups fennel bulb, thinly	and torn
sea salt	sliced	toasted pumpkin seeds
black pepper	1 cup red onion, thinly sliced	

Make the vinaigrette dressing: mix the vinegar and mustard together. Gradually add in 2 tbsp. olive oil, and season to taste with sea salt and black pepper. Set aside. Place the sectioned oranges into a bowl. Add in the fennel, red onion, and fresh basil. Add vinaigrette to bowl and toss gently to combine. Let stand 1 hour. Pile arugula onto individual salad plates; top with orange mix; sprinkle each salad with toasted pumpkin seeds. Makes 8 servings.

Nutrition per serving:	Vitamin C--------- 48 mg.	Fat ----------------- 8 g.	Magnesium ------- 69 mg.
Calories ----------- 136	Vitamin E --------- 1 IU	Cholesterol-------- 0	Potassium --------- 400 mg.
Protein ------------ 4 g.	Carbohydrates ---- 15 g.	Calcium ----------- 86 mg.	Sodium------------ 169 mg.
Vitamin A --------- 340 mg.	Fiber ------------- 4 g.	Iron -------------- 2 mg.	

Optimal Nutrition for Children

We live in the most affluent country in the world, yet many of our children's basic nutritional needs are not met. Studies show over 50% of children don't even get the recommended daily allowance (RDA) levels of nutrients. Nearly half of kids in America eat less than one serving of fruit a day; one-third eat less than one daily serving of veggies! Chips and French fries make up one-quarter of the vegetables eaten by children, and about one-third of the vegetables eaten by teenagers. The infiltration of fast food into U.S. schools is particularly insidious. Fast food hamburgers and pizzas are school lunch staples. Soda vending machines are readily available on most campuses. The result? Kids are drinking more sodas than ever—a clear risk factor for osteoporosis later in life.

Type 2 diabetes and coronary heart disease (both related to poor diet and lack of exercise) are on the rise in children. 30 – 50% of new type 2 diabetes cases are children between 9 – 19 years old! Today, one-third of all kids have high cholesterol! Autopsies show that atherosclerosis now begins in childhood. Getting childhood obesity under control through better diet and regular exercise is the best way to solve these degenerative diseases.

Why is this happening to our kids?

Because much of our agricultural soils are depleted, and most of our foods are sprayed or gassed, many micro-nutrients like vitamins and minerals are no longer sufficiently present in our foods. The most common childhood nutrient deficiencies are calcium, iron, B-1, and vitamins A, B-complex and C—the very ones that have the most impact on a child's health—slowing growth, wiping out immune defenses and impairing learning capacity!

Offer organic foods to your child whenever possible. They are higher in nutrients, and research shows children regularly exposed to pesticides have serious problems, like low stamina, underdeveloped hand-eye coordination, and poor attention span and recall. Graphically show your child what junk and synthetic foods are. Seductive TV ads and peer pressure mean that lots of kids don't really know what wholesome food is, and think they are eating the right way. Your presence as a loving parental authority is a powerful influence. Gather your family together for a meal at least once a day to establish good eating habits for your kids.

Use superfoods for kids! Superfoods are concentrated nutrients widely popular with adults today (check out the many superfoods listings in this book). They're just as good in healthy diet programs for kids. Mix them in or sprinkle them on other foods to increase the nutritional content of any meal. Superfood supplements put some great nutrients into fussy eaters. CRYSTAL STAR® RESTORE YOUR STRENGTH™ drink mix is a potent vegetarian blend of sea greens, herbs, and foods like miso, soy protein, nutritional yeast and brown rice. Add it to soups, sauces, even salad dressings. GREEN FOODS BERRY BARLEY ESSENCE has a natural raspberry-strawberry taste kids like. Kids also like bee pollen, a highly bio-active superfood often called "nature's complete nutrition," because it is so full of balanced vitamins, minerals, proteins, EFAs, enzymes, and essential amino acids. Its sweet flavor works well sprinkled on cereals or in smoothies.

Diet tips to help keep your child healthier and happier:

It's a lot easier said than done to change old dietary patterns to healthier eating… for anybody, but especially for kids. A good way to start is to find something delicious to replace whatever is being taken away.

For example:
- **If you want your kid to eat more fruits and vegetables**, start with foods that children go for, like dried fruit snacks, and smoothies for fruits. Sandwiches, tacos, burritos and pitas easily hold vegetables. Most kids like soup with vegetables. Let them add sauces or flavors they like.
- **To encourage your child to drink more water** instead of carbonated sodas or sweetened drinks, keep plenty of natural fruit juices and flavored mineral water around the house.
- **To reduce the amount of sugar your child eats,** buy sugar-free snacks. Replace sugar-filled cereals with granola or oatmeal with healthy toppings. Almost every kid likes raisins. Or try CC Pollen Co. Buzz Bars.
- **If you want to add more seafood to a child's diet**, start with favorites like shrimp, tuna fish or salmon.
- **To add healthy cultured foods to your child's diet,** keep an assortment of yogurt flavors with fruit for snacks in the fridge. Offer delicious kefir cheese for snack spreads instead of sour cream.

- **If you want more whole grains in your child's diet,** start by keeping only whole grains in the house. Kids love bagels and pastas, which come in a wide variety of whole grain options. Brown basmati rice is much tastier than white rice if your kid is a "rice kid." Stuffing is a big favorite. Popcorn is a healthy snack. Season it with low sodium soy sauce or an herb and spice seasoning blend instead of gobs of butter and salt.
- **To reduce the amount of meat and dairy protein your child is eating,** keep tasty plant protein available. Kids like tofu and grain burgers with their favorite trimmings. Most kids like beans—look for healthy chili blends. Stock peanut butter, nuts and seeds, like almonds, sunflower seeds and pumpkin seeds for snacks. Use them as toppings for soup, salad crunchies, smoothies and desserts. (Seeds and nuts give kids unsaturated oils and essential fatty acids for brain development.) Eggs are a good protein choice for kids… one of Nature's perfect foods that's gotten a bad rap. Most kids like deviled eggs, and eggs are great in honey custards, another kid favorite.

This sample diet for optimal health for your child has been kid-tested for taste

On rising: offer a protein drink like ALL 1 VITAMIN-MINERAL, especially if the child's energy or school performance is poor; or the child always seems to be ill; or 1 tsp. liquid FLORADIX KINDERLOVE MULTI-VITAMIN/MINERAL.

Breakfast: have granola with apple juice or yogurt and fresh fruit; or whole grain toast or muffins, with butter, kefir cheese or nut butter; add eggs, scrambled or baked (no fried eggs); or have hot oatmeal or puffed kashi cereal with maple syrup or yogurt.

Mid-morning: whole grain crackers with kefir cheese and fruit juice; or dried fruit leathers with yogurt or kefir cheese; or crunchy veggies with peanut butter; or a sugar-free candy bar, or trail mix stirred into yogurt.

Lunch: have a veggie, turkey, chicken or shrimp sandwich on whole grain bread, with low fat cheese. Add corn chips with a low fat dip; or bean soup with whole grain toast, and a small salad or crunchy veggies with garbanzo spread; or a vegetarian pizza on a chapati crust; or spaghetti or pasta with parmesan cheese sauce; or a Mexican bean and veggie, or rice burrito with fresh salsa.

Mid-afternoon: have juice and a dried fruit candy bar; or fresh fruit or fruit juice, or a kefir drink; or a hard boiled egg and some trans-fat free whole grain chips with a veggie or low-fat cheese dip; or some whole grain toast and peanut butter or other nut butter.

Dinner: have a veggie pizza on a chapati or egg crust, with veggies, shrimp, and low fat cheese topping; or whole grain or egg pasta with vegetables and a light tomato/cheese sauce; or a baked Mexican quesadilla with low fat cheese and some steamed veggies or a salad; or roast turkey with cornbread dressing and a salad; or a tuna casserole with rice, peas and water chestnuts.

Before bed: a glass of apple juice or a little soy milk, RICE DREAM or flavored kefir.

Should your child go veg?

Today, the American Dietetic Association says that a well planned vegetarian diet provides enough nutrients for growing kids. Strict protein combining is not necessary (as was once believed) because a variety of plant protein sources throughout the day (like beans, nut butters, soy milk and whole grains) offer the proper protein building blocks for children's needs.

I'm a big believer in the importance of EFAs for a child's developing brain. For strict vegetarians who do not eat seafood (one of the best EFA sources), consider a supplement like FLORA UDO'S PERFECTED OIL BLEND, 1 - 3 tsp. daily for children over 4 – 10, or flax seed oil, 1 tsp. daily, to maximize brain nutrition.

Choose 2 or 3 supplements to help your child rebalance and normalize faster:

- **Acidophilus, liquid or powder:** give in juice 2 to 3x daily for good digestion and assimilation. UAS DDS-JUNIOR, or SOLARAY BABY LIFE are excellent for children. NUTRITION NOW RHINO ACIDOPHILUS (chewable tablets for children ages 4 and older). Add vitamin A & D in drops if desired.
- **Vitamin C, or Ester C:** for powder form with bioflavonoids: give in juice, ¼ tsp. at a time 2x daily. For chewable wafers, use 100 mg., 250 mg., or 500 mg. potency according to age and weight of the child.
- **A sugar-free multi-vitamin and mineral supplement:** in either liquid or chewable tablet form. Some good choices are from FLORADIX, NUTRITION NOW, NEW CHAPTER, SOLARAY and TRACE MINERAL RESEARCH.

- **Cleansing, purifying herbal teas and alcohol-free extracts:** especially HERBS FOR KIDS formulas and GAIA's children's formulas. Clear child's chest congestion with CRYSTAL STAR® D-CONGEST™ SPRAY, or try herbal steam inhalations. Use eucalyptus or tea tree oil drops in a vaporizer to keep lungs mucous free, improve oxygen uptake.
- **Use a mild herbal laxative:** like NATURE'S SECRET ULTIMATE FIBER or HERBAL ANSWERS HERBAL ALOE FORCE juice in half dosage for regularity.
- **Use garlic oil:** drops or open garlic capsules into juice for natural antibiotic activity; or give CRYSTAL STAR® ANTI-BIO™ caps or extract in half dosage or WAKUNAGA KYOLIC liquid in juice.
- **Boost immunity:** open Colostrum caps and sprinkle into baby or children's food—KAL COLOSTRUM tabs.

Bodywork for kids relaxes and normalizes body pH

- **Continue with herbal baths, washes and compresses to cleanse toxins coming out through the skin.** Oatmeal baths help neutralize rashes coming out on the skin. Herbal baths help induce cleansing perspiration, too, but the child should be watched closely all during the bath to make sure he or she is not getting too hot. Make up a big pot of calendula or comfrey leaf tea for the bath water. Rub the child's body with calendula or tea tree oil, or TIGER BALM to loosen congestion after the bath.
- **Give a soothing massage** before bed.
- **Get some early morning sunlight** on the body every day possible.
- **Give a gentle enema** at least once during the detox cleanse to clear the child's colon of impacted wastes that hinder the body's effort to rid itself of diseased bacteria. A catnip tea enema is effective and safe for children.
- **Apply hot ginger-cayenne compresses** to affected or sore areas to stimulate circulation and defense response, to rid the body more quickly of infection. Alternate hot compresses with cold, plain water compresses.
  - Dab on with cotton balls, a water infusion of goldenseal, myrrh, yellow dock, black walnut, and yarrow, or CRYSTAL STAR® ANTI-BIO™ phyto-therapy gel to help heal sores and scabs.
- **Exercise for kids is a primary nutrient for body and mind.** US Public Health studies show a third of American children aren't fit. The number of obese kids has doubled in the last 20 years! Exercise is a key to weight control, growth and energy. Don't let your kid be a couch potato (the average child watches 20 – 30 hours of TV a week!), or a computer junkie. Encourage outdoor activity, and find out if your child is taking P. E. classes in school.

Overcoming Attention Deficit Disorders

Hyperactive behavior and Attention Deficit Disorder are serious problems affecting up to 2 to 3 million children today... or one child in every classroom in the U.S! A new Mayo Clinic study shows children have a 7.5% chance of being diagnosed with ADHD between the ages of 5 and 18.

But many say ADHD is over-diagnosed. Hyperactivity may be the expression of either hypoglycemia or food allergies or both. Post-traumatic stress disorder, anxiety and depression can also mimic Attention Deficit Disorder. True ADD (Attention Deficit Disorder) is marked by a chronically poor attention span, and slow learning caused by any or all of the learning disorders, and it affects children and adults. New statistics suggest that 3 to 7% of all U.S. adults may be afflicted with ADD or ADHD (Attention Deficit Hyperactivity Disorder). Short term fixes like using sugar, caffeine or stimulant drugs to improve focus worsen the disorder over the long term.

Autism is almost a "mind-blind" condition, diagnosed in the first 30 months of life. It is characterized by withdrawn behavior, lack of emotion and speech, extreme sensitivity to sound and touch. Autistic children have a brain malfunction that creates a barrier between them and the rest of the world. It is speculated that autism is related to abnormal serotonin metabolism in the brain. Children at greatest risk are male with low birth weight, and a family history of diabetes or alcoholism. Nutrition improvement and stress-calming herbs are the cornerstones of successful treatment in overcoming hyperactivity disorders.

Does your child have an attention deficit disorder? Check these signs:

- Does your child exhibit dramatic mood swings and extreme personality changes?
- Does your child exhibit aggressive, destructive behavior? Is your child extremely impatient and defiant?
- Is your child unable to follow directions? or instructions?
- Does your child have an unusually short attention span? Is he or she unable to sit still?
- Does your child have poor motor coordination, a speech impediment or dyslexia?
- Is your child an extremely slow learner? Is he or she unable to reason or think rationally?
- Is he or she abnormally accident prone? Is there evidence of self-mutilation?
- Is your child a chronic liar?
- Does your child have chronic thirst?
- Does your child have a chronic allergy symptoms like sneezing or coughing?

Is your child on Ritalin?

Prescriptions for the drug have doubled in the last 10 years!

Drug therapy with Ritalin *(Methylphenidate)* or similar drugs is the conventional approach for dealing with ADHD. Ritalin is a central nervous system stimulant used to improve concentration and reduce compulsive behavior. I believe it's all too often used as a "band-aid approach" to deal with a problem that can respond to less invasive therapies. In some parts of the U.S., 6 out of 100 children take Ritalin every day. In essence, we are drugging a whole generation with Ritalin without any thought to the long term effects.

Ritalin does not cure ADHD, and it can have serious side effects. Ritalin can cause sleeplessness, facial tics, headache, stomachache, depression, decreased appetite, high blood pressure, seizures and heart palpitations. Although a causal relationship has not been proved, many feel Ritalin affects a child's growth. It definitely should not be used in cases of severe depression, general fatigue, hypertension or epilepsy. Canadian research reveals that more than 9% of children who take Ritalin develop symptoms of psychosis like hallucinations or paranoia!

Ritalin must be used very cautiously with other drugs. There are 21 reported drug-drug interactions with Ritalin, including reactions with over-the-counter cold medicines. Like other amphetamines, Ritalin may cause small vessel damage in the heart.

Is Ritalin addictive? Ritalin is chemically similar to cocaine, and is often sold and snorted for a "quick high" on school campuses. In fact, "Ritty" is one of the top ten abused prescription drugs on the street today!

Newer drugs, Adderral and Concerta are not much better. Both drugs disrupt normal sleep patterns and can seriously depress appetite, bad news for a developing body! Like Ritalin, these drugs are habit-forming and commonly produce side effects like dizziness, anxiety, headaches, stomach aches, hallucinations and paranoia.

Parents clearly want an alternative to Ritalin and other stimulant drugs. Strattera, a new non-stimulant drug introduced in 2002, had one million prescriptions written for the just between November 2002 and June 2003. But, there's a long term price to pay for Strattera, too. Mood swings, reduced appetite, nausea and vomiting, and fatigue top the list of Strattera's side effects. Other patients have reported increased anxiety and hot flashes while on the drug, presenting a major problem for women in the throes of menopause who may be using it.

Attention Deficit Disorder Control Diet

Researchers are slowly learning more about what causes this extremely disturbing disorder. Some kids admit they "are feeling crazy" at times when they exhibit ADD behavior. (Certainly their parents and teachers are!) Most experts say a child's diet is the first place to look. Mineral and EFA deficiencies from too many chemical-filled, junk foods are always present. (Prescription drugs that block EFA conversion in the brain are culprits, too.) Food allergies to corn, wheat and additives are more than likely. Hypoglycemia, normally an unusual syndrome for a child, is usual in ADD children.

Clearly, diet improvement is the key to changing ADD behavior. Results are almost immediately evident, generally within 1 – 3 weeks. When behavior normalizes, maintain the improved diet to prevent reversion.

Watchwords:

1. **Read food labels carefully.** 70% of kids with ADD react to chemical additives. Avoid ALL food products with preservatives, BHT, MSG, BHA, additives and colors. The yellow food dye tartrazine has been clearly implicated in hyperactivity problems.

2. **Reduce sugar intake and all junk or fast foods.** Children with ADD have sensitivities to food chemicals and sugars which worsen their symptoms. The Journal of Pediatric Research reveals children with ADHD are less able to compensate for the stressful effects sugar has on the brain than other children. Use stevia instead of sugar to sweeten drinks or baked foods A diet high in trans fats and saturated fats is another known brain offender. Reduce carbonated drinks (excess phosphorus). Eliminate red meats (nitrates).

3. **Make sure the healing diet is high in vegetable proteins** (beans, soy foods, nuts and seeds), and whole grains, with plenty of fresh fruits and vegetables… organically grown if possible. Have a green salad every day.

4. **Applied kinesiology helps determine allergens** to foods like milk, wheat, corn, chocolate and citrus.

5. **Include calming tryptophan-rich foods** like turkey, tuna, wheat germ, yogurt and eggs. Add lecithin granules to whole grain cereal or yogurt for brain boosting phosphatides.

6. **Add EFA-rich foods:** sea greens, spinach and other leafy greens, soy foods, fish and seafoods. Consider NEW CHAPTER SUPERCRITICAL DHA for extra EFA support. Stay away from trans fats in fried food, baked goods and snack foods which disrupt brain function.

7. **Superfoods help.** Smoothies with additions like green superfoods such as BARLEANS GREENS or WAKUNAGA HARVEST BLEND, and LEWIS LABS high phosphatide LECITHIN and/or RED STAR NUTRITIONAL YEAST.

Choose 2 or 3 supplements to help your child rebalance without the side effects of drugs:

- **Improve behavior problems:** DMAE, 100 to 500 mg. daily in divided doses; CRYSTAL STAR® ADD-VANTAGE™ for kids or RELAX CAPS™ (adults); HERBS ETC. KIDALIN; METABOLIC RESPONSE MODIFIERS ATTENTION! gels with DMAE and phos. serine. Phosphatidylserine is used with good result by practitioners, 100 mg. daily for young children (300 mg. daily for children over 50 lbs.). Results may take up to 4 months. PLANETARY FORMULAS CALM CHILD drops as needed. Homeopathic GABA, 100 mg.; NADH 2.5 mg. daily; Rosemary tea.

- **Calming herbs:** CRYSTAL STAR® CALCIUM SOURCE™ extract in water is a rapid calmative. Valerian/Wild Lettuce extract or Catnip tea for extra calming; gotu kola or hawthorn drops for nerve stress or Taurine 500 mg. daily; CRYSTAL STAR® STRESS ARREST™ TEA (rapid); St. John's Wort extract (not if a child is on prescription drugs).

- **Enhance neurotransmitters:** Stress B-Complex; PSP MARKETING VITAL PSP PLUS (excellent results); gotu kola, or scullcap calm hyperactivity safely; Ginkgo biloba drops (older kids) 60 mg. daily also helps inner ear balance.

- **Add electrolyte minerals:** ALACER ELECTROMIX; NATURE'S PATH TRACE-LYTE minerals; Add magnesium 400 mg. and PREMIER LITHIUM .5 mg. Check the child's iron… a deficiency often results in a learning disability.

- **Correct prostaglandin imbalance with EFAs:** NEW CHAPTER SUPERCRITICAL DHA 100 (Omega-3s with DHA fatty acids); or FLORADIX UDO'S PERFECTED OIL BLEND, 1 tsp. daily; Evening Primrose oil, 500 mg.; Omega-3 flax oil; or NEUROMINS DHA 200 mg. 2x daily.

- **Homeopathic remedies help ADD:** HYLANDS CALMS AND CALMS FORTE; NATURE'S WAY RESTLESS CHILD, Camomilla.

- **Autism therapy:** Magnesium 400 mg., B-complex with extra B_6 100 mg. for nerve calm, (try UAS DDS-JUNIOR for B vitamin synthesis); Black walnut, an anti-fungal medicine (ask a practitioner for dosage); Vitamin C with bioflavs, up to 2000 mg., best in powder, ¼ tsp. every 2 hours in juice; EIDON ZINC LIQUID if high copper levels, common in autism. A gluten and casein free diet can help social behavior, cognitive skills and communication.

Bodywork for ADD kids relaxes and reduces aggressiveness

- Biofeedback treatments can reduce ADD symptoms for 85% of sufferers.
- Use full-spectrum lighting wherever possible for better mood.
- Avoid aspirin and amphetamines of all kinds if your child has any of these disorders.
- CranioSacral therapy can help if there was birth trauma or birth drug or alcohol addiction.
- Massage therapy, hypnosis and acupressure have shown some success.
- Take warm baking soda and sea salt baths.
- Use aromatherapy oils such as lavender rubbed on child's temples (highly recommended).

Maintenance Recipes for a Child's Healthy Diet

Use these recipes on an ongoing basis once the initial healing diet is producing good results.

Breakfast

Perfect Fiber Cereal

¼ cup sliced almonds	a few pinches cinnamon and cardamom powder	4 oz. dried papaya
¼ cup pumpkin seeds		2 tbsp. honey
¼ cup sunflower seeds	4 oz. pitted prunes	2 oranges, sectioned
¼ cup chopped walnuts	4 oz. dried apricots	1 banana, sliced

Preheat oven to 250°F. Toast the almonds, pumpkin seeds, sunflower seeds, walnuts in the oven. Add pinches of cinnamon and cardamom powder on top. Soak the prunes, dried apricots and dried papaya in water to cover. Add the dried fruit mix to a soup pot, and simmer over low heat to reduce liquid by half. Stir in the honey, orange sections, banana and nut mix. Serve warm or cold. Makes about 3 cups.

Nutrition per serving:	Vitamin C --------- 11 mg.	Fat ----------------- 2 g.	Magnesium ------- 22 mg.
Calories ----------- 55	Vitamin E --------- 1 IU	Cholesterol-------- 0	Potassium --------- 148 mg.
Protein ----------- 6 g.	Carbohydrates ---- 31 g.	Calcium ----------- 13 mg.	Sodium------------ 1 mg.
Vitamin A --------- 18 IU	Fiber ------------- 3 g.	Iron -------------- 1 mg.	

Piña Colada Mineral-Enzyme Smoothie

1 cup pinapple, cubed and frozen	¾ cups vanilla rice milk (or almond milk)	½ cup orange juice
1 banana, frozen	½ cup vanilla yogurt, frozen	½ tsp. vanilla extract
		3 tbsp. toasted shredded coconut

Peel and cube fruit before freezing. In a blender, mix all ingredients until smooth. Serve while frosty. Makes 2 servings.

Healing drinks

Strawberry Apple Lemonade

1½ qt. apple juice	1½ cups lemon juice	1 cup strawberries, sliced

Pour all ingredients into a large pitcher, chill and serve over ice.

Soups, salads, appetizers

Roasted Potato & Sweet Potato Sticks

2 sweet potatos, cut into sticks	2 russet potatoes, cut into sticks	2 tbsp. grapeseed oil

Preheat oven to 500°F. Oil a baking sheet. Toss potato sticks with the grapeseed oil. Place side by side, not touching on baking sheet. Bake for 10 minutes or until crispy. Season with sea salt, pepper, dulse flakes and herbal seasoning salt. Serves 4 people.

Fancy Cheese Nachos

1 lb. baked nacho chips	4 oz. kefir cheese (or low-fat	8 oz. low-fat cheddar cheese
⅓ cup plain sparkling water	cream cheese)	½ cup spinach (or chard), shredded
	8 oz. low-fat pepperjack cheese	¼ cup natural salsa

On a cookie sheet, toast the chips until crisp. In a pan over very low heat, simmer the water, kefir cheese, pepperjack cheese, cheddar cheese, spinach and salsa until cheese melts and is smooth. Spoon over toasted chips, then briefly place in the broiler to brown. Makes enough to fill a tray.

Entrées

Baby Shrimp Tostadas

8 oz. cooked salad shrimp	2 tbsp. lemon juice	1 tsp. lemon-garlic seasoning
½ ripe avocado	1 green jalapeño chile,	24 tostada chip rounds
1 tbsp. red onion, minced	minced	
3 tbsp. low-fat mayonnaise	1 tbsp. fresh cilantro, minced	

To make the topping, mix the avocado, onion, mayonnaise, lemon juice, jalapeño, cilantro, and lemon-garlic seasoning. Divide this mixture on the tostada chip rounds. Top each with the shrimp. Broil 1 minute and serve hot. Makes 24 mini tostadas.

Deep Dish Italian Pie

Like a mushroom pizza without the crust.

1 (15 oz.) jar natural pizza sauce	1 yellow onion, sliced	1 lb. mushrooms, sliced
1 small eggplant, peeled and	1 tsp. Italian herb blend	1 lb. fresh tomatoes, chopped
sliced	½ tsp. anise seed	¼ cup red wine
1½ cups grated low-fat	2 tbsp. olive oil	2 tbsp. grated parmesan cheese
mozzarella cheese	1 red bell pepper, sliced	

Prepare a 9" x 13" pan. Preheat oven to 375°F. Sauté the onion, Italian herbs and anise seed in 2 tbsp. olive oil for 5 minutes. Add the red bell pepper and mushrooms; toss until coated. Add the tomatoes and toss to coat. Spread pizza sauce to cover bottom of the pan, and cover with the eggplant slices. Cover with the mozzarella and top with the tomato/mushroom mixture. Pour on rest of pizza sauce and sprinkle with the red wine and parmesan-reggiano cheese. Bake covered for 20 minutes. Remove cover and bake for 20 more minutes. Cut in 9 big squares to serve.

Nutrition per serving:	Vitamin C 32 mg.	Fat 7 g.	Magnesium 37 mg.
Calories 160	Vitamin E 1 IU	Cholesterol 12 mg.	Potassium 464 mg.
Protein 10 g.	Carbohydrates 14 g.	Calcium 244 mg.	Sodium 330 mg.
Vitamin A 128 IU	Fiber 4 g.	Iron 2 mg.	

Hot Dog Tuna

1 (6 oz.) can white tuna	2 eggs, hardboiled and	2 tsp. yellow mustard
4 tbsp. low-fat mayonnaise	chopped	whole-grain hot dog buns
4 tsp. sweet pickle relish	2 tsp. soy sauce	alfalfa sprouts

Mix together the tuna, mayonnaise, relish, eggs, soy sauce and mustard. Spoon onto a toasted hot dog bun. Top with alfalfa sprouts. Makes 4 sandwiches.

Whole Foods Keep You Healthy

Promise yourself whole foods for your healing diet. They're the key.

First and foremost, whole foods keep you whole. Your body isn't a lot of separate parts. It's all connected. The essence of human health is body balance, establishing and maintaining whole body chemistry that resists disease and assures you energy and well-being.

Whole foods are those that come to us as nature intended, not broken down into separate "nutrients," or altered with chemicals or additives. Our bodies work best when we have whole foods to work with. Processed, refined, man-made foods make our bodies struggle to use them… and then the job is only a partial one.

Western science, and today's orthodox medicine, express diseases and health conditions in terms of different body elements. But, you are all one. Anything you do to any one part of your mind, body or spirit, affects every other part of you, too.

We are learning this same lesson about our planet, too. We have to keep the Earth healthy so she can take care of us all. It's a truth that Native Americans knew well. We are all one. The very material of our bodies comes from the Earth. Anything we do to the planet, we do to ourselves.

Almost no food we eat today comes to us as it comes from Nature

You're probably using this book because you're concerned about the health problems we face today from our diets. Our foods are refined, preserved, pasteurized, waxed, hydrogenated, canned, smoked, cured, irradiated, colored, additive-laden, chemically adulterated, even genetically altered foods. Modern processing removes many nutrients from foods. Chemically adding them back after processing doesn't make the altered food whole again. Not only are chemical additives incapable of supporting life themselves, when combined with foods, the food itself becomes chemically changed, its life-sustaining ability diminished.

Even when food values are labeled on a package, they are derived from test results of fresh, unsprayed, unprocessed produce. Further, food value measurements are outdated. They were calculated in the 1950s or earlier before the enormous amounts of pesticides agri-business uses today.

New food labeling guidelines have me very concerned

I've noticed a disturbing trend. You may have noticed it, too. Food labels may put us at the mercy of the food police with everything we eat.

Food labels were supposed to help us make better decisions about what we put in our bodies, but something else happened instead. Experts told us what we should be eating… what should be on a food label. The result is that almost every packaged food we buy today has been changed, sometimes radically, usually unfavorably, to satisfy the goals of a label so the food would sell.

In fact, we may have imbalanced the structure of our packaged foods so much to satisfy acceptable numbers on a label that our bodies no longer recognize the contents as real food with real nutrients. If we upset that natural balance too much for too long, our bodies don't know how to use the food properly.

A dramatic example:

Although we know there are good fats and bad fats, media sound bites so indoctrinated the American public to hate ALL fat that foods were redesigned so that labels could show the least possible fats. This often meant a big reduction in taste. So food manufacturers added sugars, which didn't have to register on the fat label meter, but kept some of the taste. But, consumers still didn't lose weight. Why? Raising sugar levels also raises insulin levels—the body's signal to store fat!

Then, low carb diets came along again, re-introduced after variations in the '70s and '80s. Packaged foods were redesigned again to lower carbs and fats on the label. Again, food manufacturers altered food composition to reflect what experts said should be on the label—low, or no fats, low or no sugars, no carbohydrates, and on and on, as each new diet came along, in order for them to be desirable for sale.

But, there's no doubt we're still gaining weight, and aging just as fast. And, the food we buy is tasting worse— even favorites like bottled dressings, crackers, rice and pasta mixes, just to name a few. We've lost more than taste. We're losing out on vital things for our health—essential fats, natural sugars and complex carbohydrates—things our food should be doing for us, but isn't today.

More than that, I'm convinced we're losing the connection between our food and our bodies. I believe our bodies have a synergistic relationship with the foods we eat. Mother Nature's whole foods were created for us with our best nourishment in mind, not chemically altered, fat-free or carb-free.

I've seen the phenomenon over and over again… people who found that they had to dump the "foods out of box," even packaged health foods, for their healing program to really be successful. Your body needs whole foods to heal. Whole food has essential nutrients, nutrients your body needs but can't make for itself. Our bodies don't manufacture the majority of vitamins and minerals; we must obtain them from our foods.

Are organically grown foods really better for our health?

Organically grown foods are popular and easily available today. If we look closely, Nature provides what is needed for each part of the Earth in tune with the time of year, like fruits in the summer for cooling, and root vegetables in the winter for building. It helps keep the balance around us right, reminding us that we are all part of the natural chain.

I find that a working kitchen garden can do wonders for harmony of mind and body. If you can't have a garden, eating fruits and vegetables from your own region is a wonderful way to keep a closer touch with where you are and who you are.

More than 1.2 billion pounds of pesticides (over 11 billion dollars!) are dumped yearly. 77% are used in agricultural sectors to produce our food. Pesticide by-products are even used in our water. A recent report from the Pesticide Action Network North America reveals that Americans are exposed to toxic pesticides from foods up to 70 times a day. Worse, the pesticides used today are 10 to 100 times more potent than the chemicals used just 25 years ago. Although our government has recently taken steps to reduce pesticide use by "phase out" programs, it may be too little, too late, because so many of these chemicals have already contaminated food and water supplies. Pesticides can remain in the food chain for decades. DDT, chlordane and heptachlor are found in soils more than 20 years after their use.

Over 2 million synthetic substances are known, 25,000 are added each year—more than 30,000 are produced on a commercial scale—so widespread we are unaware of them. But, they work their way into our bodies faster than they can be eliminated, and they're causing allergies in record numbers. Only a tiny fraction are ever tested for toxicity, and those that come to us from developing countries have few safeguards in place. Recent studies reveal that when *any combination of three chemicals* are taken into the body, the combined effect can be up to 5,000 times more toxic than any one by itself!

Canadian research shows that pesticide sprays encourage dangerous bacteria to grow on food crops, posing a real threat for people who eat fresh commercial produce—especially strawberries, raspberries and lettuce. Studies also link pesticides and pollutants to hormone dysfunctions, psychological disorders and birth defects. The molecular structure of many chemical carcinogens interacts with human DNA, so long term exposure can result in metabolic and genetic alteration that affects immune response.

While the use of DDT and some other harmful pollutants containing environmental hormones is illegal in America, the U.S. is still the largest producer of DDT, selling it to the rest of the world. Many food-producing countries that supply America do not support pesticide bans, so imported foods from them may still carry a toxic threat to us. Even if we ban the sprayed foods at our ports, the Earth's winds circle the globe, and all the Earth's waterways are connected, so chemical pollutants containing environmental hormones reach the entire world's food supply.

The newest statistics come from breast cancer research. The dramatic rise in breast cancer in the last decade is consistent with the increased accumulation of organo-chlorine (PCB) residues. In Long Island, for instance, women living in areas previously sprayed with DDT have one of the highest breast cancer rates in the U.S. Israel's pesticide experience offers even more dramatic evidence of the pesticide-breast cancer connection. Until twenty years ago, breast cancer rates and contamination levels of organo-chlorine pesticides in Israel were among the highest in the world. An aggressive phase-out of these pesticides has now led to a sharp reduction in contamination levels and breast cancer death rates.

Here's how the link between pesticides and breast cancer seems to work. Pesticides, like other pollutants, are stored in fatty tissue areas like breast tissue. Some, like PCB's and DDT, compromise immune function, overwork the liver and disrupt the glands like too much estrogen does. Pesticides are also full of estrogen-mimicking chemicals that affect hormone balance—a clear factor in the majority of breast cancer cases. A recent study shows up to 60% more *dichloro-diphenyl-ethylene* (DDE), DDT, and *polychlorinated biphenyls* (PCBs) in the bodies of women who have breast cancer than in those who don't. Today's older women may have higher than normal rates of breast cancer because they had greater exposure to DDT before it was banned.

Can we overcome environmental health threats? Start with the foods you eat.

It's a quandary. The healthy fruits and vegetables we're all encouraged to eat are very likely to contain *unhealthy* pesticides. (Grains have less because the milling process removes them.) *Should you stop eating fresh produce?* Of course not; fruits and vegetables clearly protect against cancer and heart disease.

Take these steps to protect yourself from chemical residues in your food.

1. **Buy organic produce whenever you can!** Organic food standards require that all foods labeled organic must be free of chemical pesticides, radiation, genetic engineering, and have no contact with sewage sludge. Recent reports find that 48% of U.S. consumers now choose organic foods as a way to protect themselves and their families against chemical overload. Studies reveal organic vegetables are higher in cancer protective antioxidants than commercially grown foods. In a study of ninety-six school children, the only child who had **no measurable pesticides** in his urine lived in a home where the family ate only organic food. Most grocery stores and markets now offer affordable organic foods to help meet the growing consumer demand.

2. **Buy seasonal, local produce whenever you can.** Avoid imported produce as much as possible. Other countries have different (usually less stringent) pesticide regulations; their produce typically contains higher levels of pesticides than locally grown. Developing countries have almost no regulations. Mexico has only recently begun phasing out DDT and chlordane—banned in the U.S. for decades. Imported produce also carries the threat of dangerous microbes, like those found in Guatemalan and Mexican strawberries in 1997.

3. **Eat fruits and vegetables that have low PCB residues**—like avocados, onions, broccoli, bananas, cauliflower, sweet potatoes, corn and watermelon. A variety of fresh foods keeps your exposure to any one pesticide low. **Wash your produce,** especially high residue foods—like strawberries, cherries, spinach, bell peppers, cucumbers and grapes.

4. **Be aware of high risk seafood.** America's coasts are in crisis. The ecosystem of our planet has been drastically upset by overfishing and by incredible amounts of waste dumped into our waters. More than one-third of U.S. shellfish beds are closed due to contamination from industrial chemicals like PCBs and methyl mercury. *Should you stop eating seafood?* Of course not. Fish, seafoods and sea greens are some of the healthiest foods our planet offers. Fish like salmon and tuna are loaded with Omega-3 fatty acids that clearly decrease our risk of heart disease and cancer. Fresh seafoods are still real, whole foods, far less affected by irradiation, genetic engineering, pesticide dumping, hormone and antibiotic loading that rob foods of their nutrients and add to toxic overload. Sea greens like nori, wakame and dulse are some of the few non-animal sources of B-12, needed for cell development and nerve function. They are rich in natural iodine to strengthen poor thyroid function (at the root of many energy and weight problems). Two tablespoons a day of dried sea greens in rice, soups or salads are enough to noticeably increase metabolism and energy.

Some seafoods are not safe to eat. At this writing, striped bass, rock cod, ocean perch, catfish, walleye, shark, caviar, lake trout, langoustinos and Maine lobster may contain high residues of DDT, chlordane, dioxin and PCBs. High mercury levels in tuna, shark and swordfish from Connecticut are not safe for pregnant women or young children. Farm-raised fish are more likely to have contaminants and may also be genetically engineered.

Wild seafood from uncontaminated waters remains the best choice. *At this printing, safe seafoods are* wild salmon, fresh tuna, halibut, Dungeness crab, shrimp, red snapper, and shellfish from uncontaminated waters.

5.   Be extra careful about your water supply. Over 100 million people in the U.S. get their drinking water from groundwater, and only half of that water is disinfected before it reaches their homes. The fact is toxic chemicals contaminate groundwater supplies on every continent! Experts say up to 50% of the U.S. water supply is contaminated with giardia, which unlike bacteria, is not killed by chlorination. Giardia waterborne bacteria sickened 300,000 people and killed more than 100 in Milwaukee in 1993. Twenty-two American cities in 1996 were served by public water systems that violated minimum safety levels for contaminants.

There are new concerns about pharmaceutical drugs polluting our water supply. Here's the problem: drugs are passed through normal body urination. Water treatment plants receive some of these wastes, but are not equipped to remove them. Hormones, caffeine, antidepressants and painkillers are all found in rivers that receive water from treatment plants. Though science has yet to determine how drug pollutants affect our health, preliminary results show clear hormone disruption in both animals and humans who live near the contaminated waters!

Should you stop drinking water? Of course not. Water is critical to your very existence. Make sure your water is as clean as possible. Drink bottled water or invest in a purification system. Reverse osmosis systems are expensive (about $1,000), but they are the best at eliminating impurities. Carafes and pitchers are much cheaper (about $25). They remove some organic pollutants and lead. Investigate your drinking water quality. Ask your water utility for its contamination review.

6.   Avoid environmental estrogens and androgens coming in from pesticide-laden foods, polluted water and personal care products. Environmental hormones critically affect your vital endocrine system of glands, hormones and cellular receptors. Nearly 40% of agriculture pesticides contain hormone-like substances, suspected endocrine disrupters that spell disaster for our health. Only in the last five years has anyone realized how common environmental estrogens are in our world. People who live in high pesticide agricultural areas, who drink from polluted water supplies, who eat a high fat diet, or hormone-injected meats, or who use placenta-containing personal care products are most at risk.

Science is just beginning to accept, (though naturopaths have known for some time), that man-made estrogens may stack the deck against women by raising their estrogen levels hundreds of times over normal. Some scientists still believe there is no significant difference between man-made and natural hormones, but it seems apparent from the evidence of thousands of women, that even if a lab test can't tell the difference, their bodies can.

Women's diseases linked to chronic exposure to synthetic estrogen mimics:
• Breast and reproductive organ cancer.
• Breast and uterine fibroids, and ovarian cysts.
• Endometriosis, and pelvic inflammatory disease (PID)

Another indication of abnormally high estrogenic activity? American girls are reaching puberty at earlier and earlier ages. Nearly half of African American girls and fifteen percent of white girls start to develop sexually by age *eight*. A 2000 study links breast development in female babies *just 6 to 24 months old* to a high number of hormone-disrupting phthalates (in plastics, personal care products, and lubricants) circulating in the blood!

Women aren't the only ones endangered by estrogen-imitating effects. Substantial evidence shows that estrogens threaten male health, too, with alarming statistics relating to sperm count and hormone-driven cancers. *Environmental androgens* in chemicals (substances that mimic <u>male</u> sex hormones) are even more widespread. Research on synthetic androgens is still too new to know all the hormonal health implications, but early indications show that these substances could have involvement in the development of some cancers. One in vitro study found that out of ten pollutants, five bound to human androgen receptors while only two bound to estrogen receptors.

Men's health problems linked to exposure from environmental hormones.

- 50% average decrease in male sperm counts over the past 50 years.
- 32% rise in undescended testes, small penis size and male fertility problems.
- Dramatic rise in prostate disease, testicular cancer and male cancer deaths.

For the first time in history, large numbers of people worldwide are having trouble conceiving children. In America today, one in six married couples of child-bearing age has trouble conceiving and completing a successful pregnancy. Chemical pollutants seem to be a factor in the birth rise of female and intersex babies where males would normally be born. Humans and animals are now being born with both male and female genitalia, a frightening sign that our hormone health, and that of future generations, is in jeopardy. Other effects include birth defects, impaired immunity, diabetes, and liver damage.

6.   Finally… consider a healthy detox. A healthy detox twice a year may be a good way to rid yourself of the dangerous chemicals in your body. See pg. 14 for my "Stress Detox Diet," a proven aid for today's environmental challenges.

The pros and cons of our 21st century food supply What about genetically-engineered foods? Are they "superfoods" or a disaster in the making?

Food technology is expanding almost at the rate of the "big bang!" In the year 2004, up to 70 percent of the foods on American grocery shelves were genetically engineered to some extent (up 90% in less than a decade). GE foods are everywhere. Most of the soy, corn, potatoes, tomatoes, dairy foods and yellow squash at your local market is genetically engineered. More than one-third of U.S. farmland is now planted with genetically-engineered seeds. *All* food is expected to be genetically engineered in the next five to ten years. Today, there may be enough GE crops to cover Great Britain, Taiwan and New York's Central Park!

Are GE foods really "franken-foods?" …should you be worried?

There are benefits from genetic engineering.

- Proponents of GE foods insist that genetic engineering can boost resistance to pests, decreasing the need for harsh pesticide sprays and incidence of plant disease.
- Genetic engineering improves shelf life by altering genes which lead to spoilage.
- GE companies want to create "super crops" that will feed the Earth's exponentially growing population for generations to come. Genetic engineering is already here for animal foods. "Super salmon" now grow to 10 lbs. in only 14 months. (Still, amazingly, a recent United Nations Food and Agriculture report reveals we will be able to produce enough food to feed the world by the year 2030 *without using* genetically modified organisms.)
- GE foods offer an easy delivery route for drugs and vaccinations. Genetically modified chickens now lay drug-enriched eggs to fight some diseases. Yet, California's Department of Food and Agriculture recently denied a biotech's company's petition to grow GE pharmaceutical rice. (For people who rely on natural therapies, drug delivery through foods is not desirable.)

There's also a downside risk to GE foods… a price to pay:

1.   New allergies could increase dramatically as we add genes into foods from substances that aren't normally in our food chain. Allergens are transferred at the molecular level, and we simply won't know which GE foods will cause reactions. Reports show that soy allergies have gone up 50% since genetically engineered soy came into the food supply in 1997.

2.   Genetically engineered foods often contain DNA from widely different species. Plant, animal, insect, even bacterial or viral DNA are used to make the new "improved" foods. Using genes in GE foods from known allergens (like peanuts) can trigger severe reactions in allergic people. Eating a GE food that contains an allergen could mean life or death for an allergic person! A 1996 study in the New England Journal of Medicine revealed that soybeans spliced with a Brazil nut gene caused the same allergy reaction as eating the Brazil nut itself.

3.   Cross-pollination means pollen from GE crops will likely transfer into organic crops located nearby, so even organic foods may be exposed to genetically altered organisms. Two Canadian organic farmers have already filed class action lawsuits against GE giants Monsanto and Aventis, claiming that their genetically engineered grapeseed has spread so rapidly across Canadian prairies that organic farmers there no longer even try to grow organic canola. As of this writing (2004), Monsanto has now voluntarily withdrawn its submissions for GE wheat in Australia, Canada, Columbia, New Zealand, Russia and South Africa, due to ongoing objections.

4.   Crops genetically engineered to build resistance to herbicides might transfer into neighboring weeds creating "superweeds" which don't yield to herbicides. Further, increasing a crop's tolerance to pesticides means commercial farmers will *use more toxic pesticides and herbicides* which ultimately pollute our environment and food.

5.   Research shows bioengineering could destroy healing properties and reduce the nutrient content of foods. A study in the Journal of Medicinal Food shows that cancer-fighting phytoestrogens in genetically engineered soybeans are 14% lower than in natural soybeans.

6.   Genetic engineering means animal by-products make their way into vegetarian foods. Fish genes (which improve shelf life) are routinely added to GE tomatoes, outraging vegetarians who assumed that their fruits and vegetables were free of animal products.

7.   Genetic engineering may prompt development of "super" insects that resist normal methods of eradication and disturb the ecosystem. We already see disruptions in insect populations from GE technology. One study shows ladybugs who eat aphids that eat genetically engineered, insect-resistant potatoes live far shorter lives and produce one-third fewer eggs. California studies report monarch butterflies dying from eating GE corn pollen!

Should we slow technology until we get a better handle on health implications?

The massive genetic pollution of our population may be the ultimate price we pay for disrupting the natural balance within plant and animal species through genetic engineering.

We know some critical GE dangers already. Once a living organism is genetically modified, it can reproduce, mutate and migrate at will. Even simple human mistakes could have disastrous consequences. For example, once you alter plant DNA you run the risk of risk of causing mutations that lead to cancer. Yet only 1% of the USDA's molecular biology budget is spent on exploring the risks of genetic engineering on our foods!

The newest GE foods developed are especially worrying because they can *create their own insecticides or herbicides*! A GE food that can kill another organism may be dangerous for consumption by both animals and people. Even its ability to kill a so-called harmful plant or insect is risky. Mother Nature has many pathways to the health and survival of the Earth's species; we know only a tiny portion of how nature really works. As Native Americans have long known, we are all one. Unnaturally changing *any* species has far-reaching consequences for others.

The "Flavr Savr" tomato introduced in 1994 is an example of GE food failure. The "Flavr Savr" produced fewer yields, and the tomatoes themselves were soft, bruising very easily. Genes in the tomatoes made people who ate them resistant to the antibiotics *kanamycin* and *neomycin*. Antibiotic marker genes are used throughout the genetic engineering process today. Yet, more than 150 genetically engineered foods were approved for sale in the year 2000, virtually none of them tested for this risk. If we keep relying on these techniques, genetic engineering could cause an increase in the rates of antibiotic-resistant bacteria coming from foods.

Darwin may have been right

His theory of natural selection showed that Nature is the world's best biochemist... it constantly makes biological adjustments that protect humans and plants from changing conditions and disease strains.

Plants and animals change naturally with time to adapt to a changing environment. We know for example, that many plant species have lengthened their growing season to better use global warming. Over time, a plant may become more resistant to a disease or the effects of pollution. Tomatoes growing in polluted areas have actually become stronger, boosting their antioxidants to protect themselves from harsh conditions, in the process, becoming a more powerful medicinal food.

Yet today, we're breaking natural laws almost without thinking about the consequences… simply because we can do it. Never before in history have we so upset the boundaries between species set by Nature as we have through genetic engineering. Some foreign markets threatened to stop buying U.S. exports until they were free of GMOs (genetically modified organisms). Europe originally rejected the new "frankenfoods," but, as of this writing (2005), has ended its 6 year moratorium on biotech crops, allowing importation of GE corn for human consumption.

At this writing (2005), no FDA labels are required on GE foods. You can't be sure if the foods you buy are genetically altered. The FDA feels GE food labels will frighten consumers. The FDA says GE foods don't need labelling because they are no different than hybrids created by cross breeding. Yet hybrids are vastly different than GE foods. Hybrids result from cross breeding two or more varieties of the <u>same</u> species. But genetically engineered foods have no species boundaries. Genes from entirely different species can be used. Animal, viral and bacterial genes can all be inserted in a GE plant or animal. In reality, the FDA has no policy on how GE foods should be regulated… they are clearly *not* natural foods, and the issue is fraught with confusion!

Our best hope may be "smart breeding." Smart breeding technology allows scientists to tap into the power of gene therapy, but restricts its use to genetic engineering *within* the same species.

Surveys show that over 80% of Americans want GE foods to be labeled. (Vermont now requires the labelling of GE seeds.) Recently, Congress has introduced a bill that may force manufacturers to label GE foods to allow consumers a choice. U.S. agricultural groups now warn farmers about the consequences of genetic engineering in terms of consumer dissatisfaction and "massive lawsuit liability."

If you want GE foods labeled, write Dr. Lester Crawford, FDA Commissioner, 5600 Fishers Lane, Rockville, MD 20857.

Americans are slowly waking up to dangers of genetic engineering. What can we do to protect ourselves?

1. **Stick with organic foods, less likely to be affected by genetic tampering.** (The Organic Standards Board *does* allow *processed* organic food to contain 5% non-organic ingredients which could theoretically be genetically engineered although the vast majority of the organic food industry opposes this. Gerber baby foods has now announced they will be "GE-free.")

2. **Buy seasonal fruits and vegetables from organic local farmers when possible.** Buying in your local community helps strengthen small farmers. Always ask if genetically engineered seeds are used.

3. **Limit *non-organic* foods containing soy and corn - foods routinely genetically engineered.** Rice, beans, tomatoes, potatoes and papayas are also regularly genetically engineered.

4. **Consider organic dairy.** Most commercial dairy is injected with rBGH, a GE hormone. *Note:* Research in the 1995 Cancer Letter shows cows treated with GE hormones have higher levels of insulin growth factor, a risk for breast and prostate cancer and child leukemia.

Getting Rid of the Junk in Your Diet

The United States is the world's richest nation, yet our population is one of the most poorly nourished. Reuters Health reports junk foods like sodas, chips and desserts now make up fully one-third of the American diet! Our diet tends to make people sick instead of strong… our cancer research institutes recognize that 40 to 60% of all cancers are related to poor diet choices.

You might think that after a decade of media attention and "food police" warnings, Americans would have changed their diets and clamored for higher nutrient foods. Yet, this is simply not the case. Food products in supermarkets and most restaurants remain chemical-laced, highly-refined, enzyme depleted and nutrient deficient. Amazingly, junk foods may even be *more* highly processed than when the warnings began; irradiation practices and virulent food-borne pathogens like *E. coli* now show up regularly in fast foods.

On a good note: I've found that most restaurants are very responsive to the requests of their discriminating clientele. Many will even prepare a fresh or low-fat dish exactly to your order at no extra cost.

Think you've heard it all before?
New reasons to eliminate problem foods from your healing diet:

Fried foods:

Maybe you love them but your arteries and heart hate them. Frying temperatures range from 400°F up to 700°F. At temperatures this high, Cis fatty acids (unsaturated fatty acids) are converted to dangerous trans-fatty acids; their molecules behave like saturated fats, raising cholesterol levels and increasing heart disease risk. Cancer studies document a high incidence of colon cancer in populations where saturated fat intake is high.

Further, when fat is *reheated* at high temperatures (like in deep fryers) the fat is likely to produce carcinogens, like acrolein and benzopyrene. Burning or overcooking fats and oils contributes to the formation of free radicals, fragmented molecules that damage your cells.

Do you suffer from indigestion? Eliminate fried foods first. They cause bloating, gas and diarrhea in many people. A tasty alternative: mix bread crumbs with your favorite seasonings, coat the food, then bake for a crispy, "fried" taste without the health risks.

Trans fats (*hydrogenated oils*):

These fats are thought to be the culprits in the recent sharp rise in LDL cholesterol levels and obesity in America. Most significant, trans fats interfere with your body's ability to metabolize natural fats, and to use the good essential fatty acids (EFAs) critical to anti-aging and beauty. Trans fats are difficult to release from the body. It may take up to 2 years to rid your blood and arteries of their deposits.

As free radical producers, trans fats can cause skin aging, and raise blood cholesterol as much as saturated fat can. A University of Texas Southwestern study shows that cholesterol drops by more than 100 points when trans fats are dropped from the diet. The American Journal of Public Health says that trans fats may be responsible for up to 30,000 heart disease deaths a year in the U.S. Further, they contribute to diabetes, obesity, rheumatoid arthritis and auto-immune diseases like fibromyalgia.

A new cancer study reveals that women with breast cancer have higher levels of trans fatty acids in their bodies than women without. Breast cancer risk increases an astounding *40%* in women with high levels of trans fats!

How do you know if trans fats are part of the foods you buy? Today trans fats are part of most snack foods, pastries and desserts because they are inexpensive, and add texture and flavor. Trans fats are present in most cooking oils, too (even some you thought were healthy, like safflower oil) because they're hydrogenated to extend shelf life. Hydrogenation or partial hydrogenation makes unsaturated fats into saturated fats. Startling studies show that even butter, once thought to be the worst of saturated fats, is better for health than hydrogenated margarine.

Trans fats aren't technically categorized as saturated or polyunsaturated, or mono-unsaturated, so food labels don't disclose the amount a food contains.

Consumer concern has mandated a trans fat content line on food labels by Jan. 2006. Until then, if you see "partially hydrogenated oil" on a label, the food DOES contain trans fats. For your best health, reduce or avoid these foods right away, and skip fast food restaurants and fried foods. Use mechanically pressed oils like olive and grapeseed oils in your recipes. Oleic acid, a mono-unsaturated fatty acid in mechanically extracted (rather than solvent extracted) olive oil, for example, retains most of its nutrients even after extraction and is less prone to oxidation. Snack foods from natural foods stores are generally free of hydrogenated oils and trans fats.

White sugar:

White sugar is the most refined carbohydrate in our food supply. A little sugar goes a long way. Did you know it takes *16 feet* of sugar cane to produce *1 teaspoon* of sugar?

Sugar entered our food supply in a big way in the middle of the last century. Today, sugar qualifies as America's favorite but most poorly understood drug. The average American now consumes 150 pounds of white sugar per year. Some say we are a nation addicted to sugar.

Eating sugary foods regularly causes abnormal insulin production that results in problems like diabetes and hypoglycemia. Sugar robs your body of B-vitamins, critical minerals like magnesium and zinc, and trace minerals like chromium (effective for weight loss and blood sugar balance). Too much sugar is linked to circulatory diseases like thrombosis, chronic gum disease and severe depression. Each of these health conditions improves when sugar is eliminated from the diet. A University of Alabama study shows dramatically reduced symptoms when sugar is removed from the diet of depression patients.

You may love sugary snacks but your skin hates them. Sugar is as bad for your skin as too much sun. Because sugar can produce more advanced glycosylation end products (AGE), it's closely associated with free radical damage and premature aging. A high sugar diet reduces skin elasticity and advances collagen cross linking—a major cause of wrinkles and sagging skin! Too much sugar initiates and adds to skin inflammation, and can even cause increased brown spots and deep wrinkles!

More bad news. Sugar wipes out immunity. Drinking just one 12 oz. can of soda reduces the ability of immune white blood cells to kill germs by 40%! This effect starts less than thirty minutes after ingestion and can last for five hours. Sugar can also trigger painful inflammation in cases of arthritis and fibromyalgia. So, watch out for sugar; it's a hidden ingredient in most processed foods.

White flour:

White flour is the most common carbohydrate in the U.S. In the 19th century, when microscopes revealed bacteria on grain, white flour became the baker's standard. It didn't spoil quickly, so was thought safer than whole grains. But white flour's long shelf life is a result of stripped nutrients; at least 22 nutrients are lost in its milling. Only *four* are replaced when the flour is "enriched." White bread lacks copper, B vitamins and zinc, and has 75% *less* fiber than 100% whole wheat. Many of us remember our grammar school days when we mixed white flour with water to form paste. White flour sticks to everything, including your intestines!

Carbohydrates are quick energy sources. Once metabolized, they supply your body with glucose for energy and brain work. Complex carbs from beans and whole grains, vegetables, fruit and nuts are generally considered to be healthful. But problems can result from eating too many carbohydrates of any kind. *Excess carbohydrates are stored in your body as fat.* Excess carbohydrates cause blood sugar levels to rise triggering insulin release from the pancreas. The insulin removes excess glucose from the blood to be stored as glycogen, and then as fat, leading the way to obesity.

Additives and preservatives:

Most of us have no idea know what we're really eating when we buy foods with additives and preservatives. We certainly can't decode the long chemical chain names. But most of our foods have them to prevent spoilage and boost looks and flavor, even in foods we might think are fresh. Many of them are not innocent, inactive ingredients. In fact, they are often harmful, taxing our immune systems and triggering hyperactive responses in children. Tests on chemical preservatives used in pet food for example, have been blamed for cancer, kidney disease, pancreatic disease, allergies, hair loss, blindness and immuno-deficiency—to name a few!

I believe we could stop using many, if not most, synthetic chemical additives. There are effective, harmless natural food preservers, which even enhance nutrition. Vitamin C for instance, is a frequently added preservative to prevent the "turning" of canned fruits or fruit juices. Vinegar, salt and wood smoke have a long history of safety when used in moderation. Vitamin E tocopherols, and rosemary extract are effective antioxidant preservers.

Beware of these food additives and preservatives...

- *Monosodium glutamate (MSG):* used to enhance the flavor of Chinese food, chips, processed meats and packet soups, causes broad allergic responses in many people. Its powerful "excitotoxins" are implicated in destroying brain and nervous system tissue. Avoid it to reduce the risk of Alzheimer's or Parkinson's disease. I advise pregnant women to avoid MSG as well.
- *Yellow Tartrazine (E102):* a widely used food coloring linked to hyperactive problems in children. If your child has ADD or ADHD, eliminate yellow tartrazine, other colorings, and all additives and preservatives from the child's diet. Most parents see improvement within a month if E102 is part of the behavior problem.

- **Nitrates and nitrites:** often added to processed meats (especially bacon, sausage and ham), and to dried fruits as color preservers. Both nitrates and nitrites convert to potentially carcinogenic nitrosamines linked to many types of cancer and thyroid problems. Choose organic meats and produce to stay clear of nitrates and nitrites.
- **Sulphur dioxide and sulfites:** used to kill sugar fermentation yeasts in food and alcoholic beverages. People with severe asthma should avoid wines, beer, soft drinks and restaurant foods that contain sulfites. Today the scare of anaphylactic shock and wide attention on salad bars that once used sulfites have reduced these chemicals.
- **Mineral hydrocarbons:** the U.S. Agriculture Dept. has advised manufacturers not to use these health hazards as non-stick additives on dried fruit. They are <u>still</u> used in non-stick sprays for baking (check labels). Mineral hydrocarbons accumulate in the lymphatic system, our body's chief detoxifier and blood waste cleanser, putting unneeded stress on your body's immune system.
- **Artificial sweeteners:** they replace sugar in sugar-free snacks, toothpaste, gum and diabetic products, but they can create even more health problems than refined sugar, and they aggravate sugar-related diseases like diabetes and hypoglycemia. Sorbitol may cause cramping and diarrhea symptoms for sensitive people. If you (or your child) are sugar sensitive, check labels for dextrose, lactose, maltose or saccharin. Synthetic sweeteners, like Nutrasweet and Equal, developed from powerful chemicals like aspartame, are everywhere. See pg. 49 for more information on the dangers of artificial sweeteners.

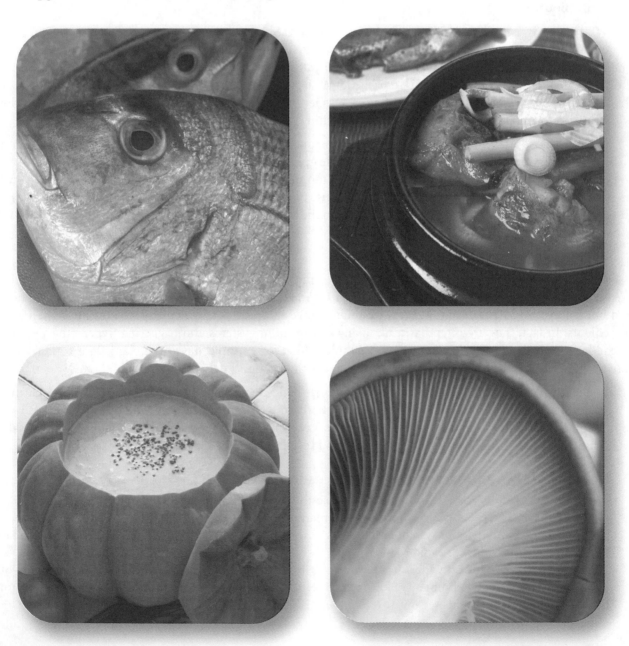

Is Your Microwave Your Cook?

Over 90% of American homes use microwave ovens for meal preparation. But microwave ovens have always posed safety questions. Original owners were even told to stand at least four feet away during use, and not to watch the food while it was cooking. New research shows that even microwave packaging is questionable for health. Testing for migration of packaging chemicals into food was only done up to 300°F. But microwave temperatures reach up to 500°F. At this high temperature microwave packaging chemicals become unstable and leach into food within 3 minutes of cooking. Uneven heating from microwaving may also release synthetic estrogens from certain plastics into the food. Further, many microwave packages contain a "heat susceptor," a piece of metallized plastic that gets hot and fries the surface of the food to crisp or brown it.

But the biggest problem with microwaving food is that it destroys enzymes.

Enzyme protection and the body's ability to use enzymes as therapy, are dramatically affected by a microwave. Enzymes are extremely sensitive to heat. Heat above 120°F. destroys them. Tests confirm that foods lose 10 percent of vitamins E and A after six minutes in a microwave; after twelve minutes they lose 40%. B-12, Vitamin C, essential minerals and fats all show less bioavailability in microwaved foods. Some experts say that if we microwaved all our food, we couldn't live.

Microwaving breast milk depletes critical immune-forming antibodies and enzymes that have an impact on a baby's proper development. A Lancet (1989) report says that microwaving infant formulas converts L-proline, a biologically active amino acid, to its d-isomer, toxic to the kidneys and nervous system.

Has the Scientific Community Responded to Concerns about Microwaves?

Swiss research shows eating microwaved food significantly decreases blood hemoglobin levels, increases leukocytes (white blood cells which can be indicative of poisoning or cell damage), alters protein molecules, and increases LDL "bad" cholesterol relative to HDL "good" cholesterol. The study authors were sued for "interfering with commerce" and a gag order prohibited them from publishing their study results. In 1992, the European Court of Human Rights ruled that the "gag order" was a violation of the scientists' right to freedom of expression, and Switzerland was ordered to pay compensation.

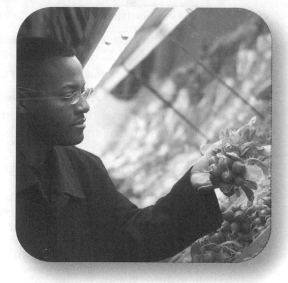

Questions still remain about microwaves. I don't microwave foods because I believe it undermines their healing properties and deadens food's natural flavors. Kinesiologists say many people show increased sensitivity to microwaved foods. From an energetic perspective, the technically derived energy from microwaves is unnaturally passed on to man when he eats microwaved foods (demonstrated in tests on microwaved foods and bacteria from test subjects.) Since our bodies are electrochemical by nature, the long term effects could be problematic.

Low blood pressure and slow pulse may be early signs of microwave overload. Later signs may include nervous system stress, headaches, eye pain, dizziness, insomnia, reproductive problems, adrenal exhaustion and heart disease. Still, very little credible modern research is available on microwaving's health effects.

If you are on a healing diet, or sensitive to chemically altered food, consider a conventional oven and include a wide variety of raw foods like fruits and vegetables to maximize your body's healing enzyme potential.

- Put foods from microwave packages into covered glass or ceramic.
- Make sure plastic wrap doesn't come in contact with food.
- Use plastic containers to store foods only, not to heat them.

Cooking Tips and Secrets
Wise ways to get healing benefits/optimum nutrition from your diet.

Sometimes it isn't just what you eat... the way you cook it can mean success for a healing diet.

Healthy Techniques with Vegetables:

...When steaming vegetables, always have water boiling first. Add 1 tsp. miso paste, or a few liquid smoke drops to the water for an outdoor grill taste if desired, then add the veggies.

...For crunchiness, color and flavor, lightly parboil vegetables in seasoned water or a light broth. Simmer liquid first, add veggies, then simmer just until color changes. Scoop veggies out quickly with a slotted spoon. Run them under cold water to set color. Then chill for a salad, or toss quickly in a hot pan with a little butter, broth or soy sauce. Squeeze on a little lemon juice over for tang. (Save cooking liquid for use in the recipe.)

...Concentrate flavors of zucchini, tomatoes and eggplant by sprinkling with sesame salt or herb salt. Let sit in a colander over the sink for 10 to 15 minutes, then press out moisture. It makes a real difference in both the tenderness and the sweetness of the vegetables.

...Dry salad greens thoroughly after washing by rolling them in paper towels, or by using a salad spinner. The greens will be crisper, and need less dressing for taste.

...Invest in a food processor. It makes your salad ingredients look and taste elegant. Today these appliances are smaller, easy to clean, and encourage you to have a salad every day.

...When stir-fry-steaming, heat the wok first; then add oil, and heat until it's very hot. Then add veggies and stir-fry fast to seal in nutrients. Turn heat to low, add sauce, cover, and steam until sauce bubbles.

...Are you juicing carrots and apples in your healing diet? Use the carrot and apple pulp from juicing in place of grated apples or carrots in baked recipes, like muffins or quick breads. You can even use the pulps in place of all or part of the sugar or honey in other baked dishes.

...Some foods release more of their nutrients when lightly cooked: Lightly steaming carrots releases bio-available carotenes (cancer preventing substances) better. Simmering tomatoes enhances lycopene activity, a cancer protective. Heating spinach leaves until just wilted improves its carotene assimilation.

Healthy Techniques for Eggs:

Note: Nutrition experts have now determined that people on a low fat diet can still eat 1 – 2 eggs daily will no ill effect. Eggs are a whole food with lecithin and phosphatides to balance out their cholesterol content.

...The secret for lightness in soufflés, dumplings, crepes, and omelets is simply gentleness. Work with a light hand when you work with eggs - no vigorous stirring or beating.

...When beating eggs to "stiff but not dry," always add a pinch of cream of tartar powder to maintain lightness and puff.

...Poach eggs in miso, chicken broth or bouillon instead of water for best flavor and to maintain shape.

Healthy Techniques with Fish:

...The two secrets to moist, tender, delicious fish are freshness and timing. Whether you broil, bake, sauté or grill it, the moment your fish turns from its natural translucent white or pink, to opaque white (like egg whites), it is done. Remove it from the heat immediately. *Even a little overcooking toughens and dries out the meat.*

...Seafood is an investment. Pay attention to it; learn to gauge its thickness correctly; test it for doneness. When you're cooking with fish, the rest of the meal should already be together. Once you put fish on to cook, it needs your undivided attention for the few minutes it takes to come to perfection.

- Use the professional 10 minute rule for best results: cook 10 minutes for each inch of thickness.
- To bake fish in foil, parchment, or simmer in sauce, 15 minutes per inch of thickness is about right.
- Bake, steam, broil or grill fish for the best health benefits. Never fry! For thick cuts, sear on a hot grill first to seal in juices, then barbecue. Cook it less and leave the meat firmer and fresher.
- Is it done? Lightly poke the fish with your finger, if it springs back it's done; or cut into the thickest part of the fish, if it is just opaque, it is just right. If it flakes easily, it is overcooked. Older recipes recommend flaking as the proper doneness point, but today's chefs know that the best flavor and texture have already gone by then.

Healthy Techniques with Poultry:

…Have poultry at room temperature before cooking. Pat meat dry.

…Oven-roast poultry bones and carcasses to enhance flavor richness. Then freeze in plastic bags to use for making homemade broth.

…When baking stuffings or cornbread separately for a roast turkey or chicken dinner, use a cast iron skillet for increased flavor and texture.

Healthy Techniques with Pasta:

…Mushy, or tough pasta can ruin a meal. Attention is the key once pasta cooking has started. Make the pasta sauce first if possible. Just keep it warm until pasta is ready.

…Use a very large pot; probably the largest one you have. Use a lot of water, so pasta can swim and separate when cooking. The more water, the less gummy the pasta. Add 1 tbsp. olive oil or grapeseed oil so water won't boil over and pasta strands will separate after cooking. Bring water to a rolling boil. Add 1 tsp. sea salt to lift pasta flavor. Your sauce should be ready before you add the pasta to the water.
- Add pasta in batches to the water slowly, so water doesn't stop boiling. Stir after each batch to keep pasta separated. Keep the water at a fast boil, covering it briefly to insure continuous boiling.
- Fresh pasta cooks fast, in 2 to 6 minutes. Watch closely. Start testing for doneness in 2 – 3 minutes. Dry pasta cooks in 8 – 20 minutes, depending on its size and shape. Start testing for doneness in 6 – 7 minutes. Remove a piece with a fork and bite it. If it isn't hard, and it isn't mushy, it's al dente (*to the tooth*) and it's done.
- Drain immediately, adding a little cold water to the pot first to stop the cooking. Draining into a colander is the easiest way. Do not rinse unless pasta is to be used for a cold salad.
- Add sauce right away and serve. If sauce can't be added right away, toss with a little oil. (To re-heat pasta before saucing, put it in a bowl of hot water, and stir to let pieces gently separate.)

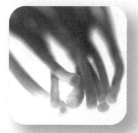 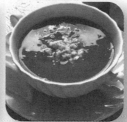 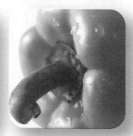 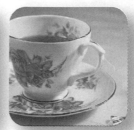 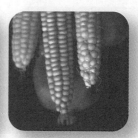

The Healthy Way to Use Oils:

Never fry when you are on a healing program.

…Use only vegetable, nut or seed oils, mechanically, expeller, or cold-pressed.

…Use oils for quick sautées, salad dressings, and as a replacement for butter in baking and sauces.

…Don't re-use cooking oils that have been heated. Store all cooking oils in the refrigerator after they have been opened. Don't use oils past their expiration date and check for rancidity by smelling before using.

Healthy Crusts, Toppings, and Coatings:

Crusts, toppings, sprinkles and coatings are an important part of a recipe. The foundation should be as healthy as the filling. A quiche, pie, or casserole is a layered dish, to be built from the bottom up.

Low-fat, thin crusts for pizzas, quiches, and vegetable tarts:

- Crushed, whole grain cracker crumbs, either plain, or sprinkled with a little low oil dressing or tamari. Bake until crispy—about 10 minutes at 375°F—then fill.
- Split chapatis or pita bread halves horizontally, or use whole wheat or corn tortillas. Toast briefly for crispiness; lay on the bottom of your baking dish and top with filling.
- Thin-slice tofu blocks horizontally. Bake with a little oil at 350°F for firmness before filling.
- Spread crispy Chinese noodles on the bottom of the baking dish. Toast in the oven; then fill.
- Sprinkle toasted nuts and seeds to cover bottom of the baking dish. Add seasoning salt and fill.
- Spread cooked brown rice to cover the bottom and sides of a lecithin-sprayed baking dish. Toast at 375° to crisp and dry slightly, then fill.
- For the ultimate easy crust, use any cooked whole grain or vegetable leftovers—whirl in the blender to a paste. Press into a lecithin-sprayed baking dish, crisp in a 400°F oven for 10 minutes, and voila! You have an original, easy crust for a new quiche, casserole, or savory pie.

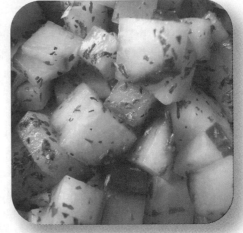

Low-fat crusts for dessert pies, tarts and custards:

Note: Whole grains produce a lighter, nutty pastry.
- Toast wheat germ in the oven. Mix with a little maple syrup or honey to sweeten, and spread on bottom and sides of baking dish. Toast again briefly and fill.
- Toast some nuts and seeds. Sprinkle with a little maple syrup or honey to sweeten. Spread on the bottom and sides of baking dish. Toast again for extra crunchiness.
- Use juice-sweetened, sugarless cookie crumbs. Press onto bottom and sides of baking dish. Toast briefly and fill.
- Sprinkle date sugar (ground up dates), or maple syrup granules, or maple sugar to completely cover bottom of a custard or dessert dish. Broil briefly to caramelize; then fill and bake as usual. Yum.

Casserole foundations—a unique cooking art:

Avoid the calories and density of a crust with a casserole foundation. Quiches and casseroles become new dishes, but still give a favorite filling something good to rest on. Cover the bottom of the baking dish with any of the following:
- Hard boiled eggs;
- Left over cooked brown rice or other whole grain;
- Spaghetti squash, cooked and briefly toasted;
- Zucchini or tomato rounds.

For both bottoms and toppings:
- Chinese-noodles, toasted;
- Whole grain granola, toasted;
- Whole grain chips, crushed slightly and toasted.

Healthy low-fat, low salt coatings for seafood, poultry and veggies:
Mix any of the following with yogurt, or egg and water; coat food and chill briefly before baking.
- Toasted wheat germ;
- Crushed whole grain chips;
- Falafel or tofu burger mix.

Looking for a healthier sugar substitute?

Just because you follow a refined-sugar-free diet doesn't mean you have to give up good taste or sweet comforts. In moderation, your body easily metabolizes whole food sugars like honey, molasses, maple syrup, fruit juice or barley malt which can satisfy your sweet tooth. Clinical tests on the herbs stevia, luohan fruit and gymnema sylvestre, are good news for sugar disorders. These natural sweeteners are heros in the effort to control sugar balance and sugar cravings. But they do not eliminate hypoglycemia or diabetes. Only a better diet and regular exercise can make a permanent difference.

Note: In your healthy sweetener quest, always look for the least processed sweetener. Most commercial sweeteners bear no resemblance to their natural counterpart. For example, before cane sugar (the worst culprit), is refined and bleached, it is rich in vitamins and minerals.

Sweet choices to consider for your healing diet:

1. **Fructose** is a commercial sugar with the same molecular structure as that in fruit. It's called fruit sugar, but it's usually made from corn starch. It has a low glycemic index, releasing its glucose into the bloodstream slowly. Fructose produces liver glycogen rapidly making it a more efficient energy supply than other sweeteners. It is almost twice as sweet as white sugar, so less is needed for the same sweetening power.

Fructose may be the sweetener of choice in a weight loss diet. In clinical tests, people who drank liquids sweetened with fructose before meals ate 20 to 40% fewer calories than normal, more than compensating for the 200 calories in the fructose. Those who drank liquids sweetened with table sugar ate 10 to 15% fewer calories; those who drank liquids sweetened with NutraSweet, Equal or aspartame (chemical sweeteners widely used in drinks and snack foods), ate the same calories as normal. Fructose also helps people pick foods with less fats, too. Dental health studies report less plaque and tarter with fructose than with sugar.

Does it have the same drawbacks as sucrose? Fructose chemical structure has highly reactive molecules which bind to protein molecules, sometimes altering the structure of critical enzymes and their proteins. This protein-fructose interaction may cause organ damage if you have diabetes. Fructose labeling can be a problem, too. Fructose products can be pure fructose, or 90% fructose, or high fructose corn syrup (55% fructose has a high percentage of glucose requiring insulin for metabolism). Fructose also inhibits copper absorption, essential to hemoglobin production. Studies in Israel reveal that rats fed a high fructose diet age faster and show deteriorating collagen changes like premature skin wrinkling. Bottom line? There are some advantages to fructose used in moderation, but if you are hypoglycemic or diabetic, fructose is still sugar and should be avoided.

1. **Stevia rebaudiana** (sweet herb), has been used as a natural sweetener in South America for over 1500 years. It is non-caloric, and about 25 times sweeter than sugar when made as an infusion with 1 tsp. leaves to 1 cup of water. Two drops of the infusion equal 1 tsp. of sugar in sweetness. In baking, 1 tsp. finely ground stevia powder equals 1 cup of sugar. If you decide to use stevia (I recommend it), experiment with it. Adding too much stevia to meals can produce a licorice-like after taste; adding too little won't sweeten adequately.

Tests show stevia helps regulate blood sugar. In South America, stevia is sold as a health aid to people with diabetes and hypoglycemia, because it helps lower high blood pressure but does not affect normal blood pressure. Stevia users say it inhibits tooth decay, aids mental alertness, counteracts fatigue and improves digestion. Most stevia users say they have less desire for tobacco and alcohol.

Clinical studies show it to be safe even in cases of severe sugar imbalance. In the 1970s, the Japanese refined the glycosides from stevia to make a product called Stevioside, 300 times sweeter than sugar. Stevioside is widely used—it enjoys a 42% share of the food sweetener market in Asia and South America. Still, stevioside does not retain the extraordinary healing benefits of whole stevia leaves and extract.

Stevia is effective for weight control because it contains no calories, yet significantly increases glucose tolerance. Stevia may block fat absorption, too. People whose weight loss problems stem from sugar cravings benefit most from stevia. They experience reduced desire for sugary foods.

Today, stevia is sold on the market as a dietary supplement after a decade-long FDA ban, heavily influenced by Nutrasweet politics.

3.   **Luohan fruit**, found largely in southern China, is a low glycemic, non-caloric sweetener 20 times sweeter than sugar. Luohan has been used for centuries in Traditional Chinese Medicine (TCM) to help treat coughs, colds, bronchitis, constipation, even diabetes. According to TCM, luohan promotes the proper flow of energy (Qi), and has a harmonizing, balancing effect on the spleen and stomach. It is rich in minerals (esp. zinc and selenium), essential fatty acids and amino acids. In addition, luohan promotes fat burning, does not affect blood sugar adversely, and is safe for diabetics and hypoglycemics. In America, the whole fruit is available in Asian food stores. Most people use convenient luohan concentrates. I've tried—and like—TRIMEDICA'S SLIM SWEET.

4.   **Date sugar** is ground, dried dates. It is the least refined, most natural sweetener. It has the same nutrient values as dried dates—about half as sweet as sugar. Use like brown sugar. In baking, mix with water before adding to the recipe to prevent burning, or add as a sweet topping after removing your dish from the oven.

5.   **Gymnema sylvestre** is an herb that curbs cravings for sweet foods and reduces blood sugar levels after sugar consumption. Gymnema's molecular structure, similar to that of sugar, can block absorption of up to 50% of sugar calories. Both sugar and gymnema are digested in the small intestine, but the larger molecule of gymnema cannot be fully absorbed. So, taken before sugar, the gymnema molecule blocks the passages through which sugar is normally absorbed.... far fewer sugar calories get assimilated. If you eat a 400 calorie, sugary dessert, only 200 of the sugar calories are absorbed. The remaining sugar is eliminated as waste.

…Take the gymnema taste test. Taste something sweet, then swish a sip of gymnema sylvestre tea in your mouth. Now taste something sweet again. You will not be able to taste the sugar, because gymnemic acid prevents the taste buds in your mouth from being activated by sugar molecules in the food. Gymnema blocks the taste of the sugar in your mouth in the same way it blocks sugar in digestion.

Gymnema has obvious uses for diabetes. It helps lower glucose significantly for diabetics, and may help lower their cholesterol and triglycerides. Studies show gymnema can actually enhance endogenous insulin production in both Type I and Type II diabetics to regenerate pancreatic cells. In fact, gymnema is regularly recommended to help control diabetes in India. Take with GTF Chromium for best results.

6.   **FOS (Fructo-oligo-saccharides)** are compounds found in foods like bananas, onions, garlic, artichokes, barley, tomatoes, rye, honey, and asparagus. They're only half as sweet as sugar. FOS are not digested in the stomach, passing untouched into the large intestine where friendly intestinal flora consume them as food. More significant, the by-products of FOS are healthy EFAs. FOS do not affect DNA nor promote cancer.

The advantages of FOS:
…FOS feed beneficial bacteria, while starving harmful bacteria
…FOS relieve constipation
…FOS stop antibiotic-induced yeast
…FOS lower cholesterol and triglyceride levels
…FOS inhibit formation of cavities
…FOS lower blood sugar levels in diabetics

Note: Use FOS as a partial replacement for sugar in recipes. Too much (more than 40 grams) can cause loose stools, since FOS are not digested. Use FOS as a nutritional enhancement. Try UAS DDS-PLUS WITH FOS.

7.   **Blackstrap molasses** is the liquid sludge left over after sucrose is extracted from cane sugar during the refining process. Rich in minerals and vitamins, molasses has more calcium, ounce for ounce, than milk, more iron than eggs, and more potassium than any other food. The amounts of B vitamins, pantothenic acid, iron, inositol and vitamin E make it an effective treatment for restoring thin and fading hair.

8.   **Barley malt and brown rice syrups** are mild, natural sweeteners made from barley sprouts, or cultured rice and water cooked to a syrup. Only 40% as sweet as sugar, barley malt's blood sugar activity is a slow, complex carbohydrate release that does not upset insulin levels. Amazake is a pudding-like sweetener made from organic brown rice. The rice is cooked, then injected with koji, the Aspergillus enzyme culture used in miso and shoyu. Amazake is 21% sugar, mainly glucose and maltose, and is high in B complex and iron.

9. **Corn syrup** is commercial glucose made from chemically purified cornstarch with everything removed except the starch. Most corn syrup has sugar syrup added to it because glucose is only half as sweet as white sugar. It is highly refined and absorbed into the bloodstream very quickly.

10. **Fruit juice concentrate** is a highly processed product with about 68% soluble sugar. It contains measurable vitamins and minerals, and promotes slower digestion. Refined sugars raise serotonin levels in the brain, which can make you feel drowsy. Unrefined fruit sweeteners have less impact on brain chemistry because natural fruit sugars do not affect serotonin levels.

11. **Honey** is a mixture of sugars formed from nectar in the bodies of bees. A natural sweetener with bioactive, antibiotic and antiseptic properties, honey contains all the vitamins, minerals and enzymes necessary for proper metabolism and digestion of glucose and other sugars. Still, honey is almost twice as sweet as white sugar. Avoid it if you have candidiasis or diabetes; use it with great care if you are hypoglycemic.

12. **Maple syrup** is made from sugar maple tree sap. It takes 30 – 40 gallons of sap to make one gallon of syrup. Unless labeled pure maple syrup, it may be mixed with corn syrup or other additives to cut its cost. Maple sugar is crystallized maple syrup.

13. **Sucanat,** (an acronym from sugar cane natural) is the trade name for a sweetener made from dried granulated cane juice, available in health food stores. Its average sugar content is 85%, with complex sugars, vitamins, minerals, amino acids and molasses retained. Use 1 – 1 in place of sugar. It is still a concentrated sweetener; use carefully if you have sugar balance problems.

14. **Turbinado sugar** is raw sugar refined by washing in a centrifuge so that surface molasses is removed. It goes through the same refining process as white sugar, just short of the final extraction of molasses, and is essentially the same as white sugar.

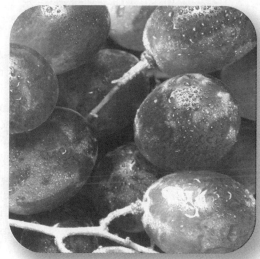

15. **Xylitol**, a sweetener derived from plums, birchwood chips, strawberries, and corn which is safe for diabetics and hypoglycemics. Just as sweet as table sugar but with ⅓ fewer calories, Xylitol works well to sweeten cereals and hot drinks, but doesn't work well for baking. Apart from its sweetening ability, Xylitol is becoming well known today for its role in fighting infections, tooth decay, and sinusitis (esp. in a nasal spray). It can cause diarrhea in susceptible people; Use Xylitol sparingly until you become used to it.

The following chart helps you convert your favorite recipes from sugar to natural sweeteners. If you have serious blood sugar problems, like diabetes or hypoglycemia, consult the appropriate diet pages in this book and your healing professional, about the kind and amount of sweets your body can handle.

Sweetener substitution amounts are for each cup of sugar:

Substitute Sweetener	Amount	Reduce Liquid in Recipe
Fructose	⅓ to ⅔ cup	....
Maple Syrup	⅓ to ⅔ cup	¼ cup
Honey	½ cup	¼ cup
Molasses	½ cup	¼ cup
Barley or Rice Syrup	1 to 1¼ cups	¼ cup
Date Sugar	1 cup	....
Sucanat	1 cup	....
Apple/Pear Juice	1 cup	¼ cup
Xylitol	1 cup	....
Stevia	2 tbsp. leaf powder	....

Need a healthy replacement for dairy foods?

Are dairy foods OK if you're <u>not</u> on a cleansing or healing diet? The answer: a little is fine—a lot is not. Most dairy products are great for taste, but questionable for optimum nutrition and highly mucous-forming. But don't despair… rich quality can be achieved without dairy. Small changes in your cooking habits and point of view are all it takes… it's mostly a matter of not having these foods around the house, and substituting dairy-free alternatives in your favorite recipes. Soon you won't feel deprived at all; and if you're like most people, you'll be delighted at the easy weight you'll lose by avoiding dairy fats.

Rice substitutes:

- **Rice Milk:** Made of brown rice, brown rice syrup, grapeseed oil, seasonings and sea greens, rice milk is my personal favorite as a dairy substitute. The taste is delicious, it's full of nutrition and it works beautifully in recipes (Use plain flavor in savory recipes, vanilla flavor in sweet dishes.)
- **Amazake Rice Drink:** a macrobiotic favorite widely available in health food stores, amazake may also be used cup for cup as a milk substitute in recipes. Simply blend ½ cup amazake with 2 cups water in a blender.
- **Rice Cheese:** Made from rice milk, rice cheese is a mild, delicious cheese replacement. With a small amount of casein, it is meltable for cooked dishes.
- **Rice Dream Frozen Dessert:** now in several flavors, sweeter with a better texture than frozen soy desserts.

Yogurt and kefir substitutes:

- **Yogurt:** smooth and creamy, yogurt is a good intestinal cleanser, beneficial for health. To use cup for cup as a replacement for milk in recipes: mix ½ cup plain yogurt with ½ cup broth, white wine, water or sparkling water for lightness. For baking, where richness is needed (like a cheesecake), or for whipped cream consistency, whip <u>one-third</u> the amount of heavy cream called for in the recipe, then fold in the remaining two-thirds with non-fat plain yogurt.
- **Yogurt Cheese, cream cheese style:** much lighter in fat and calories than sour cream or cream cheese, but with the same richness and consistency.
  …How to make it: Use a piece of cheesecloth or a sieve-like plastic funnel, (available from kitchen catalogs or hardware stores). Spoon in as much plain yogurt as you want, usually use about 16 oz. Hang the cheesecloth over the sink faucet (put the funnel over a large glass). It takes about 14 – 16 hours for the whey to drain out. Voila! you have yogurt cheese. (Use the whey as a delicious part of the liquid in soups and stews). Stored in a covered container in the refrigerator, it will keep for 2 – 3 weeks.
- **Yogurt Cheese, block cheese style:** available in health food and gourmet stores. A dairy food with yogurt, acidophilus cultures and enzymes added, yogurt cheese is a block cheese in the semi-soft Farmer cheese style.
- **Yogurt Sour Cream:** for 1 cup: mix ½ cup low-fat mayonnaise and ½ cup low-fat plain yogurt.
- **Kefir:** a cultured food made by adding kefir grains (naturally formed milk proteins), to milk and letting it incubate to milkshake consistency. Kefir has 350 mg. of calcium per cup. Use plain kefir cup for cup as a replacement for whole milk, buttermilk or half-and-half; use fruit flavored kefir in sweet baked recipes.
- **Kefir Cheese:** a delicious replacement for sour cream or cream cheese in recipes, kefir cheese is low in fat and calories, and has a slight tangy-rich flavor that enhances snack foods. Use it cup for cup in place of sour cream, cottage cheese, cream cheese or ricotta.

Soy and tofu substitutes:

- **Soy Milk:** nutritious, versatile, smooth and delicious, soy milk is vegetable-based, lactose/cholesterol free. Soy milk in your diet can help reduce serum cholesterol. Soy milk contains less calcium and calories than milk, and more protein and iron. It adds a slight rise to baked goods. Use it cup for cup as a milk replacement in cooking; plain flavor for savory dishes, vanilla for sweet dishes or on cereal.
- **Soy Cheese:** made from soy milk, the small amount of calcium caseinate (a milk protein) added allows it to melt. Mozzarella, cheddar, jack and cream cheese types are available. Use it cup for cup in place of any low-fat or regular cheese.
- **Soy Ice Cream:** frozen desserts and soy yogurt are available in many flavors.

- **Soy Yogurt Cheese:** use the recipe for yogurt cheese in the preceding section.
- **Soy Mayonnaise:** has the taste and consistency of regular mayonnaise.
- **Soy Lecithin:** low in fat and cholesterol, lecithin thickens and emulsifies ingredients to make recipes extra rich and smooth. Add 1 tablespoon lecithin granules to a sauce, custard dessert or homemade ice-y dessert.
- **Tofu:** a white, digestible curd made from soybeans, tofu is a good replacement for dairy foods, in texture, taste and nutritional content. It is high in protein, low in fat and contains no cholesterol. Available in a wealth of varieties, tofu is extremely versatile, and may be used in place of eggs, sour cream, cheese and cottage cheese.
- **Miso:** a fermented paste made from cooked aged soybeans and certain whole grains, miso is a good dairy substitute. (Light miso mixed with vegetable or onion stock is a tasty replacement for milk.)

Fruit substitutes:

- **Coconut Milk:** a semi-sweet liquid made by simmering equal parts shredded fresh coconut and water. Use in moderation in place of oil, fat and butter, (high in calories). A good complete protein source for children.
- **Frozen Fruit:** use in smoothies, shakes, dessert sauces and toppings. Simply peel, chunk and freeze fresh fruit. Then blend it in the blender. Use it as is, or combine with other ingredients and 1 – 2 tbsp. lecithin granules.
- **Fruit Juice:** may be used to replace milk in baked recipes. Apple and pear juices on cereals (either hot or cold) instead of milk are delicious.

Nut substitutes:

- **Almond Milk:** rich and nutty tasting; use one to one in place of milk in baked recipes, sauces or gravies. To make 1 cup almond milk: blend 1 tsp. almond butter, 1 tsp. honey and 1 cup water until very smooth.
- **Almond Cheese:** made from almond milk, a nutty, non-melting cheese, good in salads, spreads, dips, dressings or sandwiches.
- **Sesame Tahini:** made from ground sesame seeds. Use tahini in place of cream or sour cream in dips, sauces and gravies. Mix with water to milk consistency as a high protein milk substitute for baking. Tahini complements greens and vegetables. Mix tahini with oil and other dressing ingredients for salads. Use tahini on toast or bread instead of peanut butter, on pancakes instead of butter. Use almost anywhere you would use sesame seeds.
- **Tahini Milk:** use cup for cup as a dairy substitute in recipes: add 1 tbsp. sesame tahini and 1 tsp. honey to 8 oz. water in a blender and blend smooth.

Butter substitutes:

Although butter is a saturated fat, it is relatively stable and the body can use it in small amounts for energy. Its make-up, like that of raw cream, is a whole and balanced food, used by the body better than its separate components might indicate. If you use butter, use raw unsalted butter, never margarine, pasteurized butter or shortening. Don't let butter get hot enough to sizzle or smoke.

…For less fat saturation, simply clarify the butter by melting it and skimming off the top foam. Remove from heat. Let rest a few minutes, and spoon off the clear butter for use. Discard whey solids that settle to the bottom of the pan.

…High quality grapeseed oil (or a blend of butter and oil) may be substituted for butter without loss of taste.

…New <u>trans-fat free</u> soy spreads are OK vegetarian alternatives in baked foods and on breads and pancakes.

…Organic vegetable, chicken and onion broths are good substitutes for butter in stir fried recipes and sautées.

Other dairy substitutes:

- **Tapioca:** a sweet sun-dried starch made by crushing cassava roots with water, tapioca is natural thickener in cooking, a dessert favorite with children and easily digested by the elderly and small children.
- **Low Fat Cottage Cheese:** a low-fat, cultured dairy food, cottage cheese is well tolerated by those with only slight lactose intolerance, and is a good substitute for ricotta, cream cheese, and processed cottage cheese foods that are full of chemicals. Mix with non-fat or low-fat plain yogurt to add the richness of cream or sour cream to recipes without the fat.

Egg substitutes:

Although they contain cholesterol, eggs are also high in balancing lecithins and phosphatides, and do not increase the risk of atherosclerosis. The difference in nutrition-rich, fertile eggs from free "scratch and run" chickens and the products from commercial egg factories is remarkable; the yolk color is brighter, the flavor clearly fresher, and workability in recipes better. The distinction is noticeable in poached and baked eggs, where the yolks firm up and rise higher. Cook eggs lightly, preferably poach, soft-boil, or bake, never fry.

- **Egg Replacer:** a product made from potato starch and tapioca flour is a viable substitute for baking needs.
- **Tofu** may be used in place of eggs in quick breads, cakes, custards and quiches.
- **Flax seeds** mixed with water can replace eggs in quick breads, pancakes and muffins. Use ¼ cup flax seeds to ¾ cup water. Process in the blender until thoroughly crushed, and add to batter in place of 3 eggs.

Do you have a wheat or gluten allergy?

Here are some symptoms to watch for: Chronic headaches, moodiness, fatigue and depression are usually the first stages of sensitivity, followed by itchy, watery eyes or blurred vision, and mental fuzziness. Most people get an excessively swollen stomach and feel nauseous after eating, closely followed by gas and constipation, or diarrhea. Children become overly irritable, hyperactive, flushed in the face and get chronic ear infections. Women with wheat or gluten allergies regularly suffer from hypothyroidism, heart palpitations and osteoarthritis. Men regularly experience hypoglycemia, muscle weakness or poor coordination and excessive sweating. The elderly often get hives and ringing in the ears. Chronic congestion and unexplained obesity are universal symptoms of wheat allergies and gluten reactions.

Sensitivity to wheat and gluten was once rare. Ancient civilizations in every climate zone enjoyed wheat grains as a regular part of their daily diet. Today, commercial wheat is one of our most problematic allergen foods.

Your non-wheat options

What's left after you've eliminated wheat? Healthy options available at health food stores ease the transition. Pasta, cereals (hot and cold), whole grain flours, breads and snack foods are all available in wheat and gluten-free forms. Ancient grains like spelt and kamut can be enjoyed by 70% of people allergic to wheat. Look for spelt and kamut breads in the refrigerated section. Rice breads are a tasty option for a wheat free sandwich. (They're a little crumbly, but are well tolerated by the gluten intolerant.)

Try vegetable pastas made with quinoa or rice. Soba noodles made from buckwheat are a good wheat-free choice, but are not for people with gluten intolerance. For a wheat-free hot breakfast, cream of rice, buckwheat and oat bran are tasty. Amaranth, muesli, brown rice crisps and corn flakes are wheat-free cereals.

A short list of wheat-free, low gluten grains:

- **Kamut:** An ancient variety of wheat, used since 4000 B.C., kamut is related to durum wheat. It's available in the U.S. as a powdered drink, in cereals, pastas, and bread. It has a rich, buttery flavor that enhances recipes where you would normally use wheat, including yeasted breads. It's not a good choice for gluten sensitivity because it contains gluten. GREEN KAMUT drink by ORGANIC BY NATURE is a good choice for cleansing and is gluten-free.
- **Rice:** ok for gluten sensitivity, wheat-free. Rice is the staple grain for over half of the world's population. Available as a grain, flour, bread, pasta, cereal, and in dairy-free milk and cheese, it is one of the most versatile grains known and one of the most easily digested. Choose organic rice; commercial rice is often loaded with pesticides. For people who are also lactose intolerant, I recommend delicious rice cheeses.
- **Amaranth:** ok for gluten sensitivity, wheat-free. There are over 500 species of amaranth. Amaranth is available today as a flour for wheat-free baking. Mixing a little amaranth with grains like rice, millet or oats adds a nutty, peppery flavor. Popped amaranth makes a good snack. After toasting, popcorn-like amaranth seeds are added to soups or vegetables or eaten alone. Amaranth cereals are popular in a wheat-free breakfast.

- **Corn:** ok for gluten sensitivity, wheat-free. A staple food for Native Americans, corn still feeds much of the Americas, human and animal. It's versatile, excellent in baking, in cereals, and with quinoa in pasta. Sweet corn is the favorite America's favorite vegetable (next to the potato), great on the grill, roasted, steamed, in casseroles. Note: Corn allergies and sensitivities are quite common in people and in pets. Looks for signs like excess bloating and gas after meals for potential corn allergy.
- **Chickpea:** ok for gluten sensitivity, wheat-free. Chickpeas are not a true grain, but a legume cultivated in Mesopotamia since 5000 B.C. A nice addition to pudding and casseroles, they are best enjoyed in hummus and falafel dishes. Chickpea flour (from ground chickpeas) is gluten-free and a good thickener in soups and sauces.
- **Spelt:** ok for gluten sensitivity, wheat-free. An ancient European grain, spelt is available in the U.S. as a bread, flour and in berries. Although spelt isn't gluten-free, most people with gluten sensitivity can tolerate it. Note: Italian spelt pastas are sometimes made with whole wheat flour. If you're unsure, choose domestic products.
- **Millet:** ok for gluten sensitivity, wheat-free. An ancient grain, the Chinese used it as their staple grain before rice came along. The ancient Egyptians used millet to make bread. Millet is available today as a grain, flour, meal and in cereals. It's excellent in flatbreads, puffed in snack foods, and to add heartiness to stuffed veggies and casseroles.
- **Buckwheat:** wheat-free. Buckwheat became popular in Europe during the Middle Ages for its ability to withstand poor growing conditions. Buckwheat is available today as a flour, cereal and pasta (Soba noodles). Nutty, roasted buckwheat (kasha) is good with vegetables like onions, mushrooms and winter squash. Buckwheat is a great choice for chemical sensitivities because it's rarely treated with pesticides.
- **Oats:** wheat-free. Popular since 2500 B.C., oats are known today for their fiber providing ability. Oats are available as a grain, cereal, bran and flour. Old fashioned hot oatmeal cereal is still an American favorite. Because they are high in gluten, oats are also often used as a thickener in soups, and in meat loaf, baked goods and granola. Note: A study in the New England Journal of Medicine says celiac patients in remission can tolerate oats in moderate amounts. Another study (2004) suggests that eating oats leads to intestinal inflammation for some celiac patients. Ask your physician.
- **Barley:** ok for gluten sensitivity, wheat-free. Frequently used in the West in hearty soups, barley is a good breakfast cereal, and in bread and casseroles. Whole grain barley is the best choice. Barley is also a healing green grass.
- **Rye:** may be ok for gluten sensitivity, wheat-free. Most of Medieval Europe ate rye as a staple grain. Rye is available as a flour, berry, cereal, grits and meal. I like rye bread in a healthy Reuben sandwich with raw sauerkraut and hormone-free turkey. It's lower in gluten than wheat and may be tolerated by some people with <u>mild</u> gluten sensitivity.
- **Quinoa:** ok for gluten sensitivity, wheat-free. Considered by many a nearly perfect protein, quinoa has been cultivated in the Andes mountains for 5,000 years. It has a rich, nutty flavor and works well as a wheat free grain and pasta. Prepare quinoa just like rice; it only takes about 5 to 10 minutes before it's ready. Note: If you're allergic to wheat, make sure the quinoa pasta you buy <u>isn't</u> made with semolina flour.
- **Soy Flour:** ok for gluten sensitivity, wheat-free. Soy flour is available for baking, but because it contains no gluten, it doesn't work well by itself in raised breads. It's usually mixed with an all purpose flour (not gluten-free) in baking. Soy flour can also be used to add a creamy texture to fruit smoothies.
- *Note:* People with gluten sensitivity can also usually tolerate potato starch and tapioca, but they are not as nutritious as the grains listed above. If you're affected by wheat or gluten allergies, read product labels to make sure there is no wheat or gluten on the ingredient list. Gluten can also be found in some vitamin supplements. <u>Always </u>inquire if you are unsure.

Your non-meat protein options

Most Americans think in terms of meat and animal foods for protein. But animal protein often comes loaded with saturated fat, calories and cholesterol. Overeating these foods adds unwanted weight <u>because excess protein turns into fat</u>. Too much protein impairs good kidney function, increases calcium loss in bones, and poses a clear health risk to heart and arteries.

Our most advanced research about human needs for protein shows that mankind is a part of the ecological system of the planet like everything else, putting the question about eating meat much more into perspective.

High quality vegetable protein sources to use in your meal and diet planning.

Soy Foods: tofu, tempeh, miso, soy cheese and soy milk.

Nuts: pine nuts, walnuts, almonds, cashews, Brazil nuts and hazelnuts.

Seeds: pumpkin seeds, sesame seeds, sunflower seeds.

Beans and Legumes: peas, peanuts, lentils, pintos, lima beans, mung beans, black beans, white and red beans, turtle beans.

Whole Grains: wheat and wheat germ, brown, basmati and wild rice, millet, barley, bulgur, buckwheat, amaranth, rye, quinoa, and amazake rice drink.

Vegetables: all kinds of sprouts, mushrooms.

Sea Vegetables: all kinds of sea veggies.

Fruits: avocados, coconuts, prunes, raisins, apples, figs and dates.

Bee Pollen: Contains all the essential amino acids in one natural source.

Nutritional Yeast: Just 2 tbsp. contains as much protein as ¼ cup wheat germ, as much calcium as ½ cup orange juice, as much phosphorus as ¼ lb. haddock, as much iron as 1 cup spinach, as much thiamine as 1 cup wheat germ, as much niacin as ½ cup brown rice, as much riboflavin as 4 eggs.

Ginseng: Increases protein content in the muscles.

Get more minerals in your diet

Note: If you are a kidney patient on dialysis, work with a renal dietician or other health professional to design a diet that's right for you. Potassium, sodium, and phosphorous, and protein intake all need to be carefully monitored in order to avoid serious complications.

Foods rich in calcium: sesame seeds, salmon, sea veggies, tofu, cheese, leafy greens, nuts and legumes, olives, broccoli, brown rice, wheat germ, figs, dates, raisins, onions, leeks and chives.

Foods rich in potassium: sea vegetables, brown rice, tofu and other soy foods, beans, nuts and seeds, most dried fruits, raisins, dates, bananas, broccoli, garlic, mushrooms, potatoes and yams.

Foods rich in iron: amaranth, wheat and wheat germ, millet, fish, molasses, chard, spinach and dark greens, pumpkin and sunflower seeds, turkey, black beans, raisins, prunes and peaches.

Foods rich in chromium: potatoes, bananas, turkey and chicken, green peppers, leafy greens, nutritional yeast, organ meats, mushrooms, corn, carrots, wheat germ and fish.

Foods rich in magnesium: poultry, organ meats, mushrooms, cheese, brewer's yeast, greens, celery, water chestnuts, tofu and soy foods, nuts, seeds, sea veggies, sea foods, grains and legumes.

Foods rich in zinc: nuts and seeds, sea veggies and sea foods, liver and organ meats, eggs, nutritional yeast, legumes, leafy greens, whole grains, mushrooms, maple syrup, onions and leeks.

Foods rich in chlorine: tomatoes, celery, lettuce, sea veggies, dark leafy greens, cabbage, radishes, eggplant, cucumber, potatoes and yams, carrots, cauliflower, leeks and onions.

Foods rich in copper: oysters, liver, nuts, legumes, mushrooms, avocados, leafy greens, grains, seafoods, blueberries, raisins.

Foods rich in phosphorus: yogurt, poultry, fish, nuts, nutritional yeast, cereals, peas and beans.

Grilling great minerals

The sweetness of fresh garden vegetables intensifies on the grill. Sprinkle aromatic wood chips or herb leaves over hot coals to impart unique flavors. Blanch larger vegetable pieces like broccoli, cauliflower or potato chunks in boiling water, then plunge into cold water to stop cooking before bringing them to the grill. Precooking isn't needed for sliced vegetables like onions, bell pepper, tomatoes or eggplant. Use grilling baskets or flat skewers for vegetables. Remove all foods from the grill when they are golden, before they become charred, to avoid denaturing amino acids and DNA damage. Discard any charred portions to avoid dangerous hydro-carbons.

Cultured foods

Cultured foods are an important, even critical, part of your healing program. Cultured foods promote acid-alkaline balance (important for disease prevention), strengthen digestion with enzymes that inhibit pathogens, and build immune response. They are a specific for candida albicans, lactose intolerance and malabsorption. Cultured soy foods are full of benefits for health. Soy bean products help protect the heart by lowering cholesterol and supporting the vascular system. Further, research shows soy plays an important role in the natural treatment of osteoporosis, and hormone-related cancers like breast and prostate cancer. A rich source of phytoestrogens, soy enhances female vitality during menopause, too.

My favorite cultured foods for healing:

Yogurt: a cultured dairy food, is a key immune response stimulant. Studies show people who eat yogurt with active cultures produce four times more gamma interferon, a natural immune booster with anti-viral action. Yogurt can fight diarrhea caused by antibiotic overload, and lower cholesterol. Yogurt even normalizes vaginal pH against candida overgrowth. Research shows that eating just one cup of yogurt daily reduces candida albicans yeast living in the vagina by three times. Note: Full-fat yogurt products should be avoided by people with bladder infections and dairy intolerance. Low fat and non-fat yogurt are better tolerated.

Kefir: thought by many experts to be a better cultured dairy choice than yogurt because it contains twice as much friendly bacteria and has substantially more nutrients. Kefir is easier to digest for babies, invalids and the elderly. Kefir, like yogurt, is an immune boosting food, used with success by naturopaths to help HIV, herpes, cancer and chronic fatigue syndrome. A natural tranquilizer, kefir is a good food for children with ADD, too.

Acidophilus: a "friendly bacteria," can be used directly on foods (including pet foods) for health. Just sprinkle a teaspoon of powder, or the contents of one capsule, on your favorite foods. Acidophilus helps your body produce B vitamins, enzymes and natural antibiotics. Like all cultured foods, it counters the side effects of antibiotic therapy like diarrhea, upset stomach, and candida infections. (I've used it successfully for years in a vaginal suppository for yeast infections.) Note: Don't cook with acidophilus. It negates its healing properties.

Vinegar: used since ancient times as a preservative to extend the freshness of foods, and as an elixir for health. Vinegar was legendary as a health element for Roman soldiers. The Japanese folk remedy Tamago-su (egg vinegar) was consumed by the Samurai as a source of strength and power. Aged wine vinegar, balsamic vinegar, brown rice vinegar, apple cider vinegar, raspberry vinegar and herbal vinegars like tarragon vinegar are all good choices in a healing diet. Vinegar, like other cultured foods, helps digestive problems like heartburn and gas. It has also been effectively used in vaginal douches for feminine problems for decades. Just add 2 tsp. of apple cider vinegar to one cup of warm water for the best results.

Apple cider vinegar: well known for health benefits, apple cider vinegar is a source of over 30 important nutrients. It contains natural antibiotics and antifungals that fight ear infections, dandruff and athlete's foot, even when used externally. Cider vinegar boosts memory, fights arthritis, promotes weight loss, soothes sore throats.

Raw Sauerkraut: one of the richest sources of enzymes and lactobacillus; successfully used by natural healers to treat candida yeast disorders. Sauerkraut regenerates the blood, improves digestion and boosts metabolism. Use it in salads, on sandwiches, rice cakes, pizzas and omelettes. Commercial sauerkrauts are heated which degrades their life-giving enzymes. Try REJUVENATIVE FOODS VEGI-DELITE for the best healing results.

My favorite cultured soy foods:

Tofu: made from fermented soy milk, tofu adds richness to recipes while safeguarding you against disease. New studies show tofu even helps fight prostate cancer, research on 8,000 Hawaiian men (who traditionally have high rates of prostate cancer) shows that the men who eat the most tofu have the lowest rates of prostate cancer. Tofu is high in protein and lower in fat and calories than meat or poultry.

Still, there are concerns with eating very large amounts of tofu. A new Hawaiian study suggests that eating a lot of tofu may speed up the aging process, even affect your brain. Researchers speculate that soy's plant hormones may act as an anti-estrogen in the brain, but more research needs to be done to determine if this is true. (Note: Factors like the normal aging process itself, a history of strokes, and a good education play a much more significant role in the risk for mental decline than soy intake.)

Tempeh: a delicious, protein-packed cultured soy food, tempeh is made from whole soybeans fermented with a grain like rice or millet. It's a good choice for meat eaters evolving into vegetarians, because it's so hearty and filling. I especially like tempeh squares pre-marinated in teriyaki or Szechwan sauce.

Miso: made from fermented soybean paste, unpasteurized miso (pasteurization kills its active cultures), found in the refrigerated section of Asian food stores and health food stores is the best choice. A true superfood for health, miso is an immune system enhancer that helps neutralize toxins and repress carcinogens. I like miso in tonic broths and sauces with vegetables and immune boosting herbs.

Soy Milk: made from soaked, ground and cooked whole soybeans, soy milk is the basis for most soy foods… tofu, soy yogurt, soy frozen desserts, soy cheeses and cream cheese, and soy yuba sheets for tacos or tamales. Almost everyone likes soy milk. Some picky kids actually favor soy milk over commercial dairy milk. Soy milk is rich and creamy, and is available plain or in flavors like vanilla or chocolate. Use it in desserts, smoothies and on whole grain cereals.

Cautions: Eaten in excess (more than 4 servings a day), soy foods may disrupt thyroid function, hormone balance (especially for children who are still developing), and deplete minerals like zinc, calcium and iron. Soy beans are also routinely genetically engineered. Choose organic soy products whenever possible.

Wine is a cultured food

Wine, used since ancient times for its pain-relieving, antiseptic and relaxing properties, wine is six times more effective than Pepto-Bismol in killing the bacteria linked to traveler's diarrhea. Wine aids circulation, protects the heart, even helps the eyes! Studies show just 2 glasses of wine per day cuts heart disease risk by 50%. As little as 2 glasses <u>a month</u> may cut the risk of macular degeneration in half. Research in the journal Epidemiology reveals that 2 glasses of wine a day reduces death rates <u>from all causes by up to 30%</u>! Resveratrol, a wine component, may even help prevent cancer.

The key to using wine wisely is moderation. I recommend a glass with dinner or lightly cooking with it for the best results.

Cautionary note: research shows resveratrol has mild estrogenic effects that may aggravate hormone dependent tumors, or add to high estrogen stores in women using HRT drugs.

Sadly, the grapes which produce our wines are one of the most heavily sprayed fruits in America. And, grape skins have a high affinity for fluoride, a highly toxic substance used in pesticides and regularly added to the water supply. Choose organic wines for your healing diet. Organic wines have no added sulfites which may cause allergy reactions like congestion or stuffy nose for many people.

Bibliography

Hundreds of books and articles were reviewed during the writing of this book. Because of space constraints, the editors have chosen to list a representative sampling here.

Abernathy, Sarah. "Herb-Nutrient-Drug Interactions: Facts You Need To Know." Healthy Healing. 2003.

Abernathy, Sarah. "Iatrogenic Disease." Healthy Healing. 2003.

"ADHD Options," Choices. May 2002, Vol. 2, No. 3.

Ahmed, Aftab J., Ph.D. "Osteoporosis: Diet, Acidity and Calcium," Total Health .Vol. 24, No. 2.

Almada, Anthony L., BSc, MSc, "OTC Fire Extinguishers: Natural Options for Arthritis," Health Products Business. April 2000.

Balch, James, M.D. & Phyllis Balch C.N.C. Prescriptions for Nutritional Healing. Penguin Putnam. 2000.

"Alternative Approaches to Treating ADD," Let's Live. Sept. 1998.

"Americans Eat their Vegetables- as Long as They're French Fries." CNN.com. Sept. 30, 1998.

"Bad News: Alpha Trouble," Time. March 20, 2000.

"Bad to the Bone,"Health Sciences Institute e-Alert. April 30, 2003.

Benagh, Barbara, "Asthma Answers," Yoga Journal. July/August 2000.

Bushkin, Gary, Ph.D., CNC and Estitta Bushkin, Ph.D, C.N.C. "Children's Health, Naturally." Health Products Business. Oct. 2002.

Calbom, Cherie & Maureen Keane. Juicing For Life. Avery Pub. 1992.

Calechman, Steve, "Consumer Guide: Feel Younger Than You Are," Natural Health. April 2002.

Cancer Epidemiol Biomarkers Prev 2002; 11(8):713-8.

"Cancer Facts & Figures 2003." American Cancer Society ©2003.

"Cancer Prevention: Why Aren't We Trying," March 10, 2003.

"Can Coffee Promote Osteoporosis?" Nutrition Science News. Sept. 2000.

Carper, Jean. The Food Pharmacy. Bantam Books. ©1988.

Carper, Jean. Food- Your Miracle Medicine. Harper Collins. ©1993.

Challem, Jack, "Consumer Guide: Vitamins That Protect Against Aging," Natural Health. April 2002.

Challem, Jack, " How To Heal a Failing Heart," Letsliveonline.com. Aug. 2000.

Chek, Paul, "You Are What You Eat," FitCommerce.com. 2002-2003.

Darlington, Joy, "Beating the Blood Sugar Blues," Vegetarian Times. April 2000.

"Decade of the Brain: The Gray Area of Research on Gray Matter," Environmental Health Perspectives. Vol.102, No. 11. November 1994.

"Endometriosis," Herbs for Health. July/August 2002.

Ensminger, Konlande, & Robson. The Concise Encyclopedia of Foods & Nutrition. CRC Press. 1995.

"Fibroid Help," Herbs For Health. May/June 2002.

"Fibroid Removal and Future Pregnancy," The John R. Lee, M.D. Medical Letter. Dec. 2002.

Fischlowitz-Roberts, Bernie, "Air Pollution Fatalities Now Exceed Traffic Fatalities by 3 to 1," Earth Policy Institute. September 17, 2002.

"Flu-Related Deaths Up Sharply," CBS News. Jan. 7, 2003.

Garrison, R. & Somer, E. Nutrition Desk Reference. Keats Pub. 1995.

Gates, Donna. The Body Ecology Diet. 1996.

Gerson, Charlotte and Morton Walker, D.P.M. The Gerson Therapy. Kensington Pub. 2001.

Gittleman, Ann Louise, C.N.C. The Fat Flush Plan. McGraw-Hill ©2002.

Goldberg, Burton. Alternative Medicine: The Definitive Guide. 1993.

"Green Tea for Diabetes," Delicious Living. March 2003.

Haas, Elson M.D. The Detox Diet. Celestial Arts. 1996.

Haas, Elson, M.D. Staying Healthy With Nutrition. Celestial Arts. 1992.

Head, Kathi, N.D. "Coping with Diabetes Naturally," Letsliveonline.com. Dec. 2002.

"Heart Disease Risk and Abdominal Fat," Life Extension. Nov. 2002.

"Herb Mix Nixes Prostate Cancer in Lab," WebMD. Dec. 13, 2002.

"Hopkins Health Watch: Oh No, Not Another Cousin of Fosamax," The John R. Lee, M.D. Medical Letter. Dec. 1998.

"Hormone Replacement Therapy Poses Greatest Risk Of Heart Attack In First Year Of Use For Most Women," Brigham and Women's Hospital http://www.ahaf.org

"Hot Tub Therapy May Help Diabetics," CNN.com. Sept. 16, 1999.

Imperato, Pacal and Greg Mitchell. "Bombarding Bananas, Zapping Zucchini," The Sciences. Jan/Feb 1985. Jaffe, Harry, "New Coke," Men's Health. June 2002.

Jensen, Bernard, D.C. Tissue Cleansing Through Bowel Management. 1981.

Kahn, Sherry, M.H. P. "The Hyperactivity Puzzle," Letsliveonline.com. Aug. 2001.

"Kids at Risk for Asthma Epidemic," Healthy & Natural Journal. Vol. 7, Issue 4. Aug. 2000.

Kiely, Timothy, David Donaldson & Arthur Grube, Ph.D. "Pesticide Industry Sales and Usage 2000 and 2001 Market Estimates." U.S. Environmental Protection Agency. May 2004.

"Lack of Sleep Alters Hormones, Metabolism," Doctor's Guide, Oct. 22, 1999.

Langer, Stephen, M.D. "Keeping Environmental Toxins At Bay." Better Nutrition For Today's Living. July 1993.

La Puma, John, M.D., FACP, "Clinical Briefs: Writing Therapy to Reduce Asthma and RA Symptoms," Alternative Medicine Alert. Vol. 2, No. 6.

Maranan, Julia, "Consumer Guide: Annual Women's Health Guide," Natural Health. Dec. 2002.

Moll, Lucy & The Editors of Vegetarian Times. Vegetarian Times Cookbook. 1995.

"Obesity Nearly as Deadly as Tobacco in United States," The Associated Press. March 9, 2004.

"Overweight Prevalence," National Center for Health Statistics. 2002.

Page, Linda, N.D., Ph.D. "Look and Feel Your Best: Go Through Menopause the Natural Way Without Hormone Replacement," Institute of Health Sciences, ©2002 www.hsibaltimore.com.

Quaid, Libby, "Americans Urged to Cut Calories, Exercise," Associated Press. 2005.

Randall C, Meethan K, Randall H, Dobs F. Nettle Sting of Urtica Dioica for Joint Pain- An Exploratory Study of this Complementary Therapy. Complement Ther Med 1999 Sep;7(3):126-31.

Rea, William, M.D. "Could Chemical Overload be the Cause of Your Illness?" The John R. Lee, M.D. Medical Letter. Aug. 2000.

"Red Flag Raised Over 'Normal" Blood Pressure," CNN.com. May 14, 2003.

Robbins, John. The Food Revolution. Conari Press. 2001.

Rogers, Jean & The Editors of Prevention Magazine. The Healing Foods Cookbook. Rodale Press 1991.

"Should Ritalin be Required for Hyperactive Kids?" Natural Health Magazine. Oct./Nov. 2001.

Strauss, Edward, M.D., "Bone Density Scans-The Test Women Don't Think About," Total Health. Vol. 24, No. 3 .

"Stroke Deaths Expected to Double by 2032." WebMD. Feb 14, 2003.

"Study Finds Hay Fever Medication Worse Than Alcohol in Impairing Driver Skills," CNN.com, March 6, 2000.

"The Under-Over," Health Sciences Institute e-Alert. Feb. 6, 2003.

Tillson, Rodney, "Straighten Up," Energy Times. March 2003.

Toews, Victoria, M.P.H. "Protect Your Child from the Fat Epidemic," Letsliveonline.com. Feb. 2002.

"Treating Sinusitis Naturally," Natural Health. April 2003.

Whitaker, Julian, M.D. Health & Healing .Sept. 1998.

Williams, David, Ph.D. "Keep Your Cells Young for 100 Years or More," Alternatives for the Health-Conscious Individual ©2001.

"Women's Heart Disease, Heart Attacks, and Hormones," The John R. Lee, M.D. Medical Letter, Aug. 1998

Wood, Sharon J., "Uncovering Lesser-Known Symptoms," Digestive Health & Nutrition. March/April 2002.

www.kushiinstitute.org.

www.plasticsurgery.org

www.vaccinationdebate.com

Product Resources
Where you can get what we recommend...

The following list is for your convenience and assistance in obtaining further information about the products I recommend in Diets For Healthy Healing. The list is unsolicited by the companies named. Each company has a solid history of testing and corroborative data that is invaluable to me and my staff, as well as empirical confirmation by the stores that carry these products who have shared their experiences with us. We hear from thousands of readers about the products they have used. I realize there are many other fine companies and products who are not listed here, but you can rely on the companies who are, for their high quality products and good results.

Alacer Corp., 19631 Pauling, Foothill Ranch, CA 92610, 800-854-0249

All One, 719 East Haley St., Santa Barbara, CA 93103, 800-235-5727

Aloe Life International, 4822 Santa Monica Ave. #231, San Diego, CA 92107, 800-414-2563

Alta Health Products, Inc., 1979 E. Locust Street, Pasadena, CA 91107, 626-796-1047

Anabol Naturals, 1550 Mansfield Street, Santa Cruz, CA 95062, 800-426-2265

Arise & Shine, P.O. Box 1439, Mt. Shasta, CA 96067, 800-688-2444

Barleans Organic Oils, 4936 Lake Terrell Rd., Fern Dale, WA 98248, 800-445-3529

Baywood, 14950 N. 83rd Pl., Ste.1, Scottsdale, AZ 85260, 800-481-7169

Beehive Botanicals, Route 8, Box 8257, Hayward, WI 54843, 800-233-4483

BHI (Heel Inc.) 11600 Cochiti Road SE, Albuquerque, NM 33376, 800-621-7644

Biostrath, 75 Commerce Drive, Hauppauge, NY, 11788-3943, 800-439-2324

Body Ecology, 1266 West Paces Ferry Rd., Suite 505, Atlanta, GA 30327, 770-385-6333

Boericke & Tafel Inc.,(B & T) 2381 Circadian Way, Santa Rosa, CA 95407, 800-876-9505

Bragg/Live Food Products, Inc., Box 7, Santa Barbara, CA 93102, 805-968-1028

CC Pollen Co., 3627 East Indian School Rd., Suite 209, Phoenix, AZ 85018-5126, 800-875-0096

C'est Si Bon, 1308 Sartori Ave. Suite 205, Torrance, CA 90501, 888-700-0801

Clear Products, 4340 Vandever Ave Suite M, San Diego, CA 92120, 888-257-2532

Country Life, 28300 B Industrial Blvd., Hayward, CA 94545, 800-645-5768

Crystal Star Herbal Nutrition, 121 Calle Del Oaks, Del Rey Oaks, CA 93940, 800-736-6015

Designing Health, 28410 Witherspoon Parkway, Valencia, CA 91355, 800-774-7387

Dreamous, 2720 Monterey Ave. Suite 401, Torrance, CA 90503, 800-251-7543

Dr. Diamond/Herpanacine Associates, 145 Willow Grove Ave #1, Glenside, PA 19038, 888-467-4200

Dr. Rath's Vitamins, 2901 Bayview Drive, Fremont, CA 94538, 800-624-2442

East Park Research, Inc., 2709 Horseshoe Drive, Las Vegas, NV 89120, 800-345-8367 (orders)

Edge Labs, 470 Route 9, Englishtown, NJ 07726, 866-edgelab

Eidon Mineral Products, 9988 Hibert St. #104, San Diego, CA 92131, 800-700-1169

Enzymatic Therapy, Dept. L, P.O. Box 22310, Green Bay, WI 54305, 800-783-2286

Enzymedica, 1970 Kings Hwy., Punta Gorda, FL 33980, 888-918-1118

Earth's Bounty/Matrix Health Products, 9316 Wheatlands Road, Santee, CA 92071, 800-736-5609

Esteem Products Ltd., 15015 Main St., Suite 204, Bellevue, WA 98007, 800-255-7631

Ethical Nutrients/Unipro, 971 Calle Negocio, San Clemente, CA 92673, 949-366-0818

Fit for You, Intl., 971 S Bundy Dr., Brentwood CA 90049-5828, 800-521-5867

Flint River Ranch, 1243 Columbia Avenue B-6, Riverside, CA 92507-2123, 888-722-4589

Flora, Inc., 805 East Badger Road, P.O. Box 73, Lynden, WA 98264, 800-446-2110, (Info.) 604-451-8232

Futurebiotics, 145 Ricefield Lane, Hauppauge, NY 11788, 800-367-5433

Gaia Herbs, Inc., 108 Island Ford Road, Brevard, NC 28712, 800-831-7780

Golden Pride, 1501 Northpoint Pkwy., Suite 100, West Palm Beach, FL 33407, 561-640-5700

Green Foods Corp., 320 North Graves Ave., Oxnard, CA 93030 800-777-4430

Green Kamut Corp/Pure Planet, 1542 Seabright Ave., Long Beach, CA 90813, 800-452-6884

Grifron/Maitake Products, Inc., P.O. Box 1354, Paramus, NJ 07653, 800-747-7418

Health from the Sun/Arkopharma, P.O. Box 179, Newport, NH 03773, 800-447-2249

Herbal Answers, Inc., P.O. Box 1110, Saratoga Springs, New York 12866, 888-256-3367

Heart Foods Company, Inc., 2235 East 38th Street, Minneapolis, MN 55407, 612-724-5266

Herbal Magic, Inc., P.O. Box 70, Forest Knowlls, CA 94933, 415-488-9488

Herbal Products & Development, P.O. Box 1084, Aptos, CA 95001, 831-688-8706

Herbs Etc.,1340 Rufina Circle, Santa Fe, NM 87505, 505-471-6488

Immudyne, 11200 Wilcrest Green Drive, Houston, TX 77042, 888-2-IMMUDYNE

Imperial Elixir, P.O. Box 970, Simi Valley, CA 93062, 800-423-5176

Jagulana Herbal Products, Inc., P.O. Box 45, Badger, CA 93603, 559-337-2188

Jarrow Formulas, 1824 South Robertson Blvd., Los Angeles, CA 90035, 310-204-6936

Lane Labs, 25 Commerce Drive, Allendale, NJ 07401, 800-526-3005

Lane Labs TOKI, 1-888-AGELESS, Please mention code #6405

Liddell Laboratories, 1036 Country Club Drive, Moraga, CA 94556, 800-460-7733

MagneLyfe/Encore Technology, Inc., 80 Fifth Ave., Suite 1104, New York, NY 10011, 877-624-6353

Maine Coast Sea Vegetables, RR1 Box 78, Franklin, Maine 04634, 207-565-2907

Maitake Products, Inc., P.O. Box 1354, Paramus, NJ 07653, 800-747-7418

Mendocino Sea Vegetable Co., P.O. Box 1265, Mendocino, CA 95460, 707-937-2050

Merix Health Care Products, 18 E. Dundee Rd. #3-204, Barrington, IL 60010, 847-277-1111

Metabolic Response Modifiers, 2633 W. Coast Hwy, Suite B, Newport Beach, CA 92663, 800-948-6296

Moon Maid Botanicals, 535 Tall Poplar Road, Cosby, TN 865-217-9713, 877-253-7853

Motherlove Herbal Co., P.O. Box 101, Laporte, CO 80535, 970-493-2892

MRI (Medical Research Institute), 2160 Pacific Ave., Suite 61, San Francisco CA 94115, 888-448-4246

Mychelle Dermaceuticals, Box 1, Frisco, CO 970-668-6209, 800-447-2076

Natren Inc., 3105 Willow Ln., Westlake Village, CA 91361, 800-992-3323

Natural Balance, 3130 N. Commerce Ct., Castle Rock, CO 80104-8002, 303-688-6633

Natural Energy Plus, 4630 N. Paseo De Los Cerritos, Tucson, AZ 85745, 888-633-9233

Natural Labs Corporation (Deva Flowers), P.O. Box 20037, Sedona, AZ 86341-0037, 800-233-0810

Nature's Answer, 75 Commerce Drive, Hauppauge, NY, 11788-3943, 800-439-2324

Nature's Apothecary, 6350 Gunpark Drive #500, Boulder, CO 80301, 800-999-7422

Nature's Path, P.O. Box 7862, Venice, FL 34287, 800-326-5772

Nature's Secret/Irwin Naturals, 10549 West Jefferson Blvd., Culver City, CA 90232, 310-253-5305

Nature's Way, 10 Mountain Springs Parkway, Springville, UT 84663, 800-962-8873

Nelson Bach, Wilmington Technology Park, 100 Research Dr., Wilmington, MA 01887, 800-319-9151

New Chapter, P.O. Box 1947, Brattleboro, VT 05302, 800-543-7279

No-Miss Nail Care, 6401 E. Rogers Circle Suite 14, Boca Raton, FL 33487, 800-283-1963

Nonie of Beverly Hills, Inc., 16158 Wyancotte Street, Vans Nuys, CA 91406, 310-271-7988

NOW, 395 S. Glen Ellyn Rd., Bloomingdale, IL 60108, 800-999-8069

NutriCology /Allergy Research Group, 30806 Santana St., Hayward, CA 94544, 800-545-9960

Oshadhi, 1340 G Industrial Ave., Petaluma, CA 94952, 888-674-2344

Pacific BioLogic, P.O. Box 520, Clayton, CA 94517-0520, 800-869-8783

Penta Water, 6370 Nancy Ridge Drive Suite 104, San Diego, CA 92121, 858-452-8868

Planetary Formulas, P.O. Box 533, Soquel, CA 95073, 800-606-6226

Prince of Peace, 3536 Arden Road, Hayward, CA 94545, 800-732-2328

PSP Marketing, 23241 Areco Ct., Laguna Nigel, CA 92677, 866-777-5050

Pure Essence Laboratories, Inc., P.O. Box 95397, Las Vegas, NV 89193, 888-254-8000

Pure Form, 3240 West Desert Inn Rd., Las Vegas, NV 89103, 888-363-9817

Rainbow Light, P.O. Box 600, Santa Cruz, CA 95061, 800-635-1233

Rainforest Remedies, Box 325, Twin Lakes, WI 53181, 800-824-6396

Real Life Research, Inc., 14631 Best Ave., Norwalk, CA 90650, 800-423-8837

Rejuvenative Foods, P.O. Box 8464, Santa Cruz, CA 95061, 800-805-7957

Royal Bodycare, 2301 Crown Court, Irving, TX 75038, 972-893-4002

Solaray, Inc., 1104 Country Hills Dr., Suite 300, Ogden, UT 84403, 800-669-8877

Source Naturals Inc., 23 Janis Way, Scotts Valley, CA 95066, 800-777-5677

Spectrum Naturals, 133 Copeland St., Petaluma, CA 94952, 707-778-8900

Springlife Inc., 4630 N. Paseo De Los Cerritos, Tucson, AZ 85745, 888-633-9233

Starwest Botanicals, 11253 Trade Center Drive, Rancho Cordova, CA 95742, 888-273-4372

Sun Wellness, 4025 Spencer St. #104, Torrance, CA 90503, 800-829-2828

Superior Trading, 835 Washington Street, San Francisco, CA 94108, 415-495-7988

Transformation Enzyme Corporation, 2900 Wilcrest, Suite 220, Houston, TX, 800-777-1474

Trimedica International, Inc., 1895 South Los Feliz Drive, Tempe, AZ 85281-6023, 480-998-1041

UAS Laboratories, 5610 Rowland Road, Suite 110, Minnetonka, MN 55343, 952-935-1707

Vibrant Health, 432 Lime Rock Rd., Lakeville, CT 06039, 800-242-1835

Vitamin Research Products, 3579 Highway 50 East, Carson City, NV 89701, 800-877-2447

Wakunaga of America / Kyolic, 23501 Madero, Mission Viejo, CA 92691, 800-421-2998 / 800-825-7888

Well in Hand, P.O. Box 1200, Forest, VA 24551, 888-550-7774

Wyndmere Naturals, Inc., 153 Ashley Road, Hopkins, MN 55343, 800-207-8538

Yoanna Skin Care, P.O. Box 610072, Redwood City, CA 94061, 800-366-4617

Zand Herbal Formulas, P.O. Box 5312, Santa Monica, CA 90409, 360-384-5656

Zia Natural Skincare, 1337 Evans Ave., San Francisco, CA 94124, 800-334-7546

Index

Index of Recipes

Index of Recipes